Healthcare Policies and Systems in Europe and China

Comparisons and Synergies

Healthcare Policies and Systems in Europe and China

Comparisons and Synergies

editors

Attilio Mucelli
Marche Polytechnic University, Italy

Francesca Spigarelli
University of Macerata, Italy

World Scientific

NEW JERSEY • LONDON • SINGAPORE • BEIJING • SHANGHAI • HONG KONG • TAIPEI • CHENNAI • TOKYO

Published by

World Scientific Publishing Co. Pte. Ltd.

5 Toh Tuck Link, Singapore 596224

USA office: 27 Warren Street, Suite 401-402, Hackensack, NJ 07601

UK office: 57 Shelton Street, Covent Garden, London WC2H 9HE

Library of Congress Cataloging-in-Publication Data
Names: Mucelli, Attilio, editor. | Spigarelli, Francesca, editor.
Title: Healthcare policies and systems in Europe and China : comparisons and synergies /
by editor: Attilio Mucelli (Marche Polytechnic University, Italy),
Francesca Spigarelli (University of Macerata, Italy).
Description: New Jersey : World Scientific, 2017. | Includes bibliographical references.
Identifiers: LCCN 2017034928 | ISBN 9789813231214 (hc : alk. paper)
Subjects: | MESH: Health Policy | Delivery of Health Care | Health Care Sector |
Medicine, Chinese Traditional | Cross-Cultural Comparison | China | Europe
Classification: LCC RA418 | NLM WA 540 JC6 | DDC 362.1--dc23
LC record available at https://lccn.loc.gov/2017034928

British Library Cataloguing-in-Publication Data
A catalogue record for this book is available from the British Library.

For any available supplementary material, please visit
http://www.worldscientific.com/worldscibooks/10.1142/10742#t=suppl

Desk Editors: Dr. Sree Meenakshi Sajani/Jiang Yulin

Typeset by Stallion Press
Email: enquiries@stallionpress.com

Preface

While facing different stages of economic development, China and Europe share same demographic concerns and sustainability issues.

Europe has developed good practices of universal healthcare systems, but significant and dramatic changes that have taken place over the past two decades have led to a decrease in health expenditure and a decline in public assistance. Several European countries need to improve public services, especially for the growing aging population, while concurrently decreasing healthcare spending.

Europe has vast experience in developing and operating healthcare policies including prevention and long-term care assistance. European industries have reached a scale of efficiency, global competitiveness, and sophisticated approaches to innovation in the pharmaceutical, equipment, and para-pharmaceutical sectors.

On the other hand, China has embraced large reforms in the healthcare system to upgrade the quality and coverage of assistance provided to the Chinese people. Within this process, the universal healthcare system has been chosen as the benchmark. Multiple strategies have been promoted on both the supply and demand sides. Similar to Europe, China is experiencing the challenges associated with an increasing aging population. The geriatric population requires appropriate, specific, and long-term healthcare assistance, which costs significantly more than those services consumed by a comparatively younger population.

A Europe–China partnership in the healthcare domain could be a win–win strategy for several reasons. Potentially, Europe and China have complementarities that could help each other face their specific needs in the long run. In this scenario, China would benefit from gaining knowledge and expertise from European countries at different levels: From how to project and run a universal system and how to plan a specific care program for its aging population to the use of Western medicine (WM) to cope with new and improved medical needs of the population.

Europe could "export" to China solutions and best practices, and thus find business opportunities. At the same time, China could export to Europe practices and approaches of traditional Chinese medicine (TCM) that could be cost-saving and effective in specific pathologies.

A multidisciplinary team has contributed to this book, following the research activity and international mobility program carried out in the 4 years of the "People Marie Curie Actions Fp7-People-2013-Irses" CHETCH, i.e., *China-Europe taking care of Healthcare solutions* (GA n. 612589).

Researchers in the social science and humanities area have compared the European and Chinese healthcare systems at different levels, including value systems and ethical issues.

The economic experts have analyzed the integration reached between China and Europe in the healthcare-related industries (technologies, pharmaceutical, and other). Foreign direct investments and trade flow trends were studied at the regional and provincial levels. The typical cost–benefit tools were used to evaluate the economic impact of integrating WM and TCM practices, supporting the medical team of experts.

The legal instruments have defined obstacles and plausible solutions that can be generated by the regulatory environment, as well as appropriate solutions to enhance collaboration both at institutional, medical practice, and business levels.

The team of experts in the medical field have investigated several areas of integration. The team has developed a process of recognition and scientific validation of TCM versus complementary alternative medicine

(CAM) at different levels, as recommended by the World Health Organization Traditional Medicine Strategy 2003-2005.

A central role was played, in the whole project, by acupuncture. Indeed, in the social and historical context of Europe, the integration of acupuncture in European Healthcare Systems is an opportunity. The main motivation is the increase in the elderly population and in chronic diseases: the chronic patient is a frail patient with poor quality of life who generates costs to the healthcare system, with direct and indirect costs. The elderly patient often takes polypharmacological therapy, which reduces therapeutic compliance and causes side effects.

Evidence-based medicine (EBM) demonstrates that acupuncture is effective in treating chronic diseases, particularly pain, improves the quality of life, and helps to reduce/eliminate drug intake, significantly reducing the problem of side effects. Other fields of application of acupuncture, alone or integrated with WM, are as a support to fertility and assisted reproduction therapy (ART) and for the treatment of side effects caused by oncological therapies. Acupuncture has proven to be safe and cost-effective, and the EBM data are favorable to its integration in the National Healthcare System.

Nevertheless, to practice acupuncture, appropriate training is fundamental. The gold standard role is played by the physician (medical doctor), who has to combine western medicine training with an appropriate amount of hours of theoretical and practical learning of acupuncture and Chinese medicine.

Other professionals, apart from the medical one, must have theoretical and practical training, at least equal to that offered in China to Chinese medicine students in Chinese traditional medicine universities, to achieve a sufficient expertise in patient management.

Thanks to its multi-level analysis, the book contributes to increase the availability of interdisciplinary studies providing a comprehensive overview (including medical, legal, economic, and humanities perspectives) of Europe–China relations in the healthcare domain. This comprehensive study is also the base for further projects where the integration of WM and TCM needs to be further explored and developed, also on the basis of scientific evidence of the strong benefit that both patients and systems can get. Nevertheless, a cultural shift is needed to change the perception, in Europe, about the role and foundations of TCM. Training programs and specific public engagement activities are needed to increase the awareness of the tremendous achievements that Europe could get by deeply integrating TCM with the Western approach for the benefit of the patient and their treatments.

At the end of the 4-years cooperation within the CHETCH project, we would like to extend our deepest gratitude to some persons and organizations that really helped and supported our research program, namely:

- the China Academy of Chinese Medical Sciences (CACMS), which facilitated generously the vast clinical data from China and arranged a highly qualified team of researchers to collaborate with the CHETCH project. Our thanks go in particular to professor Yang Shuo, Director of the Research Department of the Institute of Traditional Chinese Medicine Information, for organizing the work of the research team;
- Barbara Chiucconi, project manager of CHETCH, who helped the entire team with excellent expertise and great professionality;
- Administrative staff of EU universities and Institutions for their support to the sound management of secondments and financial aspects of the project;
- Corrado Capelli, who followed all the phases of the project managing website and social media tools for dissemination;
- our group of experts that constantly provided scientific and practical support during the project. We refer to Dr. Marco Gasparroni, regional head Greater China for Exprivia Group and CEO of Exprivia IT Solutions (Shanghai) Co. Ltd; Dr. Ilan Alon, Professor of Strategy and International Marketing at University of Agder (Norway); and Stuart O. Schweitzer, Professor of Health Policy and Management at the University of California Los Angeles (UCLA).

A final word of thanks to all researchers, professors, and staff of the institution partners of CHETCH who made this project a very exciting, fruitful, and interesting experience.

Attilio Mucelli and Francesca Spigarelli

Contents

List of Contributors

Alessandra Biagini
Università Politecnica delle Marche, Italy

Alessandra Pavesi
A.M.A.B. Associazione Medici Agopuntori Bolognesi, Italy

Alessandra Poini
A.M.A.B. Associazione Medici Agopuntori Bolognesi, Italy

Andrea Ciavattini
Università Politecnica delle Marche, Italy

Attilio Mucelli
Università Politecnica delle Marche, Italy

Carlos Llopis
European Foundation of Chinese Traditional Medicine (FEMTC), Spain

Carlo Maria Giovanardi
A.M.A.B. Associazione Medici Agopuntori Bolognesi, Italy

Changmian Zhang
East China University of Political Science and Law, China

Chiara Pollio
Università di Ferrara, Italy

Claudia Skopalik
European Foundation of Chinese Traditional Medicine (FEMTC), Spain

Claudio Socci
Università di Macerata, Italy

Dan Yang
Beijing Normal University, China

Daniela Caruso
A.M.A.B. Associazione Medici Agopuntori Bolognesi, Italy

Elena Santilli
Università di Macerata, Italy

Erik Longo
Università di Macerata, Italy

Federica Monti
Università di Macerata, Italy

Federico Marmori
European Foundation of Chinese Traditional Medicine, FEMTC, Spain, the Acupuncture Department, Vithas Medimar Hospital, Spain

Francesca Spigarelli
Università di Macerata, Italy

Giacomo Tirabassi
Università Politecnica delle Marche, Italy

Giancarlo Balercia
Università Politecnica delle Marche, Italy

Gianmaria Salvio
Università Politecnica delle Marche, Italy

Giulia Sorgentoni
Università Politecnica delle Marche, Italy

Giuseppe Tallarida
A.M.A.B. Associazione Medici Agopuntori Bolognesi, Italy

Giuseppina M. Farella
A.M.A.B. Associazione Medici Agopuntori Bolognesi, Italy

He Wei
Academy of Traditional Chinese Medicine Information Institute,
China Academy of Chinese Medical Sciences, CACMS, China

Jing Wan
Nanjing University of Chinese Medicine, China

Kim Van der Borght
Vrije Universiteit Brussel, Belgium

Laura Vagni
Università di Macerata, Italy

Li Zongyou
Academy of Traditional Chinese Medicine Information Institute,
China Academy of Chinese Medical Sciences, CACMS, China

Lihong Zhang
East China University of Political Science and Law, China

Liu Xia
Beijing Normal University, China

Liu Yang
Academy of Traditional Chinese Medicine Information Institute, China Academy of Chinese Medical Sciences, CACMS, China

Manli Huang
South China University of Technology, China

Marco R. Di Tommaso
Università di Ferrara, Italy

Maria Letizia Barbanera
A.M.A.B. Associazione Medici Agopuntori Bolognesi, Italy

Matteo Serri
Università Politecnica delle Marche, Italy

Mauro Devecchi
A.M.A.B. Associazione Medici Agopuntori Bolognesi, Italy

Miriam Caffarini
Università Politecnica delle Marche, Italy

Monia Orciani
Università Politecnica delle Marche, Italy

Monica Mattioli-Belmonte
Università Politecnica delle Marche, Italy

Nina Montik
Università Politecnica delle Marche, Italy

Noemi Ferracuti
Università di Macerata, Italy

Olena Liakh
Università Politecnica delle Marche, Italy

Pamela Lattanzi
Università di Macerata, Italy

Paolo Sospiro
Università di Macerata, Italy

Ping Lv
University of Chinese Academy of Sciences, China

Qijun Fang
Nanjing University of Chinese Medicine, China

Qingle Hu
Hunan University, China

Qinhong Wu
Beijing Normal University, China

Qu Ruxiao
Beijing Normal University, China

Roberto Di Primio
Università Politecnica delle Marche, Italy

Saisai Wang
Vrije Universiteit Brussel, Belgium

Tianshu Xu
Nanjing University of Chinese Medicine, China

Tong Yuanyuan
Chinese Academy of Traditional Chinese Medicine Information Institute, China Academy of Chinese Medical Sciences (CACMS), China

Umberto Mazzanti
A.M.A.B. Associazione Medici Agopuntori Bolognesi, Italy

Xiaolin Yuan
Nanjing University of Chinese Medicine, China

Xu Zhang
Nanjing University of Chinese Medicine, China

Xueping Zhou
Nanjing University of Chinese Medicine, China

Yang Kunjie
Academy of Traditional Chinese Medicine Information Institute, China
Academy of Chinese Medical Sciences (CACMS), China

Yang Shuo
Academy of Traditional Chinese Medicine Information Institute, China
Academy of Chinese Medical Sciences (CACMS), China

Yin Renfang
Academy of Traditional Chinese Medicine Information Institute, China
Academy of Chinese Medical Sciences (CACMS), China

Yu Liang
University of Chinese Academy of Sciences, China

Yue Qi
South China University of Technology, China

Yujuan Wang
Nanjing University of Chinese Medicine, China

Zeng Yanping
Beijing Normal University, China

Zhang Huamin
Academy of Traditional Chinese Medicine Information Institute, China
Academy of Chinese Medical Sciences (CACMS), China

Zhang Lei
Academy of Traditional Chinese Medicine Information Institute, China
Academy of Chinese Medical Sciences (CACMS), China

Part 1

Healthcare System and Industry in Europe and China: Common Issues and Future Opportunities

Chapter 1

Relevance of Western Medicine and TCM in the Chinese and European Markets: An Overview

Attilio Mucelli

1. INTRODUCTION

Traditional Chinese Medicine (TCM) was developed more than 2,500 years ago as a system for studying human physiology and pathology, as well as for preventing, diagnosing, and treating illnesses. The most common TCM practices include herbal and nutritional therapy, restorative physical exercises (*qigong*), meditation, acupuncture (stimulating specific points of the body using various techniques), remedial massage (*tuina*), moxibustion (applying heat to acupuncture points by burning herbs above the skin's surface) and *tai chi* (dance-like body movements combined with coordinated breathing and mental focus).[1]

Over the period 2003–2011, it was estimated that the TCM industry sales had a 24% Compounded Average Growth Rate (CAGR), with respect to the 21% for Western Medicine (WM), indicating that it is not only one of the fastest emerging activities within the Chinese territory but also an increasingly recognized practice abroad. In value terms, TCM reached USD 14.135 million by 2014.[2]

From 2007 to 2014, the fastest growing suppliers of raw materials for TCM were Thailand (+59.7% per year) and Germany (+35.7% per year).

According to the China Chamber of Commerce for Import & Export of Medicines & Health Products (CCCMHPIE), the exports of TCM products from China had increased by 25.54% (totaling USD 3.14 billion) in 2013, thanks to the rising international demand for Chinese herbal medicine.[3] The CCCMHPIE reported that, in 2012, China's top 10 export markets included only Germany and France among the EU countries,[4] while the leading destinations of TCM exports in 2014 were Japan, Indonesia, the Philippines, Malaysia, and Thailand, which together comprised 44.8% of TCM export volume.

According to *China Daily*, the global promotion of TCM has been boosted by the establishment of an official relationship between the World Federation of Chinese Medicine Societies (WFCMS) and the World Health Organization (WHO), in order to provide technical support to the WHO as well as achieve cooperation with other nongovernmental institutions.[1]

While TCM has been expanding abroad, WM in China has become increasingly popular. An analysis of the revenue composition in TCM hospitals in China showed that, from 1999 to 2008, the percentage revenue coming from WM increased from 59.6% to 66.1%, whereas that from TCM declined from 18% to 13.7%.[5] It is obvious that WM represents a key financial source for the survival of TCM hospitals, which mainly generate revenues by providing WM services. The main reasons for this trend is related to the significant decline in government subsidies toward healthcare facilities, as well as to the fall in the demand for TCM services: 94.8% of rural residents and 84.9% of healthcare providers admitted to seeking WM care as the first choice, compared to 5.2% and 15.1%, respectively, of those opting for TCM therapies first.[5]

2. THE ROLE OF TCM IN THE CHINESE CONTEXT

The regulation on TCM is embedded into the Chinese constitution. Regulation of TCM by the People's Republic of China in 1982 affirms that the State protects, supports, and promotes the development of TCM, as well as its integration with WM (both types of medicine have equal importance, should complement each other, and improve through mutual learning and knowledge exchange). There is a TCM Department at the Ministry of Public Health,[6] and the responsibility of formulating all of the related regulations, policies, and guidelines are entrusted to the State Administration of TCM, which also has the task to build its standardized management and development.[7] TCM is fully covered under the government and private insurance schemes. Patients have the right to freely choose which type of medicine to resort to (either traditional or conventional), and TCM practitioners are able to practice in either public or private hospitals and clinics.[8]

In 2012, TCM accounted for 31.24% of the entire domestic medicine market (with expenses above USD 79.5 billion), according to the National Bureau of Statistics in China.[9]

The China Academy of the Chinese Medical Sciences assessed that, by 2013, the total output value of TCM had already reached one-third of the domestic medicine industry (estimated at USD 91.4 billion).[10] The yearly revenue growth of 18.1% (from 2008) led to a total of USD 29.6 billion during the same year, thanks to the increasing demand for these services by the patients. The top four industry competitors accounted for almost 3.1% of the entire industry revenue that year, as estimated by IBIS World (whereas the top eight participants held a combined share of less than 5%). In 2013, the number of TCM hospitals was estimated to be around 2,930, each with an average of 196 beds.[11] In terms of higher education institutions, by 2013, 45 schools were dedicated to TCM and 93 were specialized in WM.[7] In 2014, the visits to TCM hospitals accounted for 17.9% of the total hospital visits across the country (530 million visits) and the overall value of the TCM industry increased to USD 110.8 billion.[12]

The revenue of the TCM hospital industry in 2016 rose to USD 53.7 billion, which represented an 11.8% growth from 2015. On the whole, there has been an annualized revenue expansion of 16.3% from 2011 till 2016. In terms of profitability, estimates went from 0.9% in 2007 up to 4.6% in 2016.

At present, there are nearly 440,700 Chinese healthcare institutions at all levels (from general hospitals, clinics, and health stations in both urban and rural areas to TCM hospitals), offering TCM services: approximately

90% of the general hospitals include a TCM department, for inpatients and outpatients alike,[8] while the TCM institutions account for 4.3% of the total.[7] The total number of TCM hospitals in China have increased by 500 in the past five years (+15.5%): there are about 3,059 TCM hospitals to date, with 252 beds on average, employing around 831,463 people.[11] The TCM outpatient departments increased as well (by 531) and so did the TCM clinics (by 5,890).[12]

3. TCM STILL LAGS BEHIND IN EUROPE

In 2010, the WFCMS estimated that there were about 120,000 TCM practitioners and acupuncturists in Europe at the time. By that year, acupuncture as a distinct therapeutic system was recognized by law in 12 EU Member States, including Austria, Belgium, Bulgaria, Czech Republic, Denmark, Germany, Greece, Hungary, Latvia, Portugal, Slovenia, and Spain.[7]

In 2012, only 10% of China's total TCM export volume went to the EU (e.g., the exports to the UK dropped by 70%).[13] Nevertheless, over the past four years, a significant number of TCM products entered the EU market, corresponding to annual export sales of traditional Chinese herbal medicinal products to the EU of around USD 12 million (CCCMHPIE data).[14] Germany represents the main European TCM market, from which an expansion toward other EU countries can be easily achieved. In general, the EU is a high-potential market for herbal medicine trade: it is estimated to have a 47% share in the global herbal market (USD 26 billion), with more than 1,270 types of herbal medicines in circulation, and over 60% Europeans using TCM.[15]

The main trade barrier for the development of TCM in Europe is related to the EU Directive 2004/24/EC, also known as Traditional Herbal Medicinal Products Directive (THMPD), which provides the legal basis for TCM and other types of herbal medicines, in terms of entry into the EU market.[16] Its objective is the establishment of a unified regulatory regime for the medicinal products market across all the member nations (each Member State had then to apply their own rules/procedures to regulate TCM accordingly). THMPD planned to introduce a simplified registration procedure of such products, which would have been subject to the

EU quality and safety guarantees (this was particularly important as some TCM products had a very poor reputation of quality in other markets: they were either mixed with WM; contained heavy metal, rare animals, or plants; or lacked specifications regarding shelf life).[17]

The Directive stipulated that only those TCM products that had obtained the authorization could be sold within the EU (with a safety proof of utilization of 30 years, 15 of which within the EU).[18] After a transitional period of seven years (till April 2011), the products that were not registered yet could not be imported into the EU market: the products had to meet the definition of "traditional medical product" and the representative Chinese TCM producers and exporters should have applied for a marketing authorization well in advance, in order to benefit from the transitional period and be able to sell their products in the EU market as medicines (those products that were already marketed in the EU when the Directive entered into force in 2004 had an advantage, but without a marketing authorization, they could not be placed on the EU market as medicines).

However, the challenge of isolating the specific ingredients for the complex Chinese medicines on one hand (unlike WM), and the limited share of TCM in Europe on the other, made it difficult for the Chinese companies to go through the registration process.[15]

Moreover, the huge costs of obtaining approval in the EU for each specific TCM product was estimated to be around USD 650,000–800,000 (USD 160,000 to file and USD 650,000 to upgrade management and production equipment in order to meet EU's standards for Good Manufacturing Practice (GMP).[13] As a result, none of the leading TCM producers had carried out any registration procedures by the 2011 deadline, despite the fact that 350 Chinese herbal substances were licensed during the transitional period. Those products that could not be classified as "drugs", and were therefore excluded from the most lucrative markets, were often marketed in the EU under other product designations (once they met the related EU requirements), such as "food", "nutrition products" or "cosmetics".[19]

In June 2011, TCM exports dropped, as reported by the CCCMHPIE, and 99% of the 10,000 kinds of TCM that were sold as medicines in the EU before that period were prevented from accessing the EU market.

While in 2008, data on the trade of Chinese herbal medicines and extract to the EU suggest an increase in exports (the Netherlands market increased most rapidly, followed by Germany in terms of value), from 2011 to 2012, the exports of Chinese herbal medicines (CPD) declined (–14.64% in the Netherlands, –69.81% in the UK, but +32.67% in Germany, which was the first country to make registration of TM mandatory[15]) in value and volume (–13.5%).

In addition, the uneven registration pattern across the Member States shows the fragmentation (different rules applied in each territory) of the EU market as well as the incapability of the EU regime to reach market integration. In 2013, two years after the transition period, a total of only 110 applications to the registration scheme were observed in 25 European countries: some of them had more than 20 applications while in the majority, there were few to nil applications.[17]

REFERENCES

1. Burke, A., Kaptchuk, T., Lao, L., Weber, W. & Killen, J. (2013). *Traditional Chinese Medicine: An Introduction* (U.S. Department of Health and Human Services, Washington, DC), pp. 1–4.
2. IndexBox Marketing (2015). *China: Traditional Chinese Medicine — Market Report. Analysis and Forecast to 2020* (IndexBox Marketing, South Lanarkshire, Scotland).
3. Taylor, L. (2014). "China's pharma export trade growth slows," *PharmaTimes*. Available at: http://www.pharmatimes.com/news/chinas_pharma_export_trade_growth_slows_100155. Accessed 31 August 2017.
4. Wu, Q., Yang, D., Ge, J., Li, Z., Su, Z. & Mucelli, A. (2017). *Introduction and Analysis of Chinese Health Care Situation and Cooperation Opportunities between China and Europe*, CHETCH Project Material.
5. Shen, J. J., Wang, Y., Lin, F., Lu, J., Moseley, C. B., Sun, M. & Hao, M. (2011). "Trends of increase in Western medical services in traditional medicine hospitals in China," *BMC Health Services Research*, 11: 212.
6. Robinson, N., Lorenc, A., Ding, W., Jia, J., Bovey, M. & Wang, X. (2012). "Exploring practice characteristics and research priorities of practitioners of traditional acupuncture in China and the EU — A survey," *Journal of Ethnopharmacology*, 140(3): 604–613.
7. Yang, L., Cavicchi, A. & Croci Angelini, E. (2015). *Report of European firms in China and Chinese firms investing in Europe*, CHETCH Project Material.

8. World Health Organization (2013). *WHO Traditional Medicine Strategy 2014–2023* (World Health Organization, Hong Kong), p. 37.
9. Thibaud, A. (2014). *Traditional Chinese Medicine: A Profitable Worldwide Trend* (LCB Editors).
10. SSRI China (2014). "TCMs expected to play a bigger role in China's medical reform," *China Medical News*.
11. Smith, G. (2017). Traditional Chinese Medicine Hospitals in China: Industry Research Report. IBIS World.
12. SSRI China (2016). "Traditional Chinese Medicine (TCM) on the rise," *China Medical News*.
13. Cai, C. (2014). "A hard pill to swallow," *China Pictorial*. Available at: http://www.chinapictorial.com.cn/en/industry/txt/2013-11/04/content_575834.htm.
14. Wang, M. & Franz, G. (2015). "The role of the European pharmacopoeia (Ph Eur) in quality control of traditional Chinese herbal medicine in European Member States," *World Journal of Traditional Chinese Medicine*, 1(1): 5–15.
15. Yun, L. (2013). "Testing times ahead for TCM," *China Daily Europe*.
16. Dong, Z. *Present Situation and Future of TCM in Europe* (Pan European Federation of TCM Association's material).
17. Snyder, F., Lu, Y. & Yazdani G. (2013). "Traditional Chinese Medicine and European Union Law: Cultural logics, product identities, market competition, legal rechanneling, and the need for global legal and medical pluralism," *Peking University Law Journal*, 15(2). Shenzhen, research paper 15–2, pp. 2–57.
18. Yang, J. & Devapriyo, D. (2011). "Traditional Chinese medicine gains ground in Denmark," *English News*. Available at: http://news.xinhuanet.com/english2010/health/2011-05/01/c_13854000.htm.
19. HSBC (2015). "Returning to tradition: Chinese medicine regaining traction in domestic healthcare market," *Week in China*.

Chapter 2

New Horizons of Chinese Healthcare System: Reforms and Perspectives

Daniela Caruso

1. HEALTHCARE POLICY IN CHINA: A DIACHRONIC OVERVIEW

China's transformation into a major world power makes its domestic affairs and, particularly, its internal political stability, potentially important for the world. In this context, one of the most important aspects of China's recent history has been the evolution of its healthcare system. As China's economy boomed, its healthcare system nearly imploded, partly because China adopted the strategies of radical healthcare privatization. As a result, the country has faced huge healthcare problems that could pose a potential risk to China's domestic tranquility. At the same time, with governmental coffers swollen by tax revenues from the economic boom, the Chinese have opportunities for healthcare improvement that Western policymakers can only envy.

During the period 1950–1984, the Chinese government granted free healthcare service protection to every worker and, at the end of 1984, the number of people that benefited from complete assistance amounted to more than 20 million.[1] In the early 1980s, the Chinese society was also undergoing a transition from the health point of view: after a spate of epidemic diseases, the population was beginning to suffer from the diseases typical of Western societies, as cancer and cardiovascular diseases, which became the main causes of mortality.[2] Following decollectivization, privatization of the economy and the efforts to reduce centralization in favor of the local management had a serious fallout on healthcare.[3] First of all, China radically changed the method of funding assistance, and the central government reduced investments on health as well as for many other public services. From 1978 to 1999, the share of health national spending fell from 32% to 15%.[4] At the same time, the central government was transferring much of the responsibility of funding to the provincial authorities and local governments, asking them to support themselves through taxes.[5] This produced the immediate effect of supporting the richer coastal provinces to the detriment of the rural areas, laying the foundation for incredible disparity between the services offered. The government cuts facilitated the privatization of most healthcare facilities, which forced the population to rely on the sale of services in private markets. Public hospitals have ended up consider yourself entities whose operation depends primarily on their production capabilities.[6] The government allows profiting from the sale of new drugs and diagnostic technologies to the tune of a 15% profit margin and beyond. Changes have also been made to the salaries of hospital doctors, such as including productivity-based bonus and linking their income to the production (e.g medical prescription) promoting the new products. The results have shown a dramatic increase in the sales of expensive drugs and high-tech services. The complete dismantling of the cooperative system and privatizing the economy also destroyed the social safety nets in most part of the rural areas. Due to the suppressed health cooperative policy, the Chinese people did not receive government aid for medical expenses, and 900 million people were not covered by healthcare assistance. In addition to encouraging the disparity between the rural and urban areas, this policy reduced funding for public health programs in many areas. To balance, the central government allowed local departments and authority to charge for some services such as inspections on health outcomes and compliance with environmental regulations of hotels, restaurants, and industries. Between 1990 and 2002, the percentage of public funding for health dropped from 60% to 42%. The results of these investment choices affect many aspects: primarily, they affect the general system for the provision of healthcare services; second, they contribute to the growing disparities between urban and rural areas; and finally, they affect the effectiveness of the control of epidemics. Only 29% of Chinese have the health insurance (医疗保证, *yiliao baozheng*) needed to cover the cost of care, while medical costs have reached 58% in 2002 compared to 20% in 1978.[7] From 1978 to 2002, the overall health spending of citizens has increased from 3.0% to 5.5% of GDP as a result of the high profitability generated by the pharmaceutical industry and hi-tech services. Moreover, even in the medical industry, as growing foreign investment provided facilities and services in Western-style dedicated to the rich urban elite, the efficiency of the public system was reduced dramatically; with the growth of the private sector, number of health facilities, and staff, access has been precluded to the majority of the Chinese people.[8] Another way to understand the effects of China's post-1980s public assistance is comparing city and country. In a healthcare system based on market economy, consumer wealth is a selective factor for access to the service and its quality, so the citizens of urban areas with an income that was at least three times more huge that of rural areas were not far much better than their fellow farmers who still account for the most part of population. In 1999, 49% of Chinese residents in urban areas enjoyed health insurance coverage; this percentage dropped to 7% for residents in rural areas and 3% for the poorest provinces of western China.[9] Moreover, the quality of care in rural communities was lower than that in urban communities: rural communities were still depending on barefoot doctors who, in that year, based a large part of their earnings on sale of drugs and products that were not controlled. It is estimated that one-third of drugs dispensed in rural areas are counterfeit, which allows suppliers to reap huge profits.[10] These disparities are reflected in the statistics: in 1999, the infant mortality rate was 37 for every 1,000 live births in rural areas, compared to 11 per 1,000 in urban areas. In 2002, the mortality rate among children under five years of age was 39 per 1,000 in rural areas and 14 per 1,000 in urban areas.[11] A significant finding is that, in the poorest rural areas, infant mortality was increasing while it continued to decrease in urban centers. Finally, decentralization and the lack of funding for public health services have greatly weakened China's ability to mount an effective and coordinated response to potential pandemics of infectious diseases. The slow government response to SARS could also be seen as a result of this social health framework, which raised doubts about the ability of China to deal with states of emergency. Since 1998, the Government has been requiring all private and state-owned enterprises to offer a healthcare service after collecting an annual fee deposit from the worker. Under this system, the company was paying 10% of health cost and workers contributed to the service on their own, according to their annual income. Finally, to employers is offered the opportunity to purchase additional insurance to cover the higher service costs for up to 400% of the worker's salary. The central government has been slower and more reluctant but was forced to act to address the problem in rural areas. In 2002, local officials tried to test new safety nets. These schemes provided the equivalent of USD 2.50 per capita yearly to help cover a plan-based insurance for workers who must in turn pay an annual fee of USD 1.25. It was modest funding, which could only deal with the expenses of first aid and short hospitalization; meanwhile, Harvard University researchers were helping the Chinese government to identify alternative models concerning prevention, primary care, and insurance coverage.[10] Traumatized by SARS, Beijing has invested substantial funds for restoring the control of infectious diseases, however, neglecting other aspects of public health.[12] It implemented a disease-reporting mechanism at the district level and set up centers for infectious diseases, but there was large gaps in the monitoring mechanism below these levels.

1.1. *Last reforms and a new approach to the healthcare issues*

In the late 1990s, the saying "medical treatment is difficult to access and expensive" (看病难, 看病贵 *Kànbìng nán, kànbìng guì*) was very common in China; this phrase even appears prominently in the 50-page outlined in the 11th Five-Year Plan (this is the document where they are) for National Economic and Social Development of the People's Republic of China,[13] as the Chinese government became aware that healthcare access and affordability were the key components of social discontent in both urban and rural areas. China's health system reform, launched in early 2000s, has achieved better coverage of health insurance and significantly increased the use of healthcare services by the vast majority of the Chinese population. Between 2003 and 2008, insurance reforms were implemented to improve access and utilization, reduce costs, and provide higher risk protection, particularly for rural populations, primarily to redress the inequalities between rural and urban areas. Most programs were initiated as pilots to be able to accumulate lessons learned prior to scaling up nationwide. In 2003, the government implemented a pilot in four provinces and 333 counties to revamp and expand the rural cooperative medical schemes.[14] Between 2000 and 2011, the total health expenditure in China increased from Chinese yuan 319 to 1,888 (i.e., USD 51 to USD 305), with an average annual increase of 17.4%. Government and social health expenditure increased rapidly, amounting to 22.9% and 18.8% of the average annual growth rate, respectively. To increase healthcare affordability, the Chinese government re-established the rural health insurance scheme (called New Rural Cooperative Medical Scheme — NCMS) in 2003 and developed the Urban Resident Basic Medical Insurance (URBMI) in 2007, with substantial financial subsidies from central and local governments and modest premium contributions from individuals, while strengthening urban employee basic medical insurance, a social health insurance scheme jointly contributed by employees and employers in urban China.[15] For both the urban and rural populations, the greatest increase in total health expenditure was seen from 2005 onward.[16] A decade of reforms to China's healthcare system has significantly broadened government-backed insurance coverage and the availability of basic care; policy discussions regarding where to direct additional public spending and the degree of private enterprise that is desirable in China's future healthcare system are underway following a merger in early 2013 of the Ministry of Health and the National Population and Family Planning Commission to create the National Health and Family Planning Commission.[17] While the government is focusing efforts on ensuring universal access to the healthcare system, it also allowing the private sector to play a role in the delivery of healthcare services addressing the additional needs of higher-income patients.

2. 13TH FIVE-YEAR PLAN AND THE NEW OPPORTUNITIES IN THE SECTOR OF HEALTHCARE

The CPC Central Committee's Proposal on Formulating the 13th Five-year Plan on National Economic and Social Development sets out the goals, principles, and targets for China's development in the next five years and will have significant implications not only for China but also for the world, given the size and global influence of China's economy. It is the first Five-Year Plan formulated under President Xi Jinping's leadership and is considered strategically important, as the year 2020 is not only the centennial anniversary of the founding of the CPC but also the deadline for realizing China's goal to become a "moderately prosperous society" (小康社会, *xiǎokāngshèhuì*). During the annual National Party Congress meeting of 2015, Xi unveiled a set of political slogans called the Four Comprehensives (四个全面战略布局, *Sìgè quánmiàn zhànlüè bùjú*) which includes "Comprehensively build a moderately prosperous society" (全面建成小康社会, *Quánmiàn jiànchéng xiǎokāng shèhuì*). As China's population becomes older and increasingly more urban, China's growing middle class is beginning to demand higher quality healthcare. Recognizing that the Chinese government alone cannot respond to the increased demand for improved health and aged care services and products, the 13th Five-Year Plan promotes the idea of a "Healthy China" (健康中国, *Jiànkāng zhōngguó*) which aims to set up an integrated health and aged care system. Key initiatives include improving access for private investors to develop and acquire private hospitals, encouraging the development of private aged care facilities and home care services, developing more comprehensive medical insurance, expanding the scope of physicians' insurance, and establishing a more efficient mechanism for resolving disputes. In addition, the government is going to boost e-Health by encouraging investment in online healthcare products and information-sharing on cloud platforms.[18]

On March 6, 2016, the State Council issued a five-year plan on elderly care, clearly spelling out the goals and principal tasks for promoting the development of undertakings for the elderly and establishing the elderly care system during the 13th Five-Year Plan period. The plan sets the following goals for 2020 — 90% of urban workers and urban and rural residents will be covered by basic old age insurance; basic medical insurance coverage will stay above 95%; the percentage of government nursing home beds will not exceed 50%, with nursing beds accounting for at least 30%; 70% of elderly people above 65 years of age will have health management; and the coverage of grass-roots elderly people's associations in urban and rural communities will exceed 90%.

The Plan puts forward the main tasks in the following eight respects:

1. Improving and perfecting the social security system;
2. Improving the elderly care service system;
3. Improving the health support system;
4. Igniting the consumer market for senior citizens;
5. Promoting the building of a suitable living environment for the elderly;
6. Enriching the spiritual and cultural life of senior citizens;
7. Expanding senior citizens' social participation; and
8. Protecting the legitimate rights and interests of the elderly.

According to the State Council's opinion, China will continue to develop a diversified approach for medical service delivery, mainly permitting foreign joint ventures and medical partnerships. This should accelerate the development of aged care, primary care, and other diversified healthcare services and foreign investments. There is no doubt that China's enormous healthcare market will continue to expand rapidly, driven by an aging population, economic growth, and expanding basic health insurance. In 2013, healthcare expenditure in China hit RMB 3.2 trillion, maintaining an annual growth rate of 17.2% over the past nine years. Yet healthcare expenditure accounts for a mere 5.6% of GDP, in comparison with a high-income-country average of 7.7%. Given population trends and consumption patterns, it is evident that there is room for promising growth in China's healthcare market. The National Planning Guideline for the Healthcare Service System (2015–2020) represents the first comprehensive five-year blueprint targeting key areas for development by 2020; it shows that the reform of the healthcare sector is both a social and strategic priority for China. The Government's emphasis on the opening up of the private sector has attracted global interest in the development of China's healthcare sector: the 13th Five-Year Plan shows the willingness to encourage the private sector to provide healthcare services by according them the same status as public institutions.[19]

REFERENCES

1. Ding, Y. (1994). "Guanyu gongfei yiliao zhidu gaige sikao" [Considerations around the reform of the public health care system], *Shehuixue yanjiu* [*Social Sciences Studies*], 10: 11.
2. Zhōngguó wèishēng bù [Ministry of Healthcare of P.R.C] (2004). Weisheng Nanjian [China Health Yearbook], Beijing, pp. 10–12.
3. Caruso, D. (2007). "La salute della Cina: per una storia della politica sanitaria cinese dalla nascita della repubblica popolare all'economia di mercato," *Orienthalia Partenopea*, 6: 88.
4. Blumenthal, D. & Hsiao, W. (2005). "Privatization and its discontents — The evolving Chinese health care system," *The New England Journal of Medicine*, 353(11): 1165–1170.
5. Hesketh, T. & Zhu, W. X. (1997). "Health in China: The healthcare market," *British Medical Journal*, 314(7094): 1616–1618.
6. Liu, L. & Chen, N. (2000). "The Chinese experience of hospital price regulation," *Health Policy Plan*, 15(2): 157–163.
7. Liu, Y., Rao, K. & Hsiao, W. C. (2003). "Medical spending and rural impoverishment in China," *Health, Popular Nutrition Review*, 21(3): 216–222.
8. Liu, Y., Rao, K. & Hu, S. (2002). *People's Republic of China: Toward Establishing A Rural Health Protection System* (Asian Development Bank, Beijing), pp. 21–23.
9. Liu, Y. (2004). "Development of the rural health insurance system in China," *Health Policy Plan*, 19(3): 159–165.
10. Hsiao, W. C. (2004). "Disparity in health: The underbelly of China's economic development," *Harvard China Review*, 5(1): 64–70.
11. Schmitt, E. (2005). "Rumsfeld warns of concern about expansion of China's navy," *New York Times*, 18th February.
12. Cyranoski, D. (2003). "SARS triggers biomedical shake-up in China," *Nature*, 425: 333.

13. Zhou, Z., Zhu, L., Zhou, Z., Li, Z., Gao, J. & Chen, G. (2014). "The effects of China's urban basic medical insurance schemes on the equity of health service utilization: Evidence from Shaanxi Province," *International Journal for Equity in Health*, 13: 23.
14. Barber, S. L. & Lan, Y. (2010). Health insurance systems in China: A briefing note, World Health Report, Background Paper, 37, p. 8.
15. Barber, L. S. & Yao, L. (2011). "Development and status of health insurance systems in China," *The International Journal of Health Planning and Management*, 26: 339–356.
16. Long, Q. *et al.* (2013). "Changes in health expenditures in China in 2000s has the health system reform improved affordability," *International Journal for Equity in Health*, 12(40): 1–8.
17. Daemmrich, A. (2013). "The political economy of healthcare reform in China: Negotiating public and private," *Springer Plus 2*, 448: 1–13. Accessed 17 October 2017.
18. NPCC (2016). 13th Five-Year Plan, Part XIV, Better Education and Health for all Citizens, "Promote a Healthy China", p. 173.
19. Deloitte (2015). China's healthcare provider market: Riding the waves of reform, p. 2. Available at: https://www2.deloitte.com/content/dam/Deloitte/global/Documents/Life-Sciences-Health-Care/gx-lshc-china-healthcare-provider-market-en-150512.pdf. Accessed 17 October 2017.

Chapter 3

Effect of Aging on Healthcare Industry's Cooperation Opportunities Between Europe and China

Dan Yang, Qinhong Wu and Attilio Mucelli

1. INTRODUCTION

China, as one of the largest emerging markets in the world, provides tremendous cooperation opportunities with other countries in many areas. This chapter focuses specially on potential cooperation between China and Europe in the healthcare industry. In China, the healthcare industry has developed rapidly since 2005. According to the statistical data from National Bureau of Statistics of the People's Republic of China, the total expenditure on healthcare presents a growth trend, and its proportion in GDP has risen as well. In 2012, the total expenditure on healthcare was RMB 2,784.68 billion, and its percentage of GDP reached 5.36%, as seen in Fig. 1.

Figure 1. Healthcare Expenditure and Percentage in GDP in China.

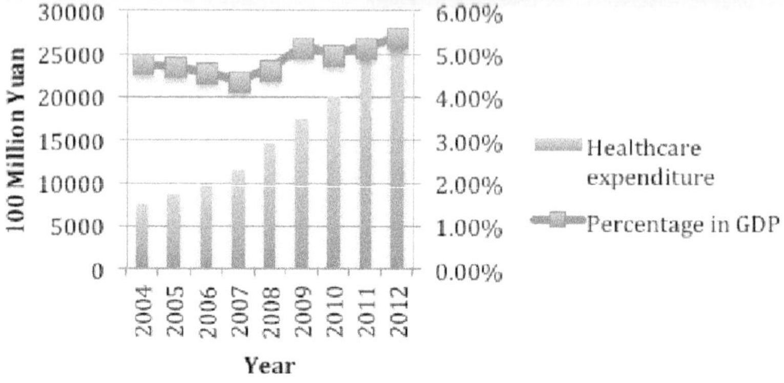

Source: National Bureau of Statistics of the People's Republic of China.

From supply–demand aspects, the supply of healthcare industry maintains steady growth in China. Up to the end of 2012, there were 9.5 million medical and healthcare institutions in China. As to the structure of the institutions, there are 0.231 million hospitals and 9.13 million primary-level medical and healthcare institutions. The primary-level medical and healthcare institutions include 0.336 million community health service centers, 0.37 million township health centers, 6.53 million village clinics, and 1.78 million clinics (dispensaries). The number of small-sized community health service centers, township hospitals, clinics, and village health centers decreased, while the scale of large-sized medical institutions expanded. An increasing number of medical institutions place greater demands of high-end medical equipment and products than before, which lay a solid foundation for the market both in China and Europe.

As for healthcare demand in the Chinese medical market, in recent years, there has been a substantial rise in the healthcare expenses of urban and rural residents. The rapid growth of healthcare expenditure represents a significant amount of per capita demand in the rural areas, driving the development of the medical industry. If we look at the structure of public health expenditure (Fig. 2), around 34.3% of

Figure 2. Change in Medical Expenditure Structure (2002–2012).

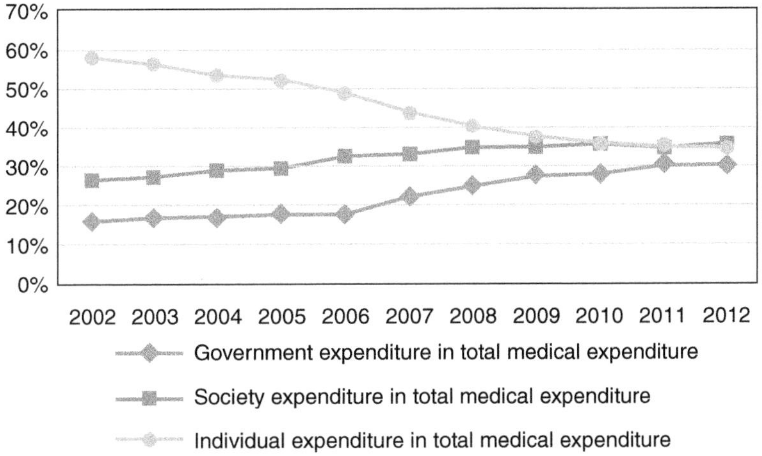

Source: National Health and Family Planning Commission of the People's Republic of China.

the total health spending was for the individual in 2012, while that in 2002 was 57.7%; the proportion of government and social expenditure in total health expenses increased from 15.7% in 2002 up to 30.0% in 2012. The new type of rural cooperative medical care system was built in 2002, and the system of medical rescue in urban and rural areas was set up in 2003. In 2007, many people benefited from the implementation because of the extension of the coverage of medical insurance.

According to the 12th Five-Year plan, the Chinese GDP will maintain a growth rate of 7% in the next five years, and the average income will increase as well. It is estimated that a comprehensive well-off society will be built until 2020. Healthcare consciousness will improve gradually, and the demand of medical institutions will increase accordingly. As a result, the demand of health protection and medical beauty therapy will be greater, and so the structure of healthcare demand needs adjustment in the future.

2. FOREIGN TRADE OPPORTUNITIES IN CHINESE HEALTHCARE

As China's economic reforms deepen, a great wave will impact various industries, especially with the adjustments of trade structure and the optimization of market structure. Chinese companies will become active in the Global Value Chain. We explore the foreign trade opportunities in Chinese healthcare in three categories: western medicines, traditional Chinese medicines, and medical devices. Table 1 summarizes the exports and imports of western medicines and traditional Chinese medicines in China in 2012. As for medical devices, customs statistical data show that, in 2013, the total trade of Chinese medical devices was valued at 34.41 billion dollars, increasing by 14.13% compared to last year. Exports reached 19.34 billion dollars, with a year-on-year growth of 9.92%, while imports reached 14.98 billion dollars, with a year-on-year growth of 20.07%. The trade surplus was 4.36 billion dollars, shrinking by 14.8% from last year. China imports medical devices from more than 100 countries and regions, with the Europe being the largest market, followed by

Table 1. Top 10 Markets for Exports and Imports in 2012 (Unit: Million Dollars).

Western Medicines				Traditional Chinese Medicines	
Country	Exports	Country	Imports	Country	Exports
USA	3,180.07	Germany	2,100.39	Japan	39,333.71
India	2,854.68	America	2,046.94	Hong Kong	29,932.50
Japan	1,379.60	France	1,333.75	America	27,961.77
Korea	1,211.28	Switzerland	1,232.26	Korea	12,994.83
Germany	1,148.17	Japan	1,130.46	Vietnam	8,318.19
Holland	978.64	Italy	1,025.84	German	7,993.19
Australia	674.22	England	844.21	India	5,600.43
Spain	608.14	Ireland	828.20	Malaysia	5,462.28
Italy	599.32	Sweden	790.35	Singapore	5,410.42
Brazil	578.53	Belgium	587.52	France	5,369.19

Source: China Chamber of Commerce of Medicines & Health Products Importers & Exporters.

North America. With regard to export of medical devices, USA, Japan, Hong Kong, Germany, and England were the top five markets of China.

3. AGING POPULATION AND HEALTH STATUS

Nowadays, population aging has attracted increasing consideration and become a hot topic in the academic and practical areas. The one-child policy promoted by the Chinese government has substantially slowed down the population growth without doubt; however, it has also contributed to population aging and many other social issues.

3.1. *Aging situation in China*

According to research from the National Bureau of Statistics of the People's Republic of China, in 2013, population aged above 60 years reached 202.43 million, comprising 14.9% of the total population while the population aged above 65 years reached 131.61 million, making up 9.7% of the total population. Population aged above 60 years represents a 1.6% increase from 2010, while the population aged above 65 years increased by 0.8%. The data shows that the degree of population aging has increased and the elderly population is growing rapidly.

In fact, there are two outstanding characteristics of aging in China.

3.1.1. *High rate of aging*

The scale of aged population in China is expanding rapidly, while the aging process continues to accelerate. In this chapter, the aging degree refers to the proportion of population aged 65 years and above. China has become an "aging society" since 1999. The first and second nationwide censuses showed that the percentage of population aged 65 years and above in 1953 and 1964 was 4.41% and 3.56%, respectively. After the 1960s, with the decline in fertility rate and death rate, the population began to age. In the period between the third and fourth nationwide censuses, the aging population increased by 30.2 million every year, with an annual growth rate of 2.85%, which is higher than the overall population growth rate. In 2000, the fifth nationwide census showed that the aging

Figure 3. Aging Degrees from 1953 to 2010 in China.

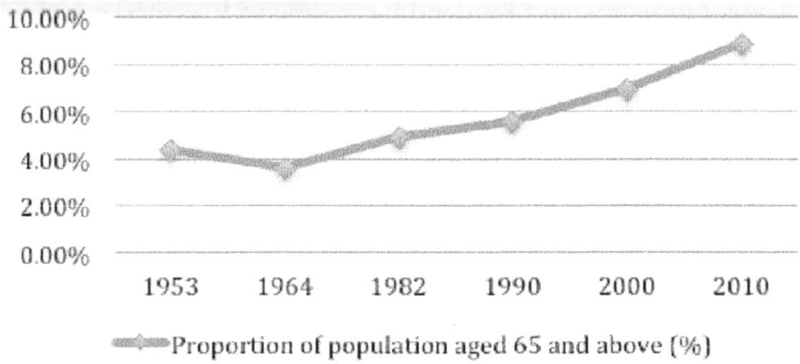

Note: Summarized by the authors.
Source: National Bureau of Statistics of China.

population was estimated at 88.1 million, accounting for 6.96% of the entire population. In 2010, the sixth nationwide census shows that aging population was 118.83 million, accounting for 8.87% of the entire population (Fig. 3).

3.1.2. *Aging degree differs in urban and rural areas*

There is a difference in the degree of aging between urban and rural areas. In many countries, the aging degree in rural areas is higher than that in urban areas. Many studies show that the main reason for this phenomenon is that the migration of the labor force from urban to rural areas, leaving behind the elders in the rural areas.[5] With regard to China, according to the data from the Statistical Yearbook, in 2010, the aging degree (population aged 65 years and above) in urban areas, towns, and villages were at 7.7%, 8.0%, and 10.1%, respectively, increasing by 1.0%, 2.0%, and 2.6% from 2000. The variation trend showed that the rural areas witnessed a higher aging rate compared to urban areas. As to the degree of aging in urban and rural areas, many studies show that the aging degree in rural areas exceeds that of urban areas since 2005 (Fig. 4).

As a result, with the decline in death rate and increase in life expectancy, the process of aging in China has grown rapidly. Large base figure, high growth rate, and high aging degree in rural areas are the main

Figure 4. Aging Degree in Urban and Rural Areas of China (1964–2010).

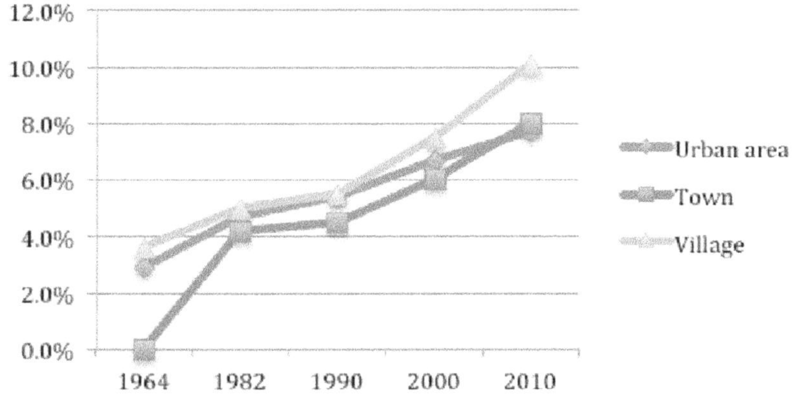

Note: Summarized by the authors.
Source: National Bureau of Statistics of the People's Republic of China.

characteristics of aging in China. Population aging brings the issue of health status of aging people, which attracts attention in related areas.

3.2. *Health status of aging population*

With increasing age, the physiological functions start to deteriorate and resistance drops, resulting in higher rates of hospitalizations and deaths in the elderly. At the same time, the elderly are affected mainly by chronic and non-infective diseases instead of acute and infective diseases. According to the data from the National Health Department, the prevalence rate of chronic diseases increases with age. The prevalence rate of chronic diseases of population aged 45 years and above increases significantly. The prevalence rate of chronic diseases in population aged 65 years and above rose to 64.54% in 2008 from 54.03% in 1993, about three to four times higher than in population aged 35 to 44 years (Table 2). The prevalence rate of chronic diseases in urban areas was found to be higher than that in rural areas. The prevalence rate of chronic diseases in urban areas was 23.96–28.58% between 1993 and 2008 while in rural areas, it was 11.84–17.05% (Fig. 5). However, the growth rate in rural areas is higher than that in urban. As to the aging population, prevalence rate of

Table 2. Prevalence Rates of Chronic Diseases (1993–2008).

	Age							
Year	0–4	5–14	15–24	25–34	35–44	45–54	55–64	65+
1993	19.2	19.2	26.0	66.4	162.0	263.4	430.5	540.3
1998	13.4	18.6	25.8	72.5	142.2	232.0	386.5	517.9
2003	6.3	9.6	18.0	58.3	117.1	219.5	362.1	538.8
2008	6.4	8.7	20.2	51.3	121.7	259.5	419.9	645.4

Note: Summarized by the authors.
Source: 2013 Statistical Yearbook of the National Health and Family Planning Commission of the People's Republic of China.

Figure 5. Prevalence Rates of Chronic Diseases in Urban and Rural Aging Population (1993–2008).

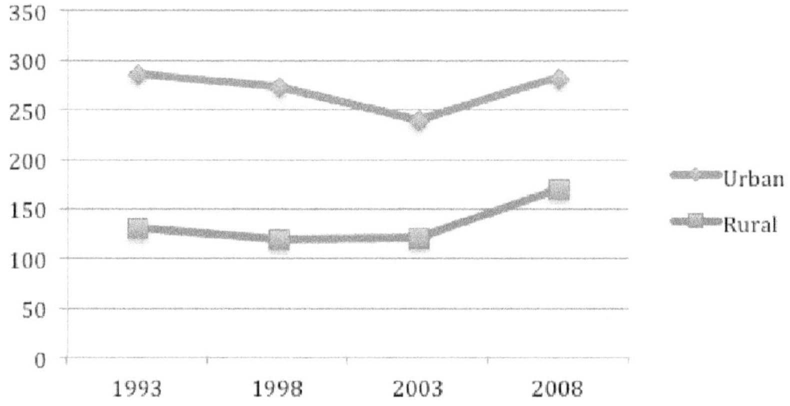

Note: Summarized by the authors.
Source: 2013 Statistical Yearbook of the National Health and Family Planning Commission of the People's Republic of China.

chronic diseases in the urban aging population is higher than that in rural areas. The former rose to 85.18% in 2008 from 78.93% in 1993, while the latter rose to 52.39% in 2008 from 39.82% in 1993. The growth rate in rural areas was higher than in urban and the difference between rural and urban areas were becoming smaller.

Normally, with the high prevalence rate, more types of diseases, and longer sick time, aging people have a higher consultation rate, hospitalization rate, and length of stay (Table 3). According to the data from the

Table 3. Two-week Prevalence Rate, Consultation Rate, and Hospitalization Rate (%).

	Age				
Rate	25–34	35–44	45–54	55–64	65+
Prevalence rate	7.5	13.6	22.7	32.2	46.6
Consultation rate	6.1	11.4	16	21.6	30.3
Hospitalization rate	6.9	4.7	6.2	9.3	15.3

Note: Summarized by the authors.
Source: 2013 Statistical Yearbook of the National Health and Family Planning Commission of the People's Republic of China.

National Ministry of Health Statistical Yearbook, the prevalence rate, consultation rate, and hospitalization rate keep growing.

4. EFFECT OF AGING ON HEALTHCARE DEMAND

In empirical analysis, healthcare devices and healthcare expenditure are always used to present healthcare demand. In theory, health status is the most substantial factor of healthcare expenditure in an aging population. The health status worsens with age, and aging people have a higher prevalence rate; as a result, the demand of healthcare services and healthcare expenditure are higher in the elderly compared to people of other age groups. From the aspect of healthcare system, a change in the population structure will lead to related healthcare demand and healthcare resources and, finally, contribute to the change in healthcare expenditures. Especially in China, the effect of aging on healthcare expenditure is more significant because of large base figure, high growth rate, and high degree of aging.

There are two main reasons that aging will significantly increase healthcare expenditure. The first one is that, with the high rate of the aging process, the aging population grows rapidly, prevalence rate increases, and healthcare expenditures increase. Second, with the development of economics and healthcare resources, the related healthcare system becomes perfect and technology advances; therefore, the satisfaction degree of healthcare demands grows gradually. As a result, only when the added demand is satisfied can aging drive healthcare expenditure.

4.1. *Features of aging and healthcare expenditure*

According to the China Health and Nutrition Survey (CHNS), in 1993, the actual healthcare expenditures of sample subjects aged over 50 years declined with age. In 2000, the actual healthcare expenditures of samples aged over 50 years declined with age, while for the age group of 60–79 years, the healthcare expenditures increased. In 2009, the actual expenditures increased with age (excluding population aged 80 years and above). The data, to some extent, reflects that in the 1990s, the healthcare demand was not satisfied and aging does not lead to the increase in healthcare expenditure, rather it even results in a decline in expenditure. Since 2000, aging and healthcare expenditure have had a positive correlation.

According to Chinese academic research, we can categorize two features of healthcare expenditure under aging. The first one is the type of healthcare expenditure that becomes nursing expenditure. With the increase in the expectant lifetime, the prevalence rate of chronic diseases and disability rate will increase; as a result, the consultation and hospitalization expenditure will decline while nursing expenditure will increase. Long-term nursing expenditure has a significant positive relationship with age.[1,2] The other feature is that healthcare expenditure of an aging population is higher than that of other age groups. According to Beijing's statistical data, the average hospitalization fee of population aged below 60 years is RMB 5,471.3 while that of population aged above 60 is RMB 9,443.5 which is 1.7 times that of the former.[3] Anderson and Hussey[4] find that the healthcare expenditure of population aged above 65 years is 2.7–4.8 times higher than that of the population aged below 65 years in some countries of OECS (Organization of Eastern Caribbean States).

Besides, the relationship between aging and healthcare expenditure differs in urban and rural areas. Because of the differences in income level, health resource supply, healthcare system, and input of government, the degrees of satisfaction of healthcare demands between urban and rural areas are different. According to the statistical data given below, healthcare expenditure of urban residents rose to RMB 1,063.7 Yuan in 2012 from RMB 25.7 Yuan in 1990. In the same period, healthcare expenditure

Figure 6. Average Healthcare Expenditure of Urban and Rural Residents.

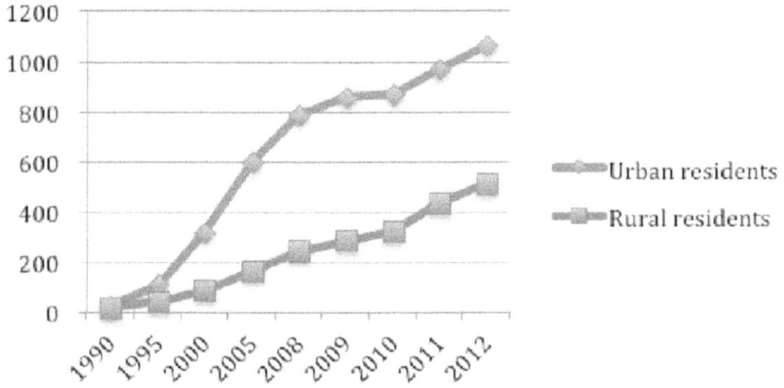

Note: Summarized by the authors.
Source: 2013 Statistical Yearbook of the National Health and Family Planning Commission of the People's Republic of China.

of rural residents rose to RMB 513.8 in 2012 from RMB 19 in 1990. The difference between the average healthcare expenditure of urban and rural residents continues to grow, and rose to 2.07:1 in 2012 from 1.35:1 in 1990 (Fig. 6). The degree of the satisfaction of demands in urban areas sis higher than rural areas, and as a result, aging in urban areas and healthcare expenditure have a more significant positive relationship.

Aging has a significant effect on healthcare expenditure and the effect cannot be ignored; especially with the increasing degree of aging population in the future, this effect will be strengthened gradually. The rapid aging process leads to a change in healthcare demand and healthcare expenditure, which poses a significant challenge for the healthcare system. Under normal circumstances, aging has a higher health depreciation rate and a stronger demand for healthcare, so healthcare expenditure will grow with the increase in aging. On the other hand, some factors, such as adequate healthcare resource supply and good economic conditions, will contribute to the allocation of healthcare resource and healthcare demand of aging. As a result, healthcare expenditure may decline while the degree of aging increases. Therefore, all the above-mentioned factors should be taken into consideration.

4.2. *Trend of healthcare demand under aging*

It is an inevitable tendency that the aging process will accelerate. The growth rate of the global elderly population is 2.6%, which is 12% higher than the overall population growth rate. It is estimated that in 2050, the percentage of population aged 60 years and above will be 22% and the population aged above 80 years will comprise 20% of the population aged 60 years and above (Fig. 7). In China, the situation is even worse. The World Bank estimates that the degree of aging in China (the proportion of people aged 65 years and above) will be 11.53% in 2020, 2.43% higher than the worldwide average level. According to the 12th Five-Year plan, from 2011 to 2015, population aged 60 years and above will rise to 221 million from 178 million and will increase by 8.6 million every year. The proportion of elderly people will reach 16% from 13.3% and increase by 0.54% every year. The scale of aging population will double by 2030.

Accordingly, compared with young people, the elderly will have a higher rate of health depreciation. Besides, decline of self-care ability in daily living, increase of prevalence rate, and long-term hospitalization will make a higher demand of healthcare service to elderly people and deepen the effect of the degree of aging on healthcare expenditure.

Figure 7. World Aging Degree (Proportion of Population Aged 60 Years and Above).

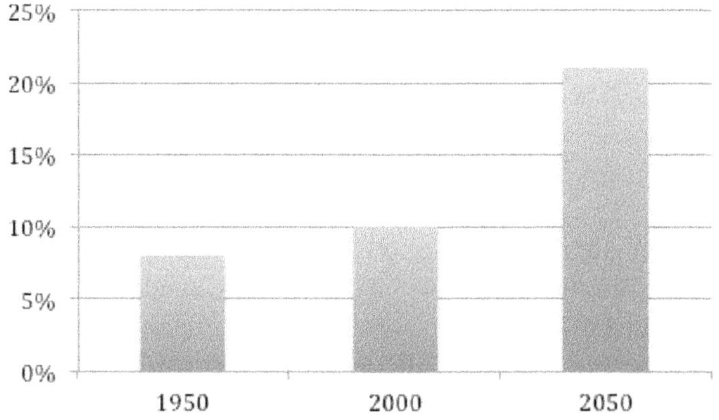

Note: Summarized by the authors.
Source: United Nations (2009).

Aging is a worldwide issue, and acceleration of aging is a definite tendency in the future. Because of the higher depreciation rate, the possibility of falling sick, and increased hospitalization time, the healthcare demand of aging population is higher than that of other age groups. Besides, since the satisfaction degree of healthcare demands in rural areas is lower than in urban areas, the market in rural areas is greater.

5. OPPORTUNITIES

5.1. *Demand of structural change in medical institutions' supply*

The structure of Chinese medical institutions is changing slowly, and the number of community health center shows an obvious increase, as hospitals and village clinics rise slowly. However, the number of township hospitals decreases every year.

There is a significant difference in devices and medicines between medical institutions, and some are not available after structural adjustment. Newly established medical institutions create more demand for medical devices and products. The decrease in community health centers and village clinics are related to policy, and this should be the case for many years to come. This will certainly increase opportunities for healthcare industry cooperation between China and Europe.

5.2. *Rapid increase in medical expenditure*

According to the data presented earlier, the total expenditures of healthcare grew rapidly and reached RMB 2.78 trillion in 2012, with an increase of 381.94 % compared to 2002, comprising about 5.36% of GDP. The rapid growth in medical expenditure has further widened the market demand in China. Further, there are two issues we need to pay attention to: one is that the improvement of the three system, including the New Rural Cooperative Medical Care System (NRCMCS), urban and rural medical assistance programs, and urban medical insurance system, extend the coverage of medical insurance. The other one is that the proportion of government and individual expenditure rises every year, and the share of personal outlays declines gradually. These two situations make the expenses of healthcare more economically affordable, and this will further stimulate the consumption of residents in China. The growth of healthcare expenditure will bring opportunities for cooperation between China and Europe.

5.3. *Expected increased imports of western medicines in China*

As mentioned earlier, in China, western medicines are mostly imported from Europe, with the growth rate of 14.16% and the import proportion of 64.48%. With the increasing healthcare expenditure share in GDP, the demand of people's medical consumption increases rapidly, which requires the growth of imported western medicines. Besides, the adjustment of county-level medical structure will drive the demand of high-quality western medicines. At the same time, the Chinese government promotes the "expanding import" policy, which will also drive the demand of western medicines.

5.4. *More competitive Chinese traditional medicines in the world market*

The Chinese government always promotes the entry of Chinese traditional medicines into the world market. Some outstanding enterprises, such as Tongrentang and Tasly, have opened many chain stores and exclusive shops overseas, bringing Chinese traditional medicines to the world with new marketing initiatives. The development of these micro-enterprises will lead the blossoming of macro-Chinese traditional medicines market, which is deemed as good news to the cooperation of China and Europe in the healthcare sector. In 2012, Chengdu Di'ao became the first enterprise to register in the European Union in traditional medicine area. "Enrichment Angelica Pills" manufactured by Lanzhou Foci successfully got through the examination of the State Drug Administration in Sweden. Besides, Yuanhu pain-kill of Foci, Rhinitis Tablet of Guangzhou Qixing, Radix isatidis of Baiyunshan, herb tablets of Jihuangpu, and some other traditional medicines have been under registration procedures in many European countries. In June 2014, the China Chamber of Commerce of Medicines & Health Products Importers & Exporters organized some Chinese traditional medicine enterprises to attend training programs on the registration of European Union traditional medicines in Sweden. They also visited the State Drug Administration of Sweden and some European medical enterprises and hospitals and discussed the process of registering in European Union markets and expanding the markets of Chinese traditional medicines.

5.5. *The growing Chinese medical devices market*

It is estimated that the Chinese medical devices market will keep growing in the next decade. Some enterprises devote themselves to using advanced technology and new materials, which will make them more competitive in the international market and promote the cooperation between China and Europe in the high-level medical devices sector. With an increasing number of large-scale enterprises entering this industry and market, the standard management will upgrade the competitiveness of the enterprises. Further, with the wide application of digital medical science, some digital medical devices, such as digital orthopedics, capsule endoscopy (an ideal tool for the treatment of gastrointestinal diseases), surgical navigation (a tool for comminuted fracture), and surgery by remote control, offer new ways to modern medical research and play significant roles in explaining medical phenomena, solving medical problems, studying the medical mechanism, and increasing the quality of life.

5.6. *Opportunities in an aging society*

On one hand, compared with young people, the elderly have higher health depreciation and higher prevalence rates of diseases. As a result, the demand of healthcare service of the elderly is greater than the others. On the other hand, the development of the economic level, perfection of healthcare system, and the increase in health recourse supply will enhance the satisfaction of healthcare demands of the elderly, especially in rural areas. It can be shown that the healthcare field has a promising prospect and a huge market. Meanwhile, as a worldwide issue, aging provides a platform for different countries to cooperate in the future and brings great opportunity for healthcare institutions.

ACKNOWLEDGMENTS

The authors acknowledge Jiahuan Ge, Zhen Li, and Zengrui Su for their assistance in information collection.

REFERENCES

1. Spillman, B. C. & Lubitz, J. (2000). "The effect of longevity on spending for acute and long-term care," *New England Journal of Medicine*, 342(19): 1409.
2. Werblow, A., Felder, S. & Zweifel, P. (2007). "Population ageing and health care expenditure: A school of 'red herrings'?," *Health Economics*, 16(10): 1109–1126.
3. Chen, K. (2000). *The Elderly Healthcare and Social Sharing* (China Labor Social Security Publishing House, Beijing).
4. Anderson, G. F. & Hussey, P. S. (2000). "Population aging: A comparison among industrialized countries," *Health Affairs*, 19(3).
5. United Nations Fund for Population Activities (UNFPA) (2009). The State of World Population 2009. United Nations.

Chapter 4

The Chinese TCM Industry: Growth, Changes, and Policies

Marco R. Di Tommaso, Manli Huang, Yue Qi and Chiara Pollio

1. THE CHINESE TCM INDUSTRY: INTRODUCTION AND LITERATURE DEBATE

Observing the development of the Chinese economy and society, there is little doubt that the increase in the capacity of Chinese health industry to provide healthcare solutions to the growing demands of the population is a key aspect.[1–6] In the same perspective, the growth capacity of the national health industry should be considered a priority for China,[7,8] as it has also been highlighted by the 12th Five-Year Plan (2011–2015). According to WHO (2013),[a] in China, there are 440,700 healthcare institutions providing Traditional Chinese Medicine (TCM) services. They have 520,600 patient beds, including all levels of TCM hospitals and general hospitals, clinics, and health ambulatories in urban and rural

[a]The WHO reports Chinese official sources: Government of China and National Bureau of Statistics of China. *China Statistical Yearbook 2011: Chinese Medicine (1987–2010). The State Administration of Traditional Chinese Medicine, China.* Available at: http://www.satcm.gov.cn/1987-2010/start.htm.

areas. The great majority of the general hospitals (90%) include at least one TCM department, and they provide TCM health services for both outpatients and inpatients. In China, government and private insurance fully cover TCM therapies and services: doctors and patients are free to follow TCM or western medicine (WM) for healthcare services. Looking at the domestic market for drugs, in 2012, the sales revenue of China's pharmaceutical industry amounted to 1,515.61 billion Yuan,[b] of which the sales revenue of TCM was 506.71 billion Yuan.[7]

In this scenario, it is also true that the Chinese TCM industry also seems to have important opportunities to grow abroad, given that the use of Traditional and Complementary Medicine[c] (T&CM) is also experiencing a clear boom outside China.[9] The large Chinese communities comprising expatriates and immigrants living abroad (in particular, in the US, Europe, and Australia) have increased the demand for TCM; in addition, foreign patients and doctors have been showing a growing interest in the so-called alternative healthcare practices. According to WHO: "...over 100 million Europeans are currently T&CM users, with one fifth regularly using T&CM and the same number preferring healthcare which includes T&CM. There are many more T&CM users in Africa, Asia, Australia and North America".[10]

For all these reasons, it seems of great importance to shed more light on this sector's performance and perspectives, underlining both the strengths, the development perspectives, and the weaknesses and obstacles it may face now and in the future.

1.1. *Definition of TCM industry in China*

The TCM industry encompasses the production, processing, services, research, and other economic activities related to TCM principles.[11]

[b] 1 USD = 6.90678 Yuan (March 2017).

[c] WHO uses the following definition: The terms "complementary medicine" or "alternative medicine" refer to a broad set of health care practices that are not part of that country's own tradition or conventional medicine and are not fully integrated into the dominant health-care system. They are used interchangeably with traditional medicine in some countries. Available at: http://www.who.int/medicines/areas/traditional/definitions/en/.

Figure 1. A Taxonomy of TCM Industry Activities.

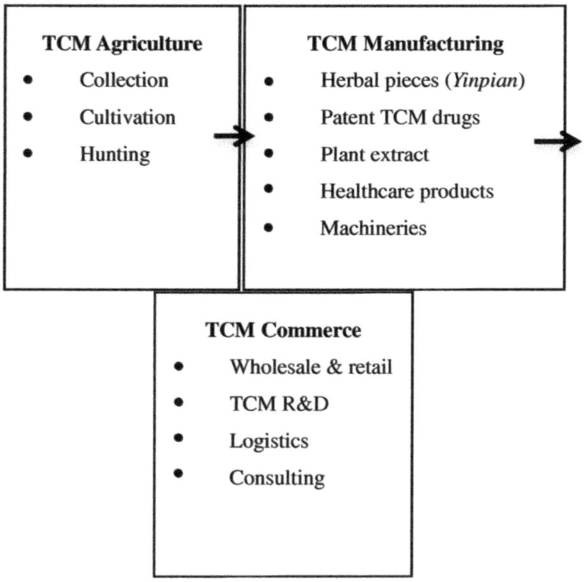

Source: Elaboration of the authors.

Based on the industrial classification by the *China Pharmaceutical Yearbook*, the TCM industry covers numerous sectors and can be divided into (1) TCM agriculture, (2) TCM manufacturing, and (3) TCM commerce (see Fig. 1):

(1) TCM agriculture refers to the collection, cultivation, and hunting of traditional Chinese medicinal materials and herbs.
(2) TCM manufacturing includes the processing of Chinese herbal pieces (also called *Yinpian*), the production of TCM prescription medicines (also known as patent TCM drugs), and the production of TCM healthcare products. More specifically, while *Yinpian* corresponds to herbal pieces prepared, stored, and distributed with the support of modern technologies, patent TCM drugs mainly consists of products — pills or concentrated powdered extracts — used for the prevention or treatment of diseases. Additionally, TCM manufacturing includes other related

activities, such as the production of TCM-specific machineries, auxiliary materials production, packaging, etc. In this chapter, we will focus on TCM manufacturing, with *Yinpian* and TCM prescription medicines as the main products under analysis.[d]

(3) TCM commerce refers to the storage, transportation, sale, and other services closely related to the TCM manufacturing activities, including exports of TCM.[12]

1.2. *The academic debate on China TCM industry*

After the TCM industry was identified as one of the strategic emerging sectors in the Chinese National 11th Five-Year Plan, it has received increasing attention from Chinese scholars coming from medicine and phytology-related disciplines. Yet, despite the long history of TCM activities and their role in China's healthcare system, the topic remains understudied by international scholars of economics and business.

1.2.1. *International contributions*

The few international studies in economics and business fields on the topic address the study of TCM industry with regard to its role in the Chinese healthcare system,[13] pharmaceutical sector,[14,15] and herbal medicine industry.[16] Some contributions focus on quality standards[16,17] and the sector's modernization,[18] which are also some of the main topics in the Chinese debate, as we shall see. Other researches focus on TCM in the European market,[19] TCM in the world,[20] TCM industry's development[21] and innovation capacity,[8] and TCM firms' performance.[7]

On the other hand, much interest on the subject has been demonstrated by medicine/phytology/phytochemistry scholars, also under the stimulus of the European Union, as it is testified, for example, by the academic publications related to the European Project "Good Practice in Traditional Chinese Medicine Research in the Post-genomic Era" (GP-TCM).

---

[d]The products taken in consideration correspond to codes 2730 (for *Yinpian*) and 2740 (for patent TCM drugs) of the National Economic Industry Classification Standards.

1.2.2. *The Chinese perspective*

As it might be expected, the economics and business debate on TCM in Chinese journals is broader and covers various topics. The debate can be framed in three main streams: the first on the modernization of TCM industry, the second on its internationalization, and the third on its competitiveness and the geographical distribution among Chinese provinces.

(1) *Modernization of TCM industry.* The modernization of the sector has been recognized as one of the main challenges for its prosperity and development.[22,23] A feature of such studies is the variety of interpretations of what "modernization" means in the context of TCM and the differences between TCM and WM.[24–26] However, in recent years, a growing number of studies have turned the attention to the factors of modernization, rather than to its interpretation. These researches focus on (a) industrial standards, (b) quality controls, and (c) independent innovation processes. As for the first, Chinese scholars complain about a non-perfect correspondence between the relevant international standards in pharmaceutical sector and TCM core characteristics.[23] However, the possibility to set independent standards to assess TCM appears to be constrained by China's still low capacity in TCM quality control and R&D.[27] Concerning quality control, the main effort of the academic contributions is to try to offer some solutions to overcome the criticized low performance in the sector. Scholars in business and economics suggest to restructure the TCM production chain,[28] to set up a full quality control and traceability system,[27] to test testing technological innovation,[29] and so forth. Finally, independent innovation processes in TCM manufacturing seems to be still lagging behind due to very weak government efforts in generating supportive infrastructure for innovation in TCM industry.[30]

(2) *Internationalization of TCM industry.* Strictly linked to that of modernization, this topic has received most attention as a part of the studies about internationalization of Chinese production. Many studies have focused on the factors fostering or hindering large internationalization processes of TCM, ranging from differences between TCM and WM, quality and

conservation issues, and property rights protection and R&D.[31–33] Other contributions suggest ways to increase the level of internationalization,[34] such as using big data or exploiting the "One Belt, One Road" National Strategy,[23] as well as promoting international cooperation at firm level, improving the standardization of TCM, and accelerating the progress in basic research and education/training and so forth.

(3) *Competitiveness and geographical distribution of TCM manufacturing among Chinese provinces*. Among the three, this topic has by far received the largest attention by Chinese scholars (see, e.g., Refs. 35–39). Such studies highlight a general increase in the competitiveness of the sector, although this evidence largely changes according to the stages of production,[40] innovation capabilities[30] and other factors pertaining to the Porter's diamonds model.[35,41]

Recently, the link between competitiveness and territories has also been stressed. While many scholars have limited their analyses to single province or territory case studies, some more comprehensive contributions have found that the degree of competitiveness of TCM industry varies widely according to regional factors, such as the availability of scientific resources and competences as well as constrains external to the sector as such.[42]

2. DEVELOPMENT OF TCM INDUSTRY IN CHINA

2.1. *Size*

TCM production in China has increasingly grown in recent years. As we can see in Table 1, the output value of TCM products has increased almost nine-fold, surging from 84 to 708 billion Yuan between 2003 and 2014. In parallel, its share in the pharmaceutical sector as a whole has increased, as WM production has grown at a slower pace than TCM: indeed, the latter has increased from 30% of the total output in pharmaceuticals in 2003 up to 35% ten years later (Table 1).

As for the different TCM product categories, patent drugs are by far the most important products in terms of economic contribution to industrial output, accounting for almost 567 billion Yuan in 2014 compared to 141.5 billion Yuan for *Yinpian* products in the same year (Fig. 2). The two categories also

Table 1. Output Value of TCM Products and WM Products, 2003–2014 (Unit: Billion Yuan).

	TCM Products		WM Products	
Year	Output Value (Billion Yuan)	As % of Total Value of Pharmaceuticals	Output Value (Billion Yuan)	As % of Total Value of Pharmaceuticals
2003	83.72	*30.58*	190.04	*69.42*
2004	92.59	*30.85*	207.53	*69.15*
2005	116.97	*30.20*	270.28	*69.80*
2006	144.57	*32.08*	306.05	*67.92*
2007	173.58	*30.91*	388.01	*69.09*
2008	208.39	*29.18*	505.81	*70.82*
2009	252.37	*29.85*	593.05	*70.15*
2010	328.16	*31.15*	725.28	*68.85*
2011	431.40	*32.41*	899.59	*67.59*
2012	490.02	*32.44*	1020.29	*67.56*
2013	607.27	*34.13*	1172.16	*65.87*
2014	708.37	*35.09*	1310.35	*64.91*

Source: Authors' elaboration on the *Chinese Pharmaceutical Yearbook* data.

Figure 2. Output by Products: *Yinpian* and Patent TCM Drugs During the Years 2003–2014 (Unit: Billion Yuan).

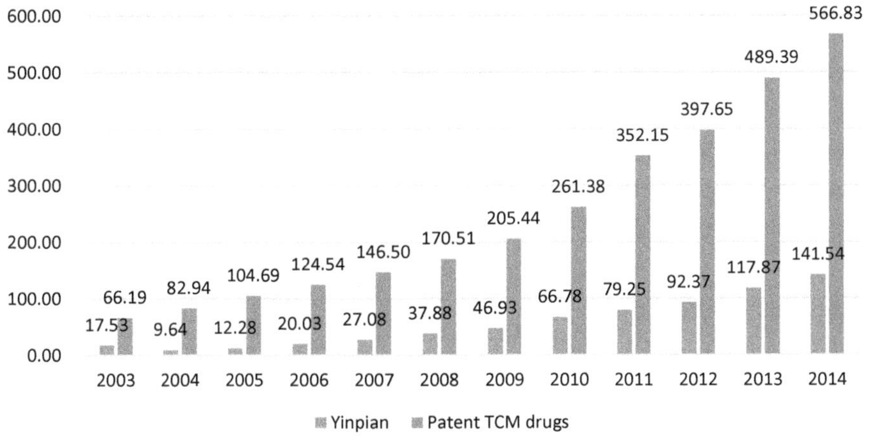

Source: Authors' elaboration on the *Chinese Pharmaceutical Yearbook* data.

Table 2. Some Indicators TCM and WM Firms, 2006–2012.

	TCM Firms			WM Firms	
	Number	Of Which Loss-Making	Average Dimension (Billion Yuan)	Number	Average Dimension (Billion Yuan)
2006	1835	*458*	0.08	—	—
2007	1948	*423*	0.09	—	—
2008	2150	*422*	0.10	—	—
2009	2256	*373*	0.11	2494	0.24
2010	2369	*319*	0.14	2525	0.29
2011	2034	*165*	0.21	2172	0.41
2012	2238	*178*	0.22	2274	0.45

Source: Authors' elaboration on the *Chinese Pharmaceutical Yearbook* and National Bureau of Statistics in China data.

show a similar growth trend across the decade from 2003 to 2014, with an average annual growth rate ranging around 64–68%, although *Yinpian* production seems to increase faster than patent drugs in the post-crisis period.

Turning to the number of firms involved in TCM production, we find that they have grown both in number and in average dimension in recent years. Their number is comparable with that of the firms producing WM products. On the other hand, it is noteworthy that the average dimensions vary hugely between the two groups, as TCM companies are systematically smaller. A closer look at the data shows that both the total number and the number of loss-making enterprises fell in 2011, with a consequent positive effect on the dimension of firms. Such rationalization might be a consequence both of the economic crisis and a change in one of the relevant policies for the sector, such as the issuing of the new GMP certification that sets higher requirements on enterprises, forcing some of the firms to exit the market (Table 2).

2.2. *Innovation*

Although TCM is a traditional industry, it is now increasingly considered as one with high technology content. Therefore, technology and innovation have assumed growing importance in this sector. In this part, we focus specifically on patent TCM drugs, as given the nature of the products, innovation processes are more difficult to quantify with respect to *Yinpian*. Technological innovation has attracted increasing attention in the TCM industry.

We summarize some indicators for innovation processes at firm level in Table 3. We proxy the resources involved in innovative processes — innovation input — by looking at the amount of R&D expenses for new products by firms producing patent TCM drugs. If we exclude the small decline in 2008, the figure maintains a growing trend across the decade of 2003–2014, increasing from less than 0.7 billion Yuan to more than 8 billion Yuan. We observe the largest increase, both in absolute and in percentage terms, in 2011, in correspondence with the already seen change in the structure of the sector in terms of number and dimension of firms.

Regarding innovation output, we report sales in new products and number of patent applications by TCM firms. Sales figures show an

Table 3. Innovation by Firms Involved in Patent TCM Drugs Production (Years: 2003–2014).

Year	R&D Investments for New Products (Billion Yuan)	Revenues from the Sales of New Products (Billion Yuan)	Number of Patent Applications
2003	0.66	12.16	347
2004	0.99	14.88	560
2005	0.97	10.46	1288
2006	1.51	12.37	1133
2007	1.77	13.66	1340
2008	1.69	17.74	1751
2009	2.10	23.42	1827
2010	2.26	29.44	2098
2011	4.19	47.84	3282
2012	5.75	65.91	4007
2013	7.47	82.96	4762
2014	8.02	101.99	5285

Source: Author's elaboration on the data based on National Bureau of Statistics in China.

impressive growth, particularly in the post-crisis period, increasing from 12.37 billion Yuan in 2003 to 101.99 billion Yuan in 2014. In addition, patents applications increased substantially, with the number of patent applications in 2014 being 15-fold larger than that in the beginning of the period. Also in the case of output, the growth appears steeper from 2011 onward.

Patents are an important indicator of innovative output. The number of patent applications by the proprietary TCM industry has maintained a certain degree of growth from 2006 to 2015, reaching 5,285 in 2014, but in 2015, there was a substantial decline, only accounting for 3,011 patents, a decline of up to 43.03% (Table 3).

2.3. *Export and import*

The total value of exports of TCM-related products was USD 1.54 billion in 2014, as shown in Fig. 3. Exports have grown in the recent years, thanks

Figure 3. Chinese Exports and Imports for TCM Products (Years: 2006–2014). Unit: Billion US Dollars.

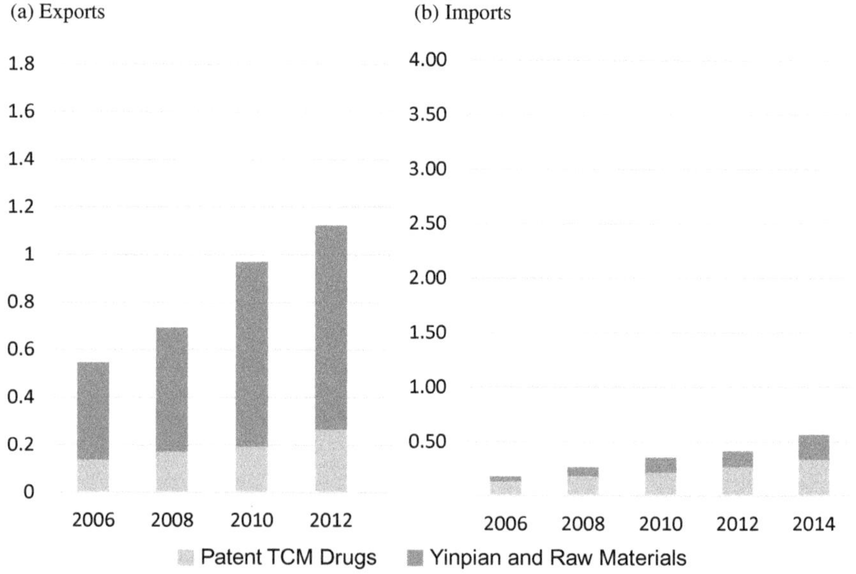

Source: Authors' elaboration on the *Chinese Pharmaceutical Yearbook* data.

in particular to the increase in demand for *Yinpian*, while the performance of patent drugs has maintained a constant trend.

The total amount of imports is much smaller, although it has also grown in the period under examination. On the other hand, we can see an opposite composition of import with respect to export: patent TCM products are the most imported, and this leads to a negative trade balance for this category of products for the majority of the years taken in consideration.

2.4. *Regional distribution of TCM production*

Due to the strong dependence on resources of the sector, its presence and dimensions varies greatly across the Chinese provinces. Figure 4 shows the industrial output value by provinces in 2014. Overall, the production seems to be concentrated in few provinces, among which Jilin, with more than 90 billion Yuan, emerges by far as the most important, followed to a large distance by Shandong and Sichuan — ranging around 50 billion

Figure 4. Output Value of TCM — *Yinpian* and Patent TCM Drugs — by Chinese Provinces (Year: 2014; Unit: Billion Yuan).

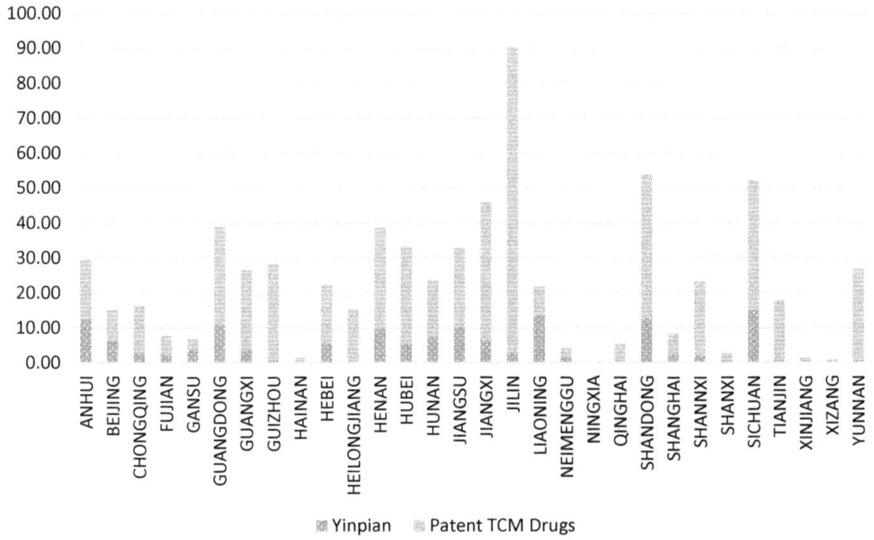

Source: Authors' elaboration based on the *Chinese Pharmaceutical Yearbook* data.

Yuan. For the case of Jilin and Sichuan, such primacy is related to the large amount of value constituted by patent TCM drugs production, while the amount of *Yinpian* is negligible for the case of Jilin. Sichuan and Shandong, on the other hand, rank among the first provinces also for *Yinpian* production together with Liaoning, although the production of the latter seems more evenly distributed across territories. According to the data, such highly performing provinces in terms of production feed mostly the domestic market: in fact, if we exclude Shandong, they are not large exporters of TCM products (Fig. 5), while other provinces such as Anhui and Guangdong rank first in export performances even with a relatively lower level of output.

The market structure — in terms of size and number of firms — is another dimension of the geographical organization of production showing high variation across provinces. Some large producers or exporters such as Jilin and Anhui have a relatively low number of firms — between 200 and

Figure 5. Exports of Herbal and TCM Products by Province (Year: 2015; Unit: Thousand Tons.).

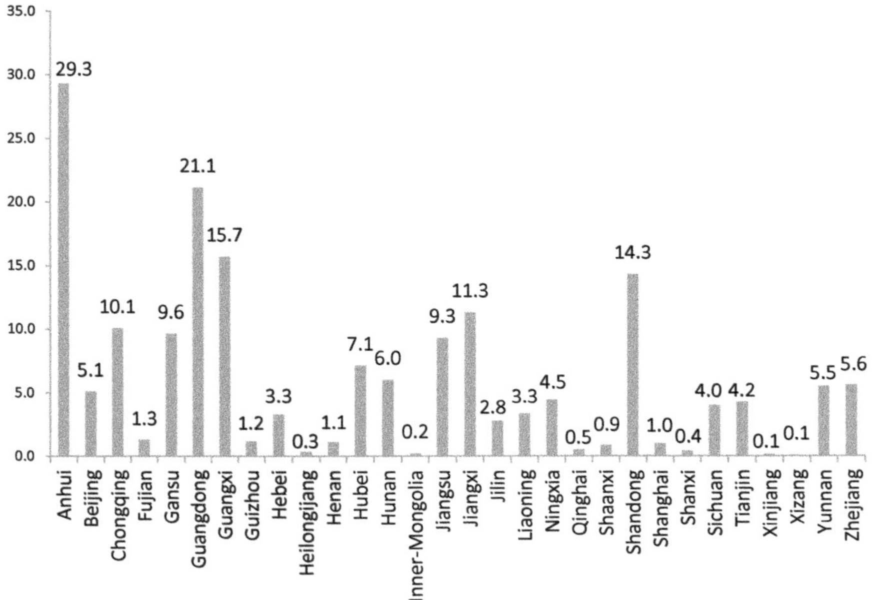

Source: Authors' elaboration based on China Custom Statistics data.

Figure 6. Number of TCM Firms by Province (Year: 2012).

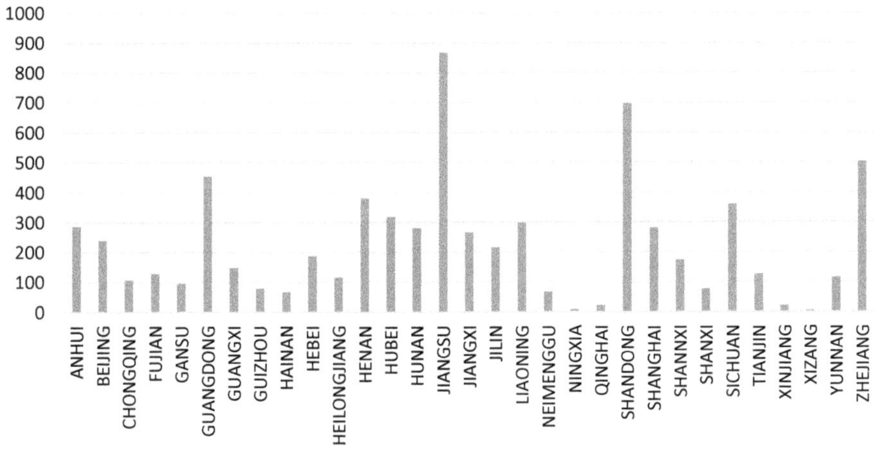

Source: Authors' elaboration based on the *Chinese Pharmaceutical Yearbook* data.

300. In other areas, such as Shandong and Guangdong, the large amount of output/exports is coupled with a large number of firms. On the other hand, we find provinces, such as Jangsu and Zheijiang, with low performances in terms of production or export but a large number of firms (Fig. 6).

Finally, regarding listed companies, Guangdong is the province where the largest number of them is located — 8 out of 61 in 2016. The companies in Guangdong also total the largest market value (as on June 30, 2016). On the other hand, few companies are located in those provinces that are in the leading positions in the industrial value of TCM production or export volume, such as Shandong, Sichuan, and Anhui (Fig. 7). This province constitutes a great potential market both for supply and demand, which should be taken into consideration by listed companies in their production and market strategies.

3. POLICIES FOR TCM IN THE LAST DECADE

Due to the complaints of market and government failures since the healthcare reforms began in the 1980s, in the last decade, TCM has received increasing attention by local and above all national policymakers as one of the most important components of China's healthcare system. At the

Figure 7. Number and Market Value of Listed Companies in TCM by Province (Year: 2016; Market Value Calculated on June 30, 2016, Unit for Market Value: Billion Yuan).

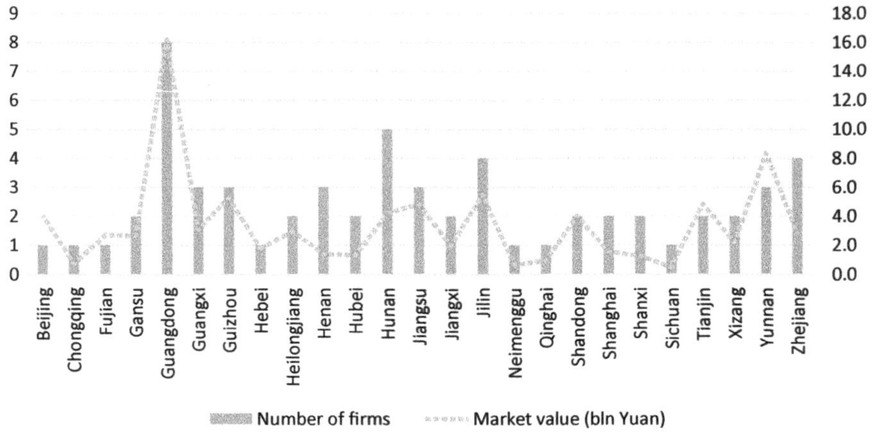

Source: Elaboration of the authors.

same time, in the light of the obstacles to the sector's internationalization and modernization, active support by the government to the sector is considered as needed not only by policymakers but also by scholars and practitioners. In this framework, in the last ten years (2006–2016), we have assisted in the issuing of a number of policy documents related to TCM by governments at different levels.

3.1. *State-level initiatives*

When analyzing the decision-making process behind the policy initiatives for TCM at the central level, different policy subjects in the Chinese hierarchical government structure appear to participate and intervene. These various subjects issue policy documents of different hierarchical levels, which also affect the amount of resources allocated as a consequence of the policy. Therefore, understanding the source of the policy, as well as the type of document issued, represents an important step toward the analysis of the objectives, targets, and potential effects of the initiative.

Before the foundation of the National Health and Family Planning Commission (NHFPC) in 2013, three levels of hierarchy intervened in health policies. From high to low, they were: the State Council, the Ministry of Health, and the State Administration of Traditional Chinese Medicine (SATCM). After 2013, NHFPC replaced the Ministry of Health in the hierarchy.

In general, the higher the institution issuing the policy, the higher the hierarchical level of the document. In addition, when a document is issued by the State Council, it will have a higher authority than those issued by the General Office of the State Council. The difference lies in that the former should be signed by the Prime Minister, while the latter should be signed either by the Prime Minister or a vice Prime Minister.

Finally, there is one exception in the hierarchy of policy documents, that is, when the policy is issued by SATCM but has been previously approved by the authority of the State Council, such policy has higher authority than the other policies issued by SATCM. In this case, the policy has higher authority than those issued by SATCM alone, and is comparable to those issued by the General Office of the State Council.

We summarize all the policy initiatives related to the TCM industry in the last decade in Tables 4 and 5. The TCM industry was selected as one of the strategic emerging industry by the 11th Five-Year Plan of the

Table 4. General Policy Documents Mentioning TCM Industry Issued by China State Council (2006–2016).

Title of the Policy Document	Issued Bureaucracy	Issued Date
1 The 13th Five-Year Plan of the National Economic and Social Development of China	The State Council	2016/3/17
2 The 12th Five-Year Plan of the National Economic and Social Development of China	The State Council	2011/3/16
3 The 11th Five-Year Plan of the National Economic and Social Development of China	The State Council	2006/3/16
4 The 13th Five-Year Plan of the National Strategic Emerging Industry Development of China	The State Council	2016/12/19
5 The 12th Five-Year Plan of the National Strategic Emerging Industry Development of China	The State Council	2012/7/20
6 China Manufacturing 2025	The State Council	2015/5/19

Source: Elaboration of the authors.

Table 5. Policy Documents Dedicated to TCM Issued by the State Bureaus of China (2006–2016).

	Title of the Policy Document	Issued Bureaucracy	Issued Date
1	Outline of Strategic Plan for the Development of TCM (2016–2030)	The State Council	2016/2/26
2	Several Opinions of the State Council on Supporting and Promoting the Development of TCM	The State Council	2009/5/7
3	Chinese Medicine Health Service Development Plan (2015–2020)	General Office of the State Council	2015/5/7
4	Strategic Plan for the Protection and Development of Chinese Herbal Medicines	General Office of the State Council	2015/4/27
5	The 13th Five-Year Plan of TCM Development	State Administration of TCM	2016/8/11
6	The 12th Five-Year Plan of TCM Development	State Administration of TCM	2012/6/11
7	The 11th Five-Year Plan of TCM Development	State Administration of TCM	2006/8/3
8	The 12th Five-Year Plan of Information Construction of TCM	State Administration of TCM	2012/7/16
9	The 11th Five-Year Plan of Information Construction of TCM	State Administration of TCM	2007/3/31
10	TCM Innovation Development Plan (2006–2020)	State Administration of TCM	2007/1/13
11	TCM Standardization Development Plan (2006–2010)	State Administration of TCM	2006/7/15

Source: Elaboration of the authors.

National Economic and Social Development of China in 2006. It was the first time that Chinese authorities announced in a Five-Year Plan the will to modernize and standardize the TCM industry. Thus, this can be identified as the first selective policy for the sector at the national level. Since then, the number of policies specifically dedicated to the TCM industry has been increasing (Table 2). Among these, the most remarkable are *the*

Outline of Strategic Plan for the Development of Traditional Chinese Medicine and the Strategic Plan for the Protection and Development of Chinese Herbal Medicines. This demonstrates that the government's attention toward the sector is increasingly becoming stronger. Not only have a larger number of documents been issued but also the authority level has increased with time. In fact, after 2013, there are three policies specified on TCM sector that were issued by the State Council. A possible explanation to such attention of policymakers toward TCM might be as follows: the healthcare system reform has encountered great difficulties in recent years, especially in making basic healthcare affordable. TCM may represent as a low-cost solution compared to WM, and its enhancement might bring consequently further steps in the reform of the healthcare system.

Regarding the contents of these policies, some of them concentrate on promoting the modernization, internationalization, standardization, and innovation of TCM industry, whereas others focus on increasing the size and the competitiveness in SMEs, while some aim at improving the upstream stages of production.

3.2. *The local-level initiatives: Guangdong Province as an example*

In 2005, Guangdong was the first among all provinces in China that officially announced its aim to become a TCM leading province in 2005. In 2006, Guangdong Provincial CPC Committee and Government of Guangdong Province issued the "Decision on Building a Strong Traditional Chinese Medicine Province," which demonstrates the determination of Guangdong's authorities to promote the province's TCM sector. Eight years later, in 2014, the Guangdong provincial government issued a new policy titled "Framework for Action of Promoting the Construction of TCM in GD (2014–2018)." Since this province is leading in terms of firms' competitiveness and export in China as we have seen, its governments underlines in this document the role of private firms in the development of the sector.

4. CONCLUSIONS

In the last decade, TCM industry has been receiving increasing attention by scholars, practitioners, and policymakers. However, it has been developing slowly compared with other contemporary industries in China. Modernization, standardization, and internationalization of the TCM industry have been dominant issues since the late 1970s until now, and China is still struggling to find the best way to overcome such obstacles. Moreover, considering its increasing role in the healthcare system, to solve such problems simultaneously with the healthcare system reform assumes increasing importance for policymakers, also in relation with the reform in the healthcare system as a whole.

REFERENCES

1. World Bank (2016). *Healthy China: Deepening Health Reform in China Building High-quality and Value-based Service Delivery* (World Bank Group, Washington, D.C.).
2. Huang, Y. (2013). *Governing Health in Contemporary China* (Routledge, Milton Park, Abingdon, UK).
3. Daemmrich, A. (2013). "The political economy of healthcare reform in China: Negotiating public and private," *SpringerPlus*, 2(1): 448.
4. Di Tommaso, M. R., Rubini, L. & Barbieri, E. (2013). *Southern China: Industry, Development and Industrial Policy* (Routledge, Milton Park, Abingdon, UK).
5. Rubini, L., Pollio, C. & Di Tommaso, M. R. (2017). "Transnational research networks in Chinese scientific production. An investigation on health-industry related sectors," *International Journal of Environmental Research and Public Health*, 14(9): 975. doi: 10.3390/ijerph14090975.
6. Rubini, L. & Pollio, C. (2017). "China and Europe networks in health. An empirical analysis on co-publications," *International Journal of Healthcare Technology and Management*. doi: 10.1504/IJHTM.2016.10004760.
7. Di Tommaso, M. R., Bonnini, S. & Qi, Y. (2017). "Focusing on the Chinese Health Industry: An empirical enquiry on the TCM listed firms. Is Large and Private Beautiful?" *The International Journal of Healthcare Technology and Management*. doi: 10.1504/IJHTM.2017.10006769.
8. Di Tommaso M. R. & Huang, M. (2010). "Knowledge transfer between universities, hospitals and industry: A case study of the traditional Chinese medicine industry," *International Journal of Healthcare Technology and Management*, 11(4): 283–295.

9. Angelino, A., Khanh, D.T., An Ha, N. & Pham, T. (2017). "Pharmaceutical industry in Vietnam: Sluggish sector in a growing market," *International Journal of Environmental Research and Public Health*, 14(9): 976.
10. World Health Organization (2013). *WHO Traditional Medicine Strategy: 2014–2023* (WHO Press, Geneva).
11. Feng, Z. & Chang, X. (2010). "Analysis of Chinese herbal medicines influence the choice of industrial organization model of economic factors," *Agricultural Technology*, 23(5): 55–63 [in Chinese].
12. Feng, Z. (2009). "The development of the Traditional Chinese Medicine industry in China and management measures, based on the theory of industrial innovation perspective," *Science and Technology Management Research*, 22(8): 6–9 [in Chinese].
13. Xu, J. & Yang, Y. (2009). Traditional Chinese medicine in the Chinese health care system, *Health Policy*, 90(2), pp. 133–139.
14. Spigarelli, F. & Wei, H. (2014). "The Chinese pharmaceutical market: Driving forces and emerging trends," *L'industria*, 35(3): 505–530.
15. Hu, C. & Feng G. (2007). "Empirical analysis of operating performance of Chinese Medicine Listed Companies," *Chinese Journal of Medical Technology, Economics and Management*, 1(6): 60–66. [in Chinese].
16. Dobos, G. J., Tan, L., Cohen, M. H. *et al.* (2005). "Are national quality standards for traditional Chinese herbal medicine sufficient? Current governmental regulations for traditional Chinese herbal medicine in certain Western countries and China as the Eastern origin country," *Complementary Therapies in Medicine*, 13(3): 183–190.
17. Wenzig, E. M. & Bauer, R. (2009). "Quality control of Chinese herbal drugs," in *Evolution of Herbal Medicinal Products*, Houghton, P. & Mukherjee, P. K. (eds.) (Pharmaceutical Press, London (UK) and Grayslake (US)), pp. 393–425.
18. Xu, Q., Bauer, R., Hendry, B. M. *et al.* (2013). "The quest for modernization of Traditional Chinese Medicine," *BMC Complementary and Alternative Medicine*, 13(1): 132.
19. Xu, J., Liu, M. & Xia, Z. (2013). "Will the European Union's traditional herbal medicinal products directive (Directive 2004/24/EC) be against traditional Chinese medicine in EU market?" *Journal of Evidence-Based Medicine*, 6(2): 104–108.
20. Chung, V. C. H., Ma, P. H. X., Lau, C. H. *et al.* (2014). "Views on Traditional Chinese Medicine amongst Chinese population: A systematic review of qualitative and quantitative studies," *Health Expectations*, 17(5): 622–636.
21. Robinson, N. (2006). "Integrated traditional Chinese medicine," *Complementary Therapies in Clinical Practice*, 12(2): 132–140.

22. Gan, S. *et al.* (1998). *Developing Strategy for the Modernization of Chinese Medicine* (Science and Technology Document Press, Beijing) [in Chinese].
23. Liu, X. (2016). "Reflections on TCM modernization and TCM international development," *China Pharmacy*, 27(11): 1441–1444 [in Chinese].
24. Wan, D. & Liu, Y. (1999). "Modernization of Traditional Chinese Medicine research," *China Pharmaceuticals*, 8(9): 30–31 [in Chinese].
25. Yan, X. (2005). "Reflections of some questions on the modernization of Traditional Chinese Medicine," *China Pharmaceuticals*, 14(4): 56 [in Chinese].
26. Li, Z. (2009). "Research on the strategy of the modernization of Traditional Chinese Medicine industry," *Pharmacy Today*, 19(1): 56–57 [in Chinese].
27. Liu, X. (2016). "Recognizing healthy development of Chinese medicine industry from resources- quality-quality markers of Chinese Medicine," *Chinese Traditional and Herbal Drugs*, 47(18): 3149–3149 [in Chinese].
28. Liu, Y., Li, Q. & Wang, X. (2014). "Analysis of complexity in Chinese Medicine industrial chain," *China Journal of Chinese Materia Medica*, 39(16): 3187–3191 [in Chinese].
29. Li, Z., Qian, Z. & Cheng, Y. (2015). "The technological innovation strategy for quality control of Chinese medicine based on Big Data," *China Journal of Chinese Materia Medica*, 40(17): 3374–3378 [in Chinese].
30. Feng, Z., Tao, Q. & Peng, D. *et al.* (2015). "Evolution, characteristics and enlightenment of self-innovation of traditional Chinese medicine industry," *China Journal of Chinese Materia Medica*, 40(11): 2252–2257 [in Chinese].
31. Wang, G. (2009). "Factor Analysis on the internationalization process of Traditional Chinese Medicine industry," *Productivity Research*, 195(10): 118–120 [in Chinese].
32. Li, Y., Yu, J. & Fan, S. (2010). "Research on the internationalization of Traditional Chinese Medicine industry," *Commercial Culture (Academic Edition)*, 8: 101 [in Chinese].
33. Jing, J. & Liao, J. (2011). "Status quo, problems and countermeasure analysis of China Traditional Chinese Medicine industry," *Guangdong Agricultural Sciences*, 38(1): 207–209 [in Chinese].
34. He, J. (2009). "Discussion on technical barrier in internationalization of Chinese Medicine," *Foreign Economic Relations & Trade*, 12(2): 33–34 [in Chinese].
35. Ma, A., Zou, Z. & Cao, Y. *et al.* (2009). "Empirical analysis on the international competitiveness of China Traditional Chinese Medicine industry," *Research on Financial and Economic*, 307(6): 34–38 [in Chinese].

36. Ma, A., Li, Y. & Yu, B. (2011). "Modernization development evaluation on Chinese Traditional Medicine industry," *Industrial Economics Research*, 52(3): 88–94 [in Chinese].
37. Fan, Y., Liu, T. & Li, J. *et al.* (2012). "Research on the international competitiveness of China Yinpian industry," *Chinese Pharmaceutical Affairs*, 26(11): 1186–1191 [in Chinese].
38. Tang, J., Li, Y. & Gao, X. *et al.* (2011). "Empirical analysis on the industrial competitiveness of provincial Patent TCM Drug industry based on Factor Analysis," *Chinese Journal of New Drugs*, 20(12): 1065–1069 [in Chinese].
39. Wang, L. & Yang, Z. (2003). "Research on the international competitiveness of China Traditional Chinese Medicine industry," *Journal of International Trade*, 2003(2): 28–32 [in Chinese].
40. He, G. & Feng, Z. (2011). "Measurement and analysis of the international competitiveness of China Traditional Chinese Medicine industry," *Chinese Health Economics*, 30(10): 60–62 [in Chinese].
41. Xue, W. (2007). "Status and evaluation of the factors of the international competitiveness of Traditional Chinese Medicine industry," *Journal of Liaoning University of Traditional Chinese Medicine*, 9(3): 40–42 [in Chinese].
42. Wan, Y. & Zhang, H. (2015). "Variance analysis on the regional differences about the industrial competitiveness of Chinese medicine," *Economic Geography*, 35(11): 138–143 [in Chinese].

Chapter 5

Trade in Medical Products Between China and EU

Qu Ruxiao, Zeng Yanping and Liu Xia

1. INTRODUCTION

As an important component of national economy, the medical industry is correlated with people's health and life quality. In recent years, Chinese consumption level in medical service has been increasing, resulting in a boom in the Chinese medical market. As one of the most important trade partners, the European Union (EU) shares the complementarity with China in the medical industry, which lays a solid foundation for the development of trade in medical products between China and EU. From 2000 to 2013, the value of trade in medical products between China and EU has realized rapid growth, from USD 1.046 billion to USD 17.446 billion. Trade in medicines increased from USD 606.2 million to USD 11.122 billion. In this chapter, first we provide the definition and classification of medical products proposed by *Commodity Classification for China Customs Statistics*. Then, we analyze the features of trade in medical products between China and EU with data of medicines and medical devices from 2000 to 2013 from UN Comtrade with HS code. Finally, we highlight the problems that impede the development of trade in medical products between China and EU and propose corresponding suggestions.

2. DEFINITION AND CLASSIFICATION OF TRADE IN MEDICAL PRODUCTS

Trade in medical products is referred as the flow of medical products across different countries or areas. Trade in medical products is developed by the international division of labor and is the result of extension and development of medical production in circulation. However, there is no unified and accurate definition and classification of medical products currently. Shen and Tong[1] proposed that medical products are composed of medicines, traditional medicines, and medical devices. While Cao, Wang, and Liu[2] thought medical service should be added into the medical products. Zhang[3] suggested medical products are related with human health and can be classified into healthcare products, medicines, healthcare cosmetics etc. Upon the research described above, it is necessary for us to give a unified classification of medical products.

In term of the function, medical products are referred to the substance that is correlated with human health, which can prevent and cure disease and adjust human physiological mechanism. According to *Commodity Classification for China Customs Statistics,* the classification of medical products can be defined as following.

(1) **Active positive ingredient:** The chemical substance for production of medicines, including medical raw materials as ingredients having therapeutic effect in medicine and medical intermediate products as the foundation for medicines production.
(2) **Medicines:** The medicines that can prevent and cure the disease or the one that can be used in medical service, surgery, and dentistry but not prevent and cure disease directly. In terms of structure and characteristics, medicines can be classified into five parts:

- Human or animal organs for medical uses, including glands and other organs for organo-therapeutic uses, dried whether or not powdered; extracts of glands or other organs or their secretions for organo-therapeutic uses; heparin and its salts; other human or animal substances prepared for therapeutic uses, prophylactic or diagnostic uses, etc.

- Human blood and other biochemical substances for medical uses, including human blood, animal blood prepared for therapeutic uses, prophylactic, or diagnostic uses; antisera and other blood fractions and modified immunological products, whether or not obtained by means of biotechnological processes; vaccines, toxins, etc.
- Medicaments, including the ones consisting of two or more constituents, which have been mixed together for therapeutic uses or prophylactic or diagnostic uses, not put up in measured doses or in packing sales, and the ones put up in measured doses or in packing sales, etc.
- Subsidiary articles for medical uses, including wadding, gauze, bandage, and similar articles such as dressings, adhesive plasters, poultices, etc.
- Other pharmaceutical goods, including dental cements and other dental fillings; first-aid boxes and kits; sterile surgical catgut; diagnostic reagent; chemical contraception preparation based on hormones, etc.

(3) **Medical devices:** According to the *EU Community Directive 93/42(medical devices)*, medical devices are classified as those including any devices, equipment, materials, or other articles, whether or not used singly or combined, even including any devices for human uses as long as they involve one of the following purposes: to diagnose, prevent, cure, or release the diseases; to diagnose, monitor, and cure patients or release the pain of patients; to use in research or as a supplement in the revision of anatomy and physiology; to control pregnancy and help to achieve some effects that cannot be fulfilled by pharmacology, immunology, and metabolism.

Above all, according to the classification described above and commodity HS code from *Commodity Classification for China Customs Statistics,* we study the state of trade in medical products between China and EU from 2000 to 2013 using the UN Comtrade database. The medical products' HS codes are listed in Table 1.

Table 1. Classification of Medical Products.

Class 1	Class 2	Representative Products
Medicines	Human or animal organs for medical uses (HS3001)	Glands and other organs for organo-therapeutic uses, dried whether or not powdered;
	Human blood and other biochemical substances for medical uses (HS3002)	Antisera, vaccines, modified immunological products
	Medicaments (HS 3003 & HS 3004)	Medicaments containing penicillins or derivatives thereof or containing other antibiotics etc.
	Subsidiary articles for medical uses (HS 3005)	Adhesive dressing, gauze, bandages
	Other pharmaceutical goods (HS 3006)	Dental cement, first-aid boxes, dental fillings
Medical devices	Instruments and appliances used in medical, surgical or veterinary sciences	Electro-diagnostic apparatus, syringes, needles, ultraviolet ray apparatus
	Mechno-therapy appliances, etc.	Massage apparatus, ozone therapy
	Other breathing appliances and gas masks, etc.	Gas masks, breathing appliances
	Orthopedic appliances, etc.	Fracture appliances, artificial teeth, hearing aids
	Apparatus based on the use of X-ray or alpha, beta or gamma radiation etc.	X-ray tubes, computed tomography apparatus Apparatus for the use of X-ray, etc.

Source: Commodity Classification for China Customs Statistics.

3. STATE OF TRADE IN MEDICAL PRODUCTS BETWEEN CHINA AND EU

3.1. *General trend of trade in medical products between China and EU*

In general, the value of trade in medical products between China and EU has increased from USD 1.046 billion in 2000 to USD 17.446 billion in 2013 (Fig. 1). Its share of total commodity trade has been growing since

Figure 1. Trade in Medical Products Between China and EU (Million US Dollar).

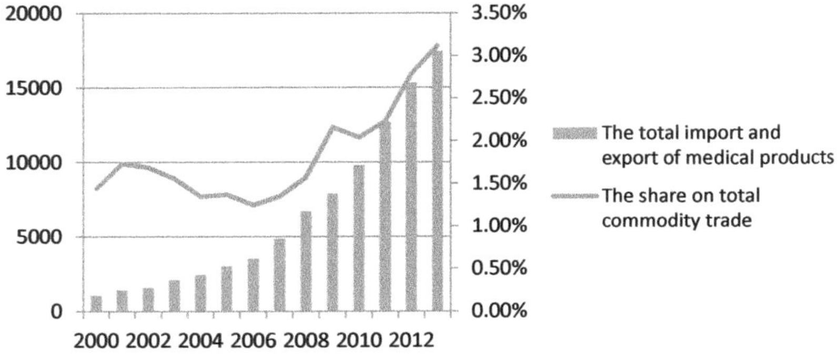

Source: UN Comtrade Database.

2006, which makes trade in medical products more exceptional. However, it is noted that, compared with trade in manufacture, trade in medical products between China and EU is still at a preliminary stage, with great potential to explore.

3.1.1. *Import and export in medical products between China and EU*

In Fig. 2, we find that although both export and import of medical products between China and EU increased, trade deficit of China has grown year by year from USD 544 million in 2000 to USD 9.32 billion in 2013. Besides, the growth rate of import share on total commodity trade exceeds that of export, obviously. In 2000, the import share and export share reached 2.55% and 0.60%, respectively, but in 2013, the rates of both increased to 6.13% and 1.05%, respectively. The gap between import and export has become much wider. Two possible reasons could provide an explanation . First, in terms of product structure, exports from China to EU consist of labor-intensive goods such as gauze, bandage, etc., whose export value is much lower than the import value. However, the imports to China from EU center on technology-intensive and high-value-added goods such as X-ray tubes and medicaments, whose value is much higher. Second, China's growing economy has increased Chinese

Figure 2. Export and Import of Medical Products Between China and EU (Unit: Million US Dollar).

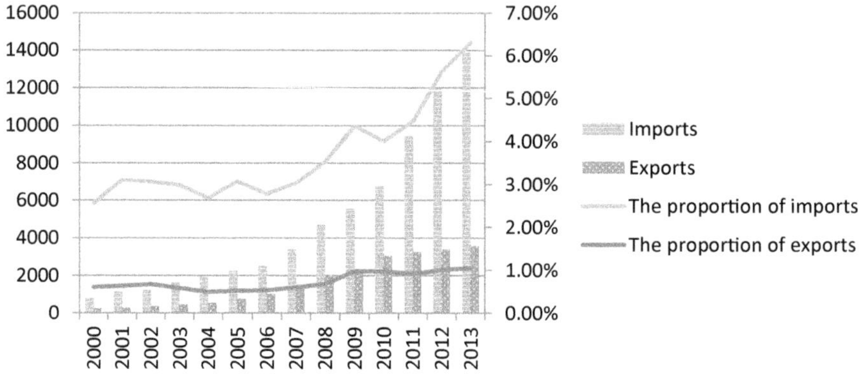

Source: UN Comtrade Database.

consumption for medical services, which has raised the demand for medical products, especially high-end medical products from developed countries.

3.1.2. *Growth trend of trade in medical products between China and EU*

In terms of trade growth, we find that the technological complementarity between China and EU and great potential for demand in Chinese medical market promote trade in medical products between China and EU to grow rapidly from 2000 to 2013. The growth rates during this period were almost above 15%, except for the years 2000 and 2013. The lowest growth rate of import was 8.26% in 2002. It was the year China joined the World Trade Organization (WTO), hence it required time to learn and adapt to the WTO rules and the market mechanism. On the contrary, in 2008, the growth rate of trade reached 38.48%, with import rate and export rate peaking at 39.17% and 36.90%, respectively (Fig. 3).

Figure 3. Growth Rate of Trade in Medical Products Between China and EU.

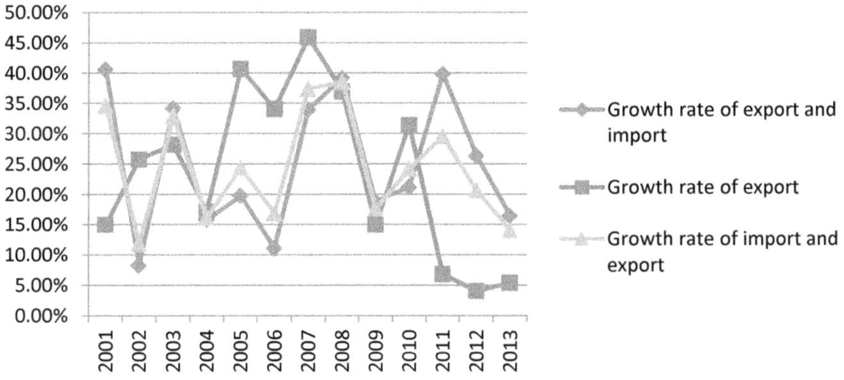

Source: UN Comtrade Database.

3.2. *Structure of trade in medical products between China and EU*

3.2.1. *Structure of trade in medicines between China and EU*

From 2000 to 2013, trade in medicines between China and EU increased steadily from USD 606.2 million in 2000 to USD 11.13 billion in 2013 (Fig. 4). Besides, the import and export of medicines between China and EU increased as well. Compared with export, import has always shown a positive growth rate. In terms of exports, the demand for Chinese medicines diminished due to the SARS disease outbreak in 2003 and EU debt crisis in 2012, thereby showing a decline in exports by a small margin in those two years. The trade gap of China's medical medicines has risen from USD 177.81 million in 2000 to USD 2.09 billion, which showed a serious imbalance of China's medicines trade. Such imbalance could be caused by the structure of trade in medicines between China and EU. Therefore, the trade structure in medicines must be analyzed.

Figure 4. Trade in Medicines Between China and EU (Unit: Million Dollar).

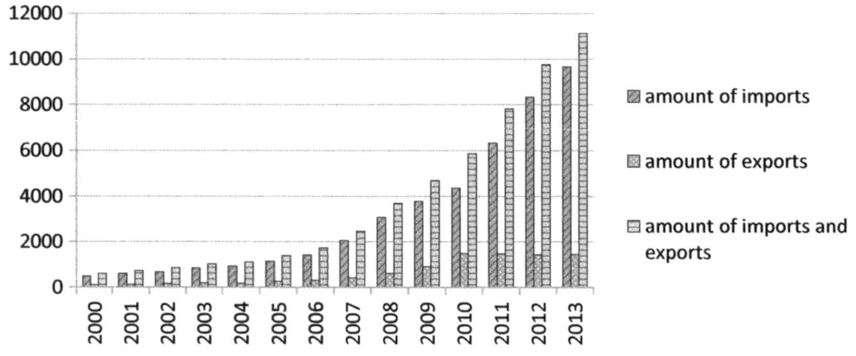

Source: UN Comtrade Database.

Figure 5. Trade in Medical Devices Between China and EU (Unit: Million Dollar).

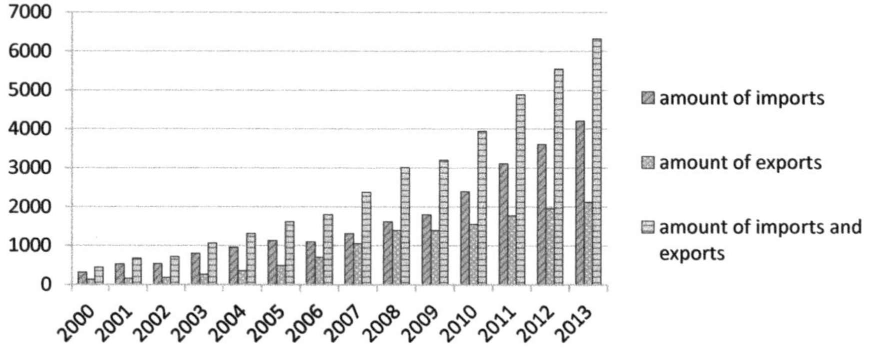

Source: UN Comtrade Database.

3.2.2. *Structure of trade in medical devices between China and EU*

Similar to trade in medicines, the import of medical devices by China from EU exceeded its export. The value of trade increased from USD 439.74 million in 2000 to USD 6.33 billion in 2013. The import of medical devices by China from EU maintained rapid growth except for the year

2002. Compared with import, the export of medical devices from China to EU has maintained a steady state. Therefore, China's trade deficit in medical devices with EU has been negative for many years, and its gap is expanding consistently, which indicates a serious imbalance existing in the trade in medical devices between China and EU (Fig. 5).

3.3. *Destination of China's medical products trade with EU*

3.3.1. *Importers of China's medical products trade in EU*

Figure 6 shows the top 10 importers in EU of China's medical products in 2013. In 2013, Germany, Belgium, France, United Kingdom, and Italy were the top five importers among the 28 EU members. The import shares of those five countries were 27%, 23%, 13%, 13%, and 7%, respectively. Among those five countries, Germany is the biggest importer of medical products from China, with imports valued at USD 959.49 million.

Figure 6. Top 10 Importers of Medical Products from China to EU in 2013.

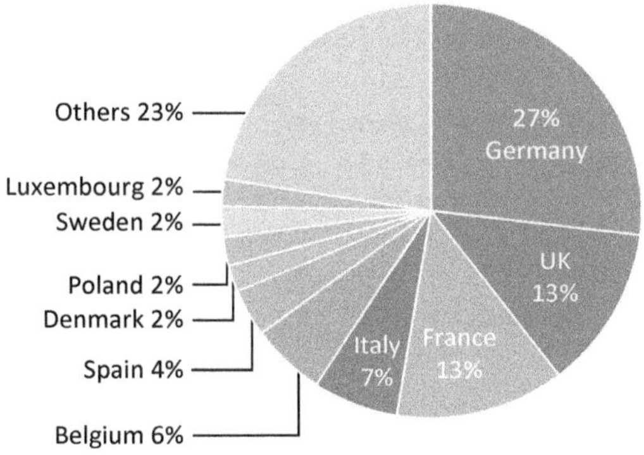

Source: UN Comtrade Database.

3.3.2. *Exporters among EU to China*

According to Fig. 7, Germany, Italy, France, United Kingdom, and Sweden are the top five exporters of medical products from EU to China. The export shares of these five countries are 38%, 12%, 11%, 9%, and 5%, respectively. Similar to the import scenario described earlier, Germany was the biggest exporter of medical products to China in 2013. The exports from Germany to China reached USD 5.23 billion in 2013. Germany has become the biggest and most important trade partner in medical products of China.

3.3.3. *Structure of trade in medical products between China and its main trade partners*

According to the above analysis, we find that United Kingdom, Germany, France, and Italy are the main trade partners of China in medical products. Therefore, in this part, the structure of trade in medical products between China and these four countries has to be analyzed. The result is shown in Table 2.

According to Table 2, except for UK, the trade between China and other three countries all presents trade deficit. The trade deficit in medicaments consisting of mixed or unmixed products (HS3004) is largest among all medical products. In 2013, the net trade between China and those four

Figure 7. Top 10 Exporters in Medical Products from EU to China in 2013.

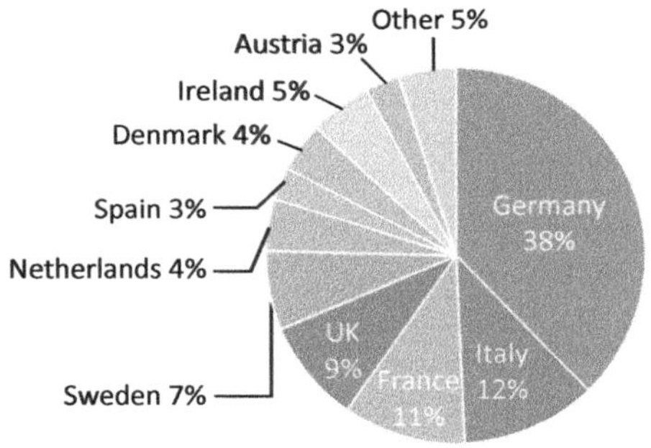

Source: UN Comtrade Database.

Table 2. Trade in Medical Products Between China and Main EU Partners in 2013 (Trade Unit: USD 10,000).

	France					Germany				
HS	Export	Share	Import	Share	Net Trade	Export	Share	Import	Share	Net Trade
3001	15794.79	34.53%	0.00	0	15794.79	13129.65	13.68%	0.00	0	13129.65
3002	1128.31	2.47%	26209.18	17.93%	–25080.86	909.22	0.94%	104757.74	20.03%	–103848.52
3003	331.14	0.72%	2249.90	1.54%	–1918.76	1440.40	1.50%	2523.79	0.48%	–1083.39
3004	4495.35	9.82%	87490.60	59.85%	–82995.26	2384.00	2.48%	184173.65	35.21%	–181789.66
3005	4488.55	9.81%	385.93	0.26%	4102.62	11219.55	11.69%	813.40	0.15%	10406.15
3006	216.61	0.47%	4069.56	2.78%	–3852.95	3155.22	3.28%	13669.15	2.61%	–10513.93
9018	6064.29	13.25%	6162.84	4.21%	–98.55	32826.18	34.21%	96965.81	18.54%	–64139.63
9019	3669.75	8.02%	547.39	0.37%	3122.36	11606.89	12.09%	9322.46	1.78%	2284.43
9020	10.50	0.02%	457.87	0.31%	–447.37	155.57	0.16%	714.59	0.14%	–559.02
9021	1872.68	4.09%	5595.35	3.83%	–3722.68	7894.32	8.23%	21449.25	4.10%	–13554.93
9022	7673.20	16.77%	12993.33	8.89%	–5320.13	11229.59	11.70%	88634.46	16.95%	–77404.86

(Continued)

Table 2. (*Continued*)

	UK					Italy				
HS	Export	Share	Import	Share	Net Trade	Export	Share	Import	Share	Net Trade
3001	896.19	1.98%	4.17	0%	892.02	5361.43	22.77%	2.75	0%	5358.68
3002	516.41	1.14%	4469.51	3.66%	–3953.10	136.03	0.57%	4601.08	2.86%	–4465.05
3003	154.73	0.34%	2120.67	1.74%	–1965.94	583.59	2.48%	4359.32	2.71%	–3775.74
3004	6451.78	14.23%	90748.77	74.27%	–84296.99	119.17	0.51%	127674.96	79.44%	–127555.79
3005	8285.75	18.28%	1037.39	0.84%	7248.36	4367.35	18.56%	72.75	0.04%	4294.60
3006	1985.55	4.38%	616.83	0.50%	1368.72	45.74	0.19%	249.92	0.16%	–204.18
9018	8538.62	18.84%	4793.07	3.92%	3745.55	8127.26	34.52%	15378.31	9.58%	–7251.06
9019	5249.20	11.58%	352.91	0.29%	4896.29	1962.00	8.33%	998.10	0.62%	963.90
9020	193.28	0.42%	114.61	0.09%	78.67	18.25	0.07%	22.18	0.01%	–3.92
9021	6686.57	14.75%	2651.60	2.17%	4034.97	485.76	2.06%	3444.07	2.14%	–2958.31
9022	6369.92	14.05%	15273.48	12.50%	–8903.56	2336.80	9.92%	3918.08	2.44%	–1581.29

Source: UN COMTRADE Database.

countries were valued at USD –829.95 million, USD –1.82 billion, USD –842.96 million, and USD –1.275 billion, respectively. The large trade deficit represents the fact that there exists great demand in the Chinese medical market, especially the medicaments market. Besides, it reflects the gap in medical industry advancement between China and EU. At present, Chinese medical products lack international competitiveness, especially the high-value-added and technology-intensive products. The exports from China to EU concentrate on low-value-added and labor-intensive products, which can be shown in Table 2. In 2013, the net trade in subsidiary articles (HS3005), blood and animal organs (HS 3001), and orthopedic appliances, etc. (HS9019) was positive. Take blood and animal organs (HS3001) as an example. In 2013, the export shares from China to France, Germany, UK, and Italy were 35.54%, 13.68%, 1.98%, and 22.77%, respectively. However, the import shares from these four countries to China are very small, especially France and Germany, the import shares of which approach 0%. In terms of the product features, those four types of medical products are resource- and labor-intensive, low-value-added products. The advantage of their exports derives from plentiful medical resources and cheap labor cost, which is inconsistent with the direction of China's trade policy. In particular, in recent years, the labor cost in China and pressure on environment protection are rising, which will push up the production cost of medical products in China and weaken its existing advantage.

4. PROBLEMS IN MEDICAL PRODUCTS TRADE BETWEEN CHINA AND EU

This section lists the problems in medical products trade between China and EU from the perspectives of EU's policy, external environment, and the state of medical industry in China. The problems can be summarized as follows:

(1) EU policies such as *EU Directive-26* and *EU Traditional Herbal Registration Program Instruction* raise the threshold standard of medical products imported into the EU market and hinder the development of trade in medical products between China and EU.

(2) The high standard of environmental protection, rising cost of Chinese labor, and appreciation of RMB push up the cost of medical products. The trade between China and EU is challenged by some emerging countries such as India and Brazil.
(3) The medical industry of China can be characterized as labor- and resource-intensive. The medical products exported to EU are of low-end value, which is inconsistent with the policy on Chinese industrial transformation.

4.1. *Problems of EU policy*

The EU policies on medical products raise the standard of medical products exported to the EU market, which hinders the development of trade in medical products between China and EU. The representative policies on medical products are *EU Directive-26* and *EU Traditional Herbal Registration Program Instruction.*

EU Directive-62[a] requires that since July 2, 2013, the active positive ingredients supplied by exporters should satisfy one of the following requirements before they are sold in EU market: first, the regulation institution must make sure that the products exported to EU should satisfy the EU's Good Manufacturing Practice (GMP) standards. Second, only if the companies are on the list announced by EU can their products be exempted from offering the certification provided by the local regulation institution. Also, they have to satisfy the first requirement described above. The implementation of this policy is of great significance to the protection of public health and enhances the international competitiveness of Chinese companies which produce and export active positive ingredients to the EU market. But as one of main exporters to EU, the implementation of this policy undoubtedly raises the threshold for Chinese medical companies to enter the EU market. Despite the efforts made by the Chinese government to revise its national GMP standard in accordance with the GMP standard

[a] *European Union Directive 2011/26* was implemented by the Committee of European Union in June 2011. The *Directive-62* requires that any active ingredient exported to EU should be offered with certificate ratified by regulators from the exporting countries.

of EU, there still exists a gap between China and EU. Parts of Chinese Active pharmaceutical Ingredient (API) exporters still do not satisfy the *EU Directive-26*, which impedes exports from China to EU.

Besides, the *EU Traditional Herbal Medical Products Registration Program Instruction 2004/2*[b] put forward in 2004 also impedes the trade of medicines between China and EU, especially the trade in traditional medicines. According to the *EU Traditional Herbal Registration Program Instruction 2004/24,* the producers of traditional herbal medicines could register through a simplified procedure. The procedure requires a certification that the medicines are harmless to the patients instead of clinical and safety tests and also demands that the traditional Chinese medicines should be in use for at least 30 years in China and for 15 years in the EU market before the registration. The Chinese medical companies entered the EU market in the 1990s, and some companies entered even later, which qualifies only a part of them for the standard required by *EU Traditional Herbal Registration Program Instruction.* Besides, although traditional Chinese medicines have a history of thousands of years, it is still hard for Chinese medical companies to show the certification because most of the traditional medicines comprise health products, food additives, etc. Apart from this, the high cost for registration has forced some Chinese medical companies to withdraw from the EU market.

4.2. *Problem from external environment*

From the aspect of China, in recent years, the labor cost of China and standards of environmental protection are increasing gradually. Chinese medical companies, especially those producing resource- and labor-intensive medical products, are confronted with huge production costs, which pose a great challenge. Some of the medical companies in China

---

[b] *European Union Traditional Herbal Products Registration Program Instruction 2004/24 (abbreviated as EU2004.24)* is carried out by European Union Parliament and Council on 31 March 2004. EU2004/24 aims to simply the registration process and requires that the certificates that herbal products are harmless should be provided. The details are described in this paper.

that cannot improve their production modes on time and satisfy the related requirements for environmental protection will be on the edge of closing down. Meanwhile, the appreciation of the Chinese currency RMB will weaken the international competitiveness of the Chinese medical industry. Besides, new emerging economies are also occupying the EU medical market successively, which hinders the development of trade between China and EU. Compared with China, countries like Vietnam, Brazil, and India also own bountiful medical resources. The increasing production cost of medical products has led to the shifting of parts of the medical industry to the above-mentioned countries. Take India as an example: since the export prices of active positive ingredients in China are lower than the local prices, medical companies in India import them from China at a lower price. Then they process them into downstream products and export them to the EU market. Apart from these issues, the tightening of fiscal and monetary policies of EU following the EU debt crisis could have a negative effect on the economic growth of EU countries, reduce their consumption level, and drag down their import demands for Chinese medical products.

4.3. *Problem in medical industry*

According to the analysis in Sec. 3, we find that the trade in medical products between China and EU is in a serious imbalance. The exports from China to EU comprise resource- and labor-intensive products with low export value. However, the imports from EU to China comprise high-end medical products that are technology-intensive and high-value-added. Such great disparities reflect the flaws and problems of the medical industry in China. First, the structure of the medical industry in China is unsustainable. Most of the medical companies are engaged in the production of low-end medical products and lack innovation and core technology. The exports from China to EU comprise homogeneous and low-value-added medical products, which obstruct the upgrade of trade in medical products between China and EU. Second, most of the companies in the Chinese medical industry are small- and medium-sized. Most of these companies lack core technology and become the main suppliers of low-end medical products. In order to earn more profits than others, many small- and medium-sized companies adopt low pricing strategy to push up their exports. Such a strategy results in China's circle of competition industry falling into the vicious circle of competition. Besides, in recent years, the Chinese government has strengthened its investment on the development of the domestic medical industry and implemented a series of favorable medical policies for Chinese medical companies. Many medical companies described earlier made use of this opportunity to expand their medical production, which has resulted in excessive investment and production.

5. SUGGESTION ON TRADE IN MEDICAL PRODUCTS BETWEEN CHINA AND EU

In this section, we will propose some suggestions based on the features of medical products trade between China and EU to enhance its development. The suggestion can be summarized as follows:

(1) China and EU should intensify their economic cooperation, especially the cooperation on the high-end medical products, and realize the effective configuration of medical resources between China and EU.
(2) Chinese medical enterprises should focus on the research and development of medical technology and increase their capabilities of self-innovation.
(3) The Chinese government should strengthen its support for domestic medical companies to help them realize the upgrading of medical technology and provide them assistance on registration and regulation of medicines so as to reduce the possibilities of the medicines not complying with the requirement of EU policies.

First, from the aspect of the development of medical industries between China and EU, it is obvious that the medical industry of EU is endowed with advanced medical technology while the medical industry of China is endowed with bountiful medical resources and great demand for medical services. Such complementarity in both medical industries creates chances for cooperation and paves the way for the development of trade in medical products between China and EU. Therefore, economic cooperation is essential to the development of trade in medical between China and EU. On one hand, economic cooperation could facilitate a more efficient flow of factors in medical industry. On the other hand, it could prove useful for Chinese medical companies to absorb more advanced medical technology and enhance the level of its medical industry. Therefore, in the future, China should strengthen its economic cooperation on medical products with EU, especially cooperation on advanced medical products, and encourage more local medical companies to participate in the competition and cooperation on global medical products. Besides, through cooperation, Chinese medical companies should learn and absorb the advanced medical technology and mature management experience of EU medical countries so as to speed up the pace of internalization of the Chinese medical companies.

Second, from the aspect of the medical industry, at present, the conspicuous feature of medical industry in China can be described as low-cost and resource-intensive. The medical industrial structure is in imbalance, and the medical industry in China suffers from overcapacity and lack of innovation. Besides, the majority of the medical products exported from China to EU are homogeneous and of low- and medium-end, which hinders the upgrading of trade in medical products between China and EU. Therefore, in the future, China should encourage its local medical companies to increase their inputs in the research and development of medical technology and emphasize self-innovation on medical products. Besides, the medical companies should improve the production of medical products and expand the production on biochemical products, chemical medicines, and medical apparatus with sophisticated technology in order to improve the trade structure between China and EU and push up the development of bilateral trade in medical products.

Third, in terms of government, the Chinese government should strengthen its support for local medical companies to improve their medical technology and achieve the upgrading of the Chinese medical industry. Local governments in China should use various ways, including providing production permission, checking registration, and granting permission of GMP, to help the medical companies enhance their medical technology. Meanwhile, to deal with the negative effects on Chinese medical companies from *EU26 Directive*, the Chinese government should establish the quality management system in accordance with EU GMP and carry out related training on international certification of medical products for local medical companies. Meanwhile, in order to avoid the possibility that the orders are cancelled because the medical products do not meet the criteria of EU, the Chinese government should help local companies to examine some related materials for international registration and permission of medical products to enhance the development of trade in medical products between China and EU further.

REFERENCES

1. Shen, J. & Tong, Z. (2005). "Classification and coding of pharmaceutical products," *China Medical Devices*, 20(11): 45–47.
2. Cao, Y., Wang, X. & Liu, B. (2006). "Analysis of the economic characteristics of pharmaceutical products," *Medicine and Society*, 19(11): 62–64.
3. Zhang, H. (2013). *Basic knowledge of practical pharmaceutical products*, (China Medical Press, Beijing).

Chapter 6

The Healthcare Industry in the Chinese Economy: Insights from Input–Output Analysis

Noemi Ferracuti, Claudio Socci and Francesca Spigarelli

1. INTRODUCTION

In the context of urbanization and rapidly aging population, China faces the need to improve and modernize its domestic healthcare system. The Chinese government has identified the improvement of quality of healthcare services and the adoption of new technologies as key priorities in the future to overcome service disparities.[1] Government reforms affect pharmaceutical, medical equipment, and diagnostics industries in the country.

In this chapter, after a brief description of market trends and general characteristics of trade flows between Europe and China, we implement a dispersion effects analysis using an Input–Output model in order to determine whether healthcare industry is a "key" sector in the Chinese economy compared to the upstream and downstream connections with all the other sectors.

2. REFORMS AND INDUSTRY GROWTH

In 2012, the People's Republic of China became the largest exporter in the world.[2] This remarkable leadership is based on an upward trend that began in the late 1970s. Economic reforms undertaken since 1978 by Deng Xiaoping, economic policies that promoted the attraction of foreign direct investments (FDI), and an export-oriented policy drove Chinese surge in the global economy.[3]

Rapid industrialization and urbanization, growing pollution, as well as an accelerating aging population require China to face complex issues related to the health conditions of its citizens: from the potential threat of the emerging and traditional diseases, security and safety of food, to full coverage of services for all provinces. Hence, there is the need to develop a model in which both the demand and the supply of healthcare services are regulated in a timely manner.[4]

The government has been embracing an expansive healthcare reform to improve the quality and coverage of healthcare assistance by promoting multiple strategies, both on the demand and the supply sides. The 12th Five-Year Plan for Health Sector Development has set a fundamental step in this process, remarked by the 13th Five-Year Plan.[5]

According to "US–China Economic and Security Review Commission," the current healthcare reforms represent opportunities and challenges for healthcare companies abroad, generating demand for better healthcare services, with opportunities for private and foreign investments.[6]

The Chinese market has been growing at double-digits over the past 10 years, at different rates for different subsectors, such as Medicinal and Pharmaceutical products, Medicaments including veterinary medicaments, Traditional Chinese Medicine (TCM), Electro-diagnostic Apparatus for medical sciences, and Instruments and Appliances. Nevertheless, weaknesses are still huge in terms of firms' competitiveness as well as the effectiveness of reforms: significant challenges remain to be addressed. In particular, the Ministry of Health (MOH) and other government departments have recognized the need for reform and the existence of problems such as the inefficiency of medical services, high costs of treatments, corruption, and lack of high quality standards.[7]

Figure 1. Breakdown of China's 2009 Healthcare Investment Package.

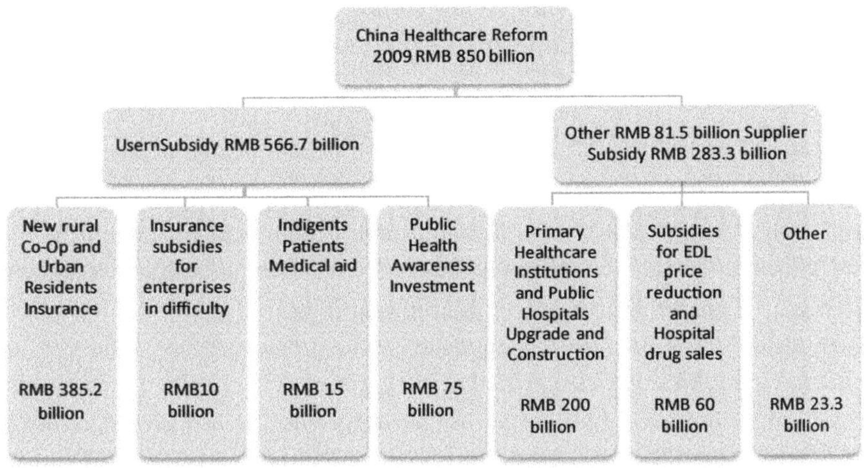

Source: J.P. Morgan (2011). "Implementation Plan for the Recent Priorities of the Healthcare System Reform (2009–2011)," *Shanghai Pharma Prospectus*, p. 2.

To face such issues, China has been pushing for further progress in the healthcare reform, which was supported, in the last decade, by the launch of an ambitious RMB 850 billion (USD 124 billion) three-year investment plan.

The distribution of this fund is shown in Fig. 1.

3. CHINA–EUROPE TRADE FLOWS IN THE HEALTHCARE SECTOR

In this general picture, it is interesting to analyze the status of trade cooperation between Europe and China.

Europe is an important trading partner for China: according to the data provided by the United Nations, China's total imports from Europe with regard to healthcare products are on average 44% of the total imports taking place with the rest of the world, with an average annual growth of about 17%.[8]

In particular, two healthcare industry subsectors, i.e., Medical Devices[a] and Medicinal and Pharmaceutical products,[b] are still relatively undeveloped and have a large growth potential.

3.1. *Medical devices*

China is now the world's second largest market for medical equipment. It offers significant potential for EU companies interested in expanding into the Chinese market, with huge demand for better healthcare services, driven by an increasing aging population and improved medical insurance coverage.[9] While the Chinese medical device companies provide low- to mid-range technology and products, they generally lack the expertise and experience deemed appropriate by Western standards. Foreign medical device companies are considered as more reliable than their Chinese counterparts,[10] so China has relied on imports of medical equipment.

As shown in Fig. 2, it is clear that imports outweighed exports. In particular, in 2012, China's import of medical devices from Europe was

Figure 2. Medical Devices Trade Between China and European Union (EU28).

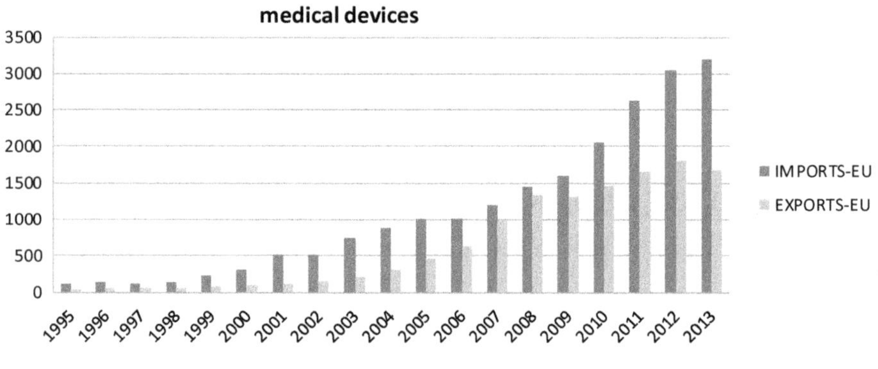

Source: Authors' own calculation based on UNCTAD data available at: http://unctadstat.unctad.org/wds/ReportFolders/reportFolders.aspx.

---

[a] Medical devices include electro-diagnostic apparatus for medical sciences, as well as instruments and appliances.

[b] For a detailed classification of healthcare products included in the two subsectors, refer to Table A.1 in Appendix A.

valued at a total of USD 3.036 billion, while exports to Europe accounted for USD 1.804 billion.

3.2. *Medicinal and pharmaceutical products*

The pharmaceutical market offers a different picture. China is the world's third largest pharmaceutical market in term of sales[11] and is expected to attain the second place by 2020, behind only the United States. The market is becoming increasingly attractive to Western firms.[12]

As for Europe, besides driving medical progress and improving health within Europe and worldwide, the research-based pharmaceutical industry is a key asset to the EU economy, providing one of Europe's best performing high-technology sectors.[13] The profile of China within the pharmaceutical industry is still far from leading position. The Chinese market has shown impressive growth since the mid-1980s, at a rate far exceeding the annual GDP growth. Nevertheless, the Chinese market is still comparatively small, given the country's population.[14]

International Trade Imports of pharmaceutical products in China have grown rapidly in recent years and are predicted to follow an upward trend.

EU is at present an important Chinese trade partner in pharmaceuticals, with a positive trade balance of EUR 4.866 billion in 2013 (see Fig. 3 in

Figure 3. Medicinal and Pharmaceutical Trade Between China and European Union (Unit: USD Millions).

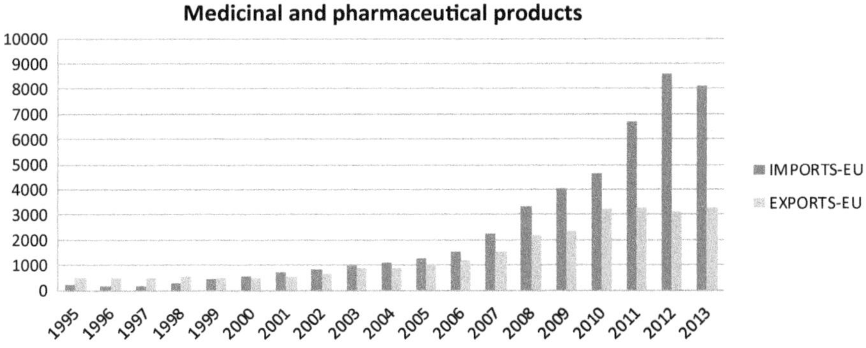

Source: Own calculation based on UNCTAD data available at: http://unctadstat.unctad.org/wds/ReportFolders/reportFolders.aspx.

Ref. 8). The European pharmaceutical industry has been very active in the Chinese market during the past years and is also one of the main foreign investors.

4. THE INPUT–OUTPUT MODEL

The increase in healthcare expenditure emphasizes the relevance of healthcare industry in the world production and confirms its importance within national economies.[15] The healthcare industry is characterized by the absorption and creation of a complex set of goods and services[16] and require a detailed analysis of connections among healthcare and the other industries.[17]

In this section, we present an I–O analysis for China that represents an important source of information for the investigation of the interrelations existing among different industries. In particular, it provides the tools to assess structural changes in the economy, in terms of linkages between economic sectors. The healthcare industry, in these terms, must be considered interacting with all the other industrial productions and all the institutional sectors, which make up the economic system. For this reason, we will apply a dispersion effects analysis in order to highlight the healthcare interindustry links in terms of both supplier and user (when it receives or provides inputs from/to other industries in the production process). Based on the general picture provided in the first paragraphs, we seek to understand the relative importance of the Chinese healthcare industry in its articulation. We use the analysis of direct and indirect effects on the economic system due to a shock that is typical of I–O model.

I–O analysis is the traditional tool for assessing and measuring the contribution of healthcare industry to a region's economy. This is one of the most useful techniques to measure economic impacts, with the most important advantage being the ability to numerically measure indirect and induced impacts.[18] The study requires an objective-oriented database that is able to highlight, in multisectorial terms, the links between the healthcare industry, productive processes, and end-users.

In this study, we decided to use the World Input–Output Database (WIOD). All data in the WIOD are obtained from official national statistics and are consistent with the National Accounts.[19] The WIOD classification list has 35 industries based on NACE rev 1 (ISIC rev 2) in which Healthcare is enclosed in the industry called "Health and Social Work." Each industry includes figures related to intermediate demand, final demand, value added, and imports.[20]

The I–O table can assume various structures useful to highlight the links between the interindustrial production processes activated in the economic system for the production of several types of industries, including Healthcare industries. The I–O table records the flows of intermediate goods and primary factors (in value) required for production, which are able to meet the intermediate and final demand. The database used in this study is China's I–O table for the year 2011 with symmetrical structure Industry by Industry, divided into 35 production sectors (WIOD database, September 2012 release).

The table offers a systematic and consistent picture of goods and services flows traded with the rest of the world and used within the country during a given year, which flows alongside the services rendered by labor and capital to the industries (see Ref. 21).[c]

In particular, the column contains information on the total amount of resources used in the system according to the industry's classification. A product can be imported or domestically produced. The columns indicate the values of all intermediate goods and primary inputs used in production. The vector of input shares in output is often referred to as the technology for domestic production. The compensation for labor and capital services together make up "value added," which indicates the value added by the use of domestic labor and capital services to the value of the intermediate inputs. Total supply of the product in the economy is determined by domestic output plus imports. Rows indicate the use of products, for intermediate or final use. Each product can be an intermediate in the production of other products (intermediate use). Final demand includes

[c]The System of National Accounts, 2008 (2008 SNA) is a statistical framework that provides a comprehensive, consistent and flexible set of macroeconomic accounts for policymaking, analysis and research purposes. It has been produced and is released under the auspices of the United Nations, the European Commission, the Organization for Economic Co-operation and Development, the International Monetary Fund and the World Bank Group. It represents an update, mandated by the United Nations Statistical Commission in 2003, of the System of National Accounts, 1993, which was produced under the joint responsibility of the same five organizations.

domestic use (private or government consumption and investment) and exports. The final element in each row indicates the total use of each product according to the industry's classification.

An important accounting identity in the I–O table is that total output by industry is equal to the use of output from the industry so that all flows in the economic system are accounted for.[20] The I–O table reflects the principle of double entry of every transaction in the system of national accounts, which guarantees the balance between rows and columns. In this way, given a period, each expenditure of one entity is a resource of another one and the expenditures of every institutional sector, recorded along columns, are equal to its resources, registered in rows.[22]

In the I–O table, healthcare expenditure is included in industry 33 (Health and Social Work).

The "Health and Social Work" total output in 2011 is USD 338,296 million, given by the use of USD 221,104 million (66%) for intermediate consumption (domestic and foreign) and USD 116,100 million (34%) for factors of production (expressed by the value added) excluding international transport margins. From Fig. 4, we can see the Health and Social Work production positioning within the entire Chinese economy in terms of value added.

On the other hand, in Fig. 5, we can observe the Health and Social Work industry's production within the entire Chinese economy, in terms of intermediate consumption of goods.

Since 1995, the "Health and Social Work" industry has been steadily increasing and grew by 94.67% between 1995 and 2011, together with imports of products designed for the healthcare production (pharmaceutical products and medical devices). Moreover, as shown in Fig. 6, in the reference period, imports increased by the 93.75%.

The total value of intermediate goods comprises USD 200,134 million (90%) of health products of domestic origin and USD 20,970 million (10%) of imported products.

Examining the dependence of the Healthcare industry from material inputs, we focus on the production function composition, in terms of domestic and foreign intermediate consumption.

Figure 4. Value Added by Industry (Unit: USD Millions).

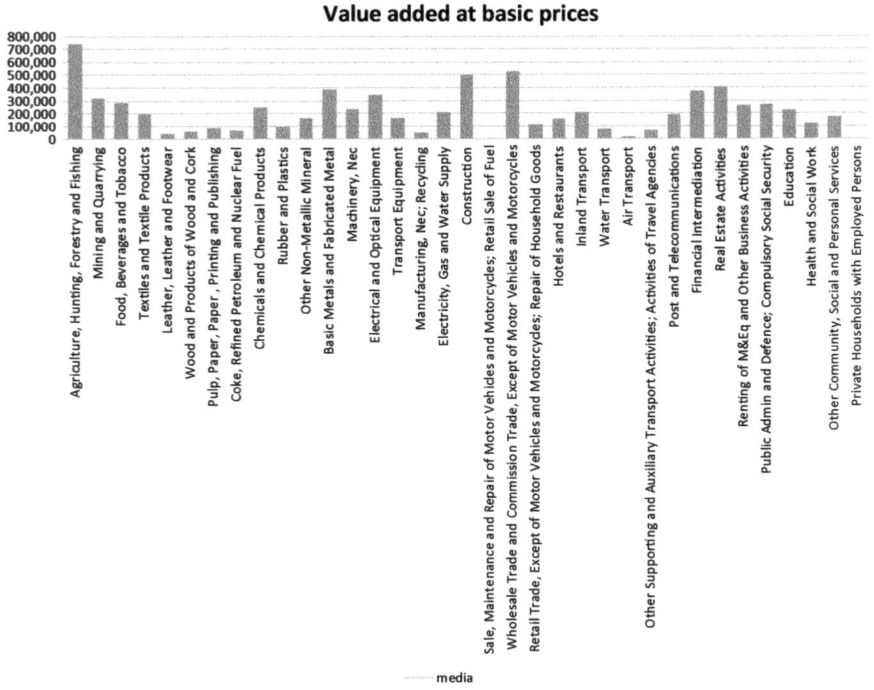

Source: Authors' own calculation based on WIOD Input–Output Table, available at: http://www.wiod.org/new_site/database/niots.htm.

Most of the inputs used in "Health and Social Work" industry, came from the "Chemicals and Chemical Products" industry, as medicines, pharmaceutical products, remedy, and vet products.[d] In particular, "Health and Social Work" absorbs domestic chemical industry products valued at USD 91,631 million (41% of total intermediate consumption) and imports chemical and pharmaceutical products of over USD 14,015 million, corresponding to about 6% of the total material goods absorption and 67% of total Healthcare's imports.

[d]For more details on the correspondence between the industries in the table and the imported goods, see Table A.1 in Appendix A.

Figure 5. Total Intermediate Consumption by Industry (Unit: USD Millions).

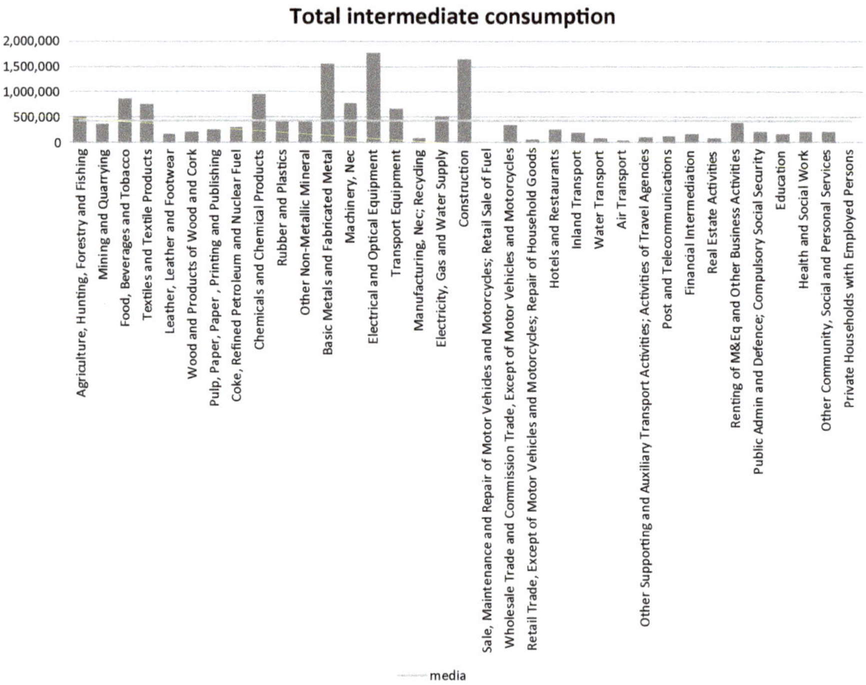

Source: Author's own calculation based on WIOD I–O Table, available at: http://www.wiod.org/new_site/database/niots.htm.

Figure 6. Health and Social Work Total Output (Unit: USD Millions).

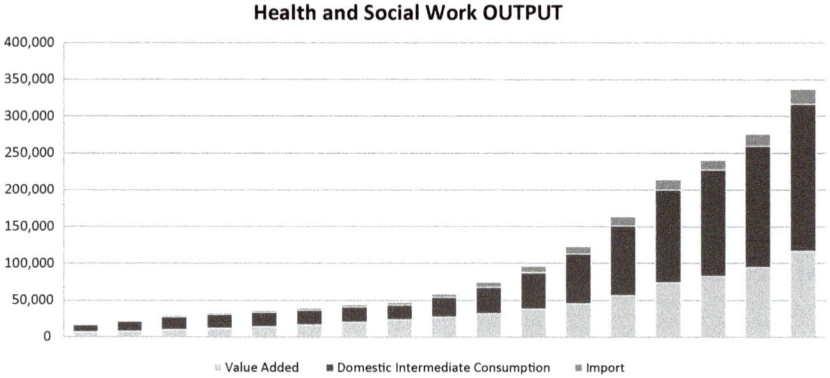

Source: Authors' own calculation based on WIOD I–O Table, available at: http://www.wiod.org/new_site/database/niots.htm.

In China, 7.7% of the chemical industry total output is related to healthcare products and 9.14% of the chemical's imports from the rest of the world are allocated to the "Health and Social Work" industry.

In relation to other domestic inputs, products belong to the following industries: "Machinery" for USD 15,565 million (7% of total intermediate consumption), "Wholesale Trade and Commission Trade, Except of Motor Vehicles and Motorcycles" with a value of USD 17,046 million (7.71%), and "Construction" with USD 9,489 million (4.29%).

Analyzing the imports, we note that most of them belong to "Machinery," and "Electrical and Optical Equipment" categories, valued at USD 3,166 million, which represent 15% of total imports bound to the healthcare industry.

Final consumption by the government and households has increased by far in the last decade, as well as the use of intermediate goods from healthcare industry. The amount of exported Health and Social Work's services remains very limited even while maintaining a high level of growth in the recent years.

As for the "Health and Social Work" industry, the export level exceeds that of import, but we should take into account that, in the I–O table, we do not have the breakdown by partner, so we are considering imports and exports from China with the rest of the world (Fig. 7).

Figure 7. Health and Social Work: Imports and Exports (Unit: USD Millions).

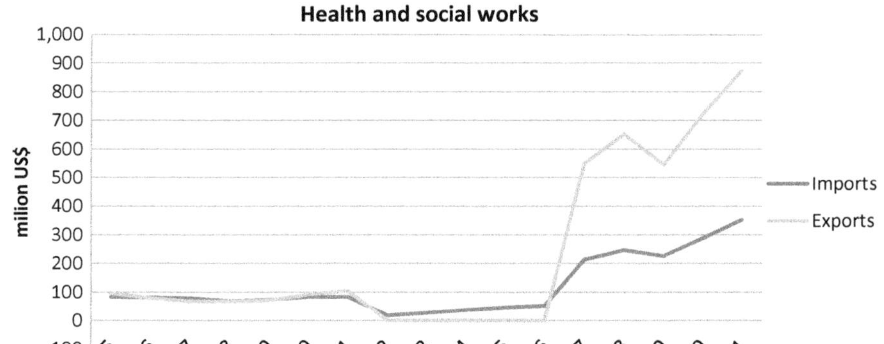

Source: Authors' own calculation based on WIOD Input–Output Table, available at: http://www.wiod.org/new_site/database/niots.htm.

5. A DISPERSION EFFECTS ANALYSIS FOR THE CHINESE HEALTHCARE SECTOR

Implementing a policy requires the availability of information on the links between economic agents, so it is necessary to have synthetic indicators, qualitative and quantitative, to support the policy maker.

For this reason, we implemented a dispersion effects analysis in order to determine the importance of healthcare industry relative to the upstream and downstream connections with all other industries, in China. The interdependence measured through this analysis[23] is restricted to demand pull and supply push effects of changes in final demand. The indices are an expression of the way that input and output relations diffuse demand changes for the final products of a given industry j to other industries in the economic system, as the amount of inputs they provide to the directly affected industry j are dependent on the final demand for the products produced by industry j. Thus what is studied is the systemic character of an economy: no unit (industry) exists in isolation from the other units in the system.[24]

In fact, each new industrial investment offers opportunities for other suppliers (*backward*) and provide inputs for utilization by other users (*forward*). In other words, the provision of healthcare is important not only for the degree of coverage of the territory and the quality of the service but also because it could be one of the "key" industries in the development, in direct or indirect terms. It defines a strategic asset for all other industries.[25]

Taking into account the multisectoral model,[e] we can derive two vectors of indices:

Power of dispersion: $$\pi_{\cdot j} \frac{\frac{1}{m} r_{\cdot j}}{\frac{1}{m^2} \sum_{j=1}^{m} r_{\cdot j}}$$

It describes the relative extent to which an increase in final demand for the jth industry is dispersed throughout the system of industries (*backward*). When $\pi_{\cdot j} > 1$, it shows that an increase in the jth exogenous final

---

[e] For the specification of the model, see Appendix B.

demand determines a larger increase in output and vice versa when ($\pi._j <$ 1) if compared to the industries in general.

$$\text{Sensitivity of dispersion:} \quad \pi._i \frac{\frac{1}{m} r._i}{\frac{1}{m^2}\sum_{i=1}^{m} r._i}$$

This second index, taking into account the average increase in the *i*th industry's output given by a unitary increase of all exogenous final demand's elements, indicates the extent to which industry *i* is effected by an expansion in the system of industries (*forward*). When it assumes a value greater than one ($\pi._i > 1$), it indicates that the increase of the *i*th output is greater than any other, given a unit increase of the exogenous final demand of all and vice versa when $\pi._i < 1$. It suggests that the increased investment in industry *i* would induce output increases in all using industries, as users take advantage of the increased availability of inputs.[34]

The term *backward* is used to indicate this kind of interconnection of a particular industry to those industries from which it purchases inputs. On the other hand, increased output in industry *j* also means additional amounts of product *j* available to be used as inputs to other industries for their own production. That is to say, there will be increased supplies from *j* (as a seller) for the industry, which use good *j* in their production. This is the direction of causation in the supply-side model. The term *forward* is used to indicate this kind of interconnection of a particular industry to those sectors to which it sells its output. The results of the analysis allow us to understand whether healthcare industry is a "key industry" for the Chinese economy. The matrix *R* is used to perform a dispersion effects analysis, which is able to assess the importance of "Health and Social Work" in the economic system in terms of activation of production and contribution to the production of other industries.

Among the major investors in healthcare, Germany is the first with EUR 247 million, followed by Italy (EUR 119 million) and France (EUR 82 million).[26] For this reason, the analysis of dispersion is achieved on the I–O table of China and on the I–O tables of the main European investors and trading partners: Germany, France, and Italy. All tables used

Figure 8. China: Backward and Forward Index (2011) I–O Tables.

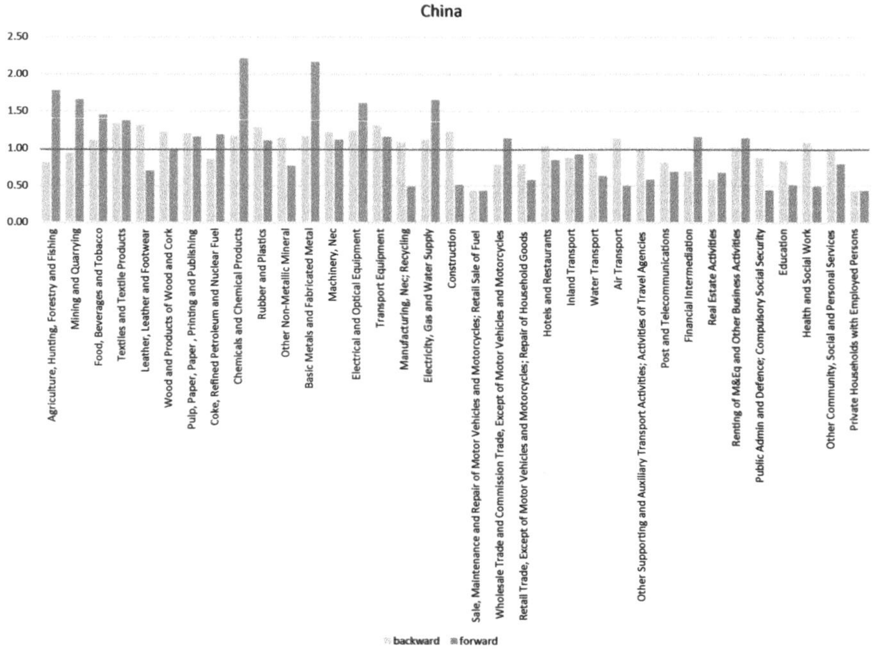

belong to the WIOD database, with symmetrical structure Industry by Industry, divided into 35 sectors. The results are presented in Table C.1 in Appendix C, in which industry 33 "Health and Social Work" represents the services provided by Healthcare. From the results, we can see that China's productive structure is very different from the other countries.

In Fig. 8, China's index values are shown for all sectors.

From a backward point of view, the *power of dispersion* index for "Health and Social Work" is bigger than one (1.08), so it leads us to consider that this is a key sector, as it plays a strong upstream connection. A sales increase in Healthcare industry will produce a wider increase in all the other supplier industries in the system. The high amount reflects the nature of healthcare involving the utilization of many different products purchased from a large number of industries.

From the forward side, the *sensitivity of dispersion* index reported in Table C.1 in Appendix C, is lower than one; for China it is 0.49. This result highlights how services provided by the Healthcare industry are not so significant like suppliers if we stimulate all purchasers' activities.

"Chemicals and Chemical Products" industry presents, in I–O China's table, values bigger than one both from the backward and forward sides; to be exact, the power of dispersion is 1.17, and the sensitivity of dispersion is 2.21. The empirical result leads us to believe that this industry, to which medicinal and pharmaceutical products belong to, is an area that strongly activates other supplier production if there is an increase in chemicals sales. At the same time, the chemicals industry provides a very important contribution to the other industries like suppliers, whereas there is an increase in all the final demand of the other industries. Thus the chemical industry is a key sector for China.

Another industry that presents both backward and forward indices higher than 1 is "Electrical and Optical Equipment." Medical devices belong to this industry, which presents a power of dispersion index of 1.24 and a sensitivity of dispersion index of 1.60.

"Chemicals and Chemical Products" and "Electrical and Optical Equipment" are both "key industries" for China's economy. In fact, new industrial investment in this country could offer an important opportunity to potential suppliers to get into the market (*backward*) and widened its offer to an increased range of users (*forward*).

The same analysis for Germany, France, and Italy highlights different results. As shown in Figs. 9–11, Health and Social Work index values are lesser than 1.

For Germany (Fig. 9), services supplied by the healthcare industry are not critical for upstream and downstream connections with all the other industries: in fact, the power of dispersion index is 0.83 and the sensitivity of dispersion index is 0.65.

For "Chemicals and Chemical Products," it is the same: from a backward perspective, the index is 0.98, and from the forward side, it is 0.84. Also for the Electrical and Optical Equipment industry, indices are less than 1 (backward: 0.94; forward: 0.84).

In Fig. 10, France's power of dispersion and a sensitivity of dispersion indexes are shown. Health and Social Work linkages are less than 1; the power of dispersion 0.72, and the sensitivity of dispersion is 0.63.

Considering "Chemicals and Chemical Products" and "Electrical and Optical Equipment" sectors, these have backward values greater than 1

Figure 9. Germany: Backward and Forward Index (2011) I–O Tables.

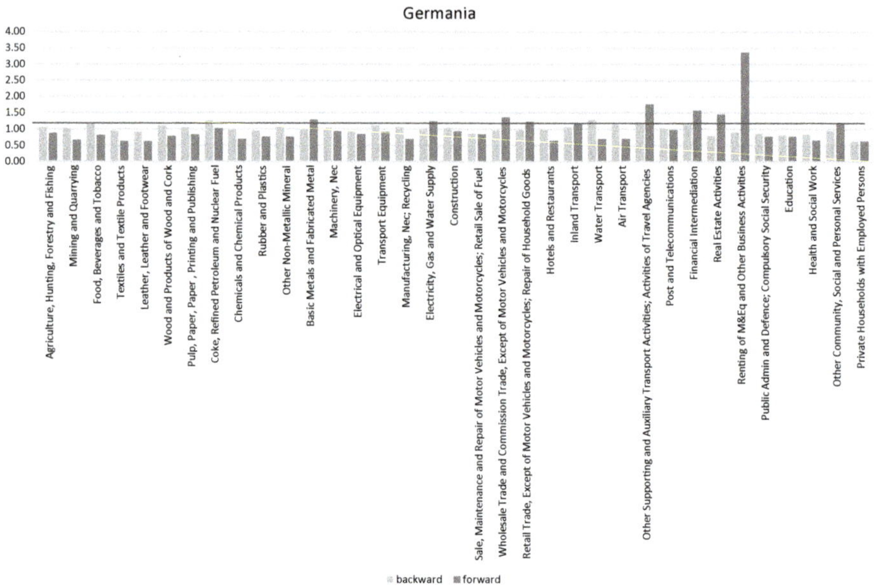

Figure 10. France: Backward and Forward Index (2011) I–O Tables.

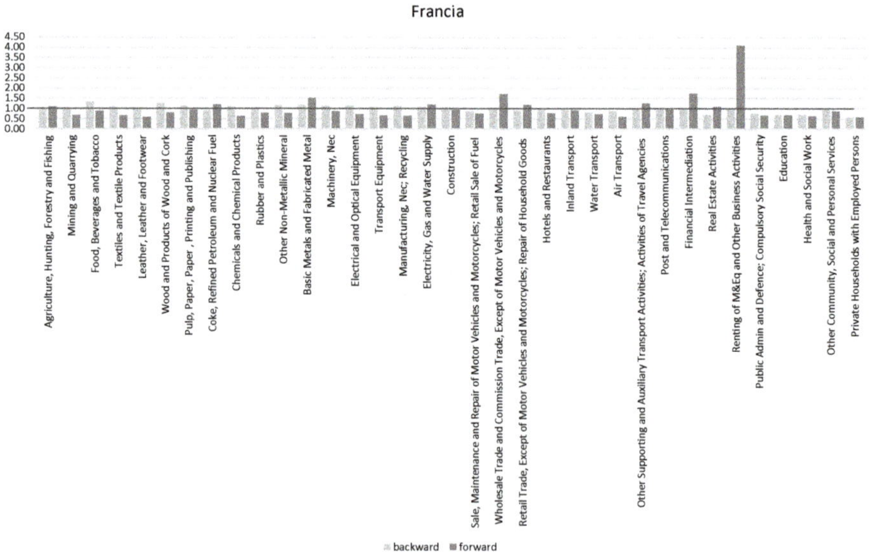

Figure 11. Italy: Backward and Forward Index (2011) I–O Tables.

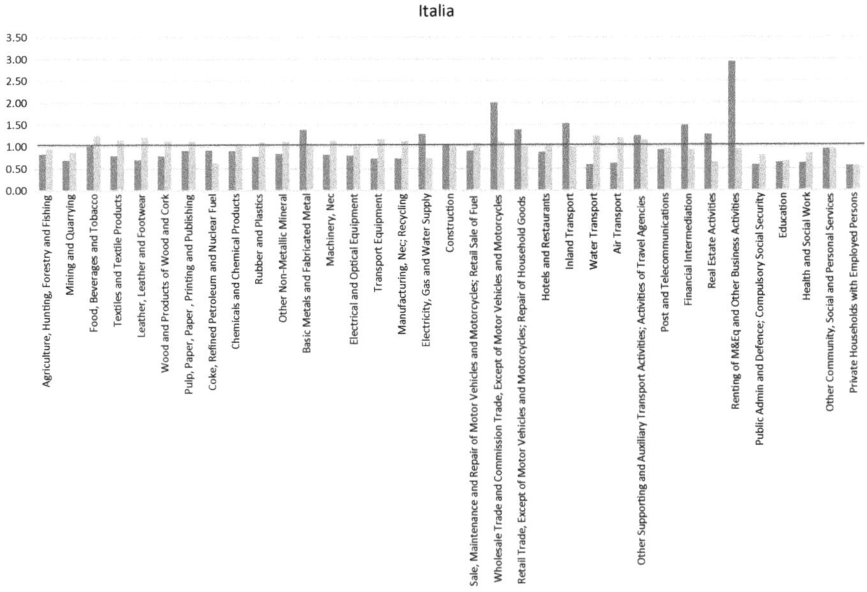

(1.10 and 1.15, respectively). This result implies that, for France, they are "key industries." An increase in their final demand causes a major increase in the total industries' output.

From the forward side, as in the case of Germany, these industries are not relevant because they present values less than 1 (Chemicals and Chemical Products: 0.63; Electrical and Optical Equipment: 0.74).

In Fig. 11, the results of the dispersion effects analysis for Italy are displayed.

Also in this case, "Health and Social Work" indices are less than 1. In fact, power of dispersion is 0.85 and sensitivity of dispersion is 0.62. As for France and Germany, healthcare services are not a key sector from a dispersion analysis point of view, while for Italy, "Chemicals and Chemical Products" (1.07) and "Electrical and Optical Equipment" (1.02) are key industries from the backward side. This means that, in Italy, healthcare services act like purchasers stimulating own suppliers industries.

6. CONCLUSIONS

This chapter was intended to provide an analysis of the importance of the healthcare industry in the Chinese economy, based on a multisectorial approach. We focused on the impact that the healthcare industry has on the main economic aggregates of the country.

The multisector analysis applied to the healthcare industry allowed us to understand the interdependency networks between the healthcare industry and the production activities and connections with institutional sectors.

The aim of the I–O model that we used was to define the importance of the Chinese healthcare industry's production within the economic system. First, we analyzed whether an increase in healthcare final demand plays a significant (or nonsignificant) role in the activation of all the other industry production (backward), and then whether an exogenous shock in the whole final demand would produce a modification in the healthcare output (forward).

Through the dispersion effects analysis, we observed that China's power of dispersion index for healthcare industry is significant, higher than 1, while for Germany, France, and Italy, it is less than 1. This first result allows the belief that healthcare is a key industry for China's economy because of the relevant upstream link in the production process. A different consideration was reached, instead, by observing the sensitivity of dispersion index. These indexes were less than 1 for all countries considered. This result suggests that healthcare services are not significantly activated from other industries' production.

In more general terms, some conclusions can be derived from our study.While China is moving toward a new universal healthcare system and a huge government budget is allocated to implement reforms, the Chinese population is increasingly demanding Western standard services and products for their health.[27]

For foreign companies, for example, those in the medical device and pharmaceutical product fields, reforms in China could prove to be a great advantage. While the European medical device market has been hit by the financial crisis, the Chinese market has seen a vertical growth, making it a potential growth factor for foreign companies.[28]

The increase in healthcare services demand, in addition to creating a great opportunity for European companies, involves a strong advantage that is reflected in the Chinese economic system. The multisectoral analysis confirmed that an increase in the final demand for healthcare services corresponds to a larger increase in all productive industries that act as suppliers.

Recent healthcare reforms have produced enormous social, economic, and sectoral changes. This means that companies are addressing a highly specialized and competitive sector due to an increase in the attractiveness of the local market to foreign investors.[29]

China can therefore offer enormous opportunities for European firms. Entrepreneurs and policymakers should be aware of the trends highlighted in the Chinese healthcare market and seize this opportunity.

REFERENCES

1. Hew, C. (2006). *Healthcare in China: Towards Greater Access, Efficiency and Quality*, (IBM Global Services, NY), pp. 1–16.
2. Morrison, W. M. (2013). "China's economic rise: History, trends, challenges, and implications for the United States," *Current Politics and Economics of Northern and Western Asia*, 22(4): 461.
3. Dias, E. B. & Makalengva, K. (2013). "China inward FDI and Chinese exports to high-income countries (HICs): A historical perspective based on bibliometric method," *International Business Research*, 6(12): 17.
4. Gong, P., Liang, S., Carlton, E. J., Jiang, Q., Wu, J., Wang, L. & Remais, J. V. (2012). "Urbanisation and health in China," *The Lancet*, 379(9818): 843–852.
5. Wan J. (2014). "Healthcare reform in China," *Pharmaceutical Technology Europe*, 26(9): 21–22.
6. Congress, U. S. & Congress, O. H. S. (2014). USCC 2014 Annual Report, U.S.-China Economic and Security Review Commission, November 2014.
7. Daemmrich, A. (2013). "The political economy of healthcare reform in China: Negotiating public and private," *SpringerPlus*, 2(1): 448.
8. UNCTAD (2014). *World Investment Report 2014: Investing in the SDGs: An Action Plan* (United Nations Publication, New York, Geneva, and Beijing).
9. EUSME Centre (2012). The Healthcare Sector in China. Available at: http://www.ccilc.pt/sites/default/files/docs/setor_da_saude_en_eusmecenter.pdf. Accessed 17 October 2014.

10. PriceWaterhouseCoopers (2009). *Investing in China's Pharmaceutical Industry*, 2nd Edn. Available at: http://www.pwc.com/gx/en/pharma-life-sciences/investing-china/index.jhtml. Accessed 20 June 2012.
11. Economic Research Institute (2013). *China's Pharmaceutical Market 2012* (Social Sciences Academic Press, Beijing).
12. Spigarelli, F. & Wei, H. (2012). *The Rising Chinese Pharmaceutical Industry: Local Champions vs Global Players*, c.MET Working Paper 06/2012.
13. Blanc, L. (2014). The European Pharmaceutical Industry in a Global Economy: What drives EU exports of pharmaceuticals? (Department of European Economic Studies, College of Europe, Bruges).
14. European Commission (2006). *Pharmaceutical Sector: Forward-Looking Perspective of EU-China Trade & Investment Relations* (Trade EU Publications, Brussels, Belgium).
15. Works, K. R. H. (2003). *The Economic Impact of the Local Health Care System on the Anderson County Economy* (University of Kentucky-College of Agriculture, KY, USA).
16. Harris, T. R., Griswold, T., Segurson, M., Packham, J. & Ford, C. (2004). *Economic Impact and Linkages of the Local Health Sector on the Economy of Lander County* (University of Nevada, Reno, NV, USA).
17. Socci, C., Ciaschini, M., Pretaroli, R. & Severini, F. (2010). "Health services as a key sector for income and employment change," *Bulletin of the Transilvania University of Braşov*, 3: 52.
18. Ciaschini, M., Pretaroli, R. & Socci, C. (2010). "Multisectoral structures and policy design," *International Journal of Control*, 83(2): 281–296.
19. Dietzenbacher, E., Los, B., Stehrer, R., Timmer, M. & De Vries, G. (2013). "The construction of world input–output tables in the WIOD project," *Economic Systems Research*, 25(1): 71–98.
20. Timmer, M., Erumban, A. A., Gouma, R., Los, B., Temurshoev, U., de Vries, G. J. & Pindyuk, O. (2012). *The World Input-output Database (WIOD): Contents, Sources and Methods (No. 20120401)* (Institute for International and Development Economics, University of Groningen).
21. United Nations (2008). *System of National Accounts* (UNSO, New York).
22. Socci, C. & Pretaroli, R. (2008). "Produzione e distribuzione del reddito in una SAM biregionale." In *Modelli Computazionali per la Valutazione dell'impatto del Federalismo Fiscale sulla finanza locale* cap. 3 (Ministero dell'Interno, Roma), pp. 29–71 [in Italian].
23. Rasmussen, P. N. (1956). *Studies in Inter-Sectoral Relations* (E. Harck, Copenhagen and Amsterdam), p. 15.

24. Drejer, I. (2002). "Input–output based measures of interindustry linkages revisited — a survey and discussion," *14th International Conference on Input–Output Techniques*, Montreal, Canada.
25. Fiorillo F., Pretaroli, R. E. & Socci C. (2005). *La Sanità e le Interdipendenze Produttive: Un Approccio Multi-Settoriale* (Società Italiana di Economia Pubblica Dipartimento di Economia Pubblica e Territoriale — Università di Pavia, Italy) [in Italian].
26. EUROSTAT (2013). *International Trade and Foreign Direct Investment*, 2013 Edn. (Eurostat Pocketbooks, Luxembourg).
27. Rein, S. (2009). "China's New Purchasing Powerhouse: Women," *Forbes. com*. August 5, 2009. Available at: http://www.forbes.com/2009/08/05/china-women-marketing-leadership-managing-retail.html. Accessed 2 September 2009.
28. AMCHAM Shanghai (2011). *Healthcare, Medical Equipment and Devices*, White Paper Industry-Specific Issue.
29. Deloitte (2011). Survey of Health Care Consumers in China. Key Findings, Strategic Implications. Available at: https://www2.deloitte.com/content/dam/Deloitte/de/Documents/Country%20Services%20Group/CSG%20China/Industry%20News/12-LSHC-2011-survey.pdf. Accessed 18 October 2014.
30. Leontief, W. (1956). "Factor proportions and the structure of American trade: Further theoretical and empirical analysis," *The Review of Economics and Statistics*, 38(4): 386–407.
31. Ciaschini, M. & Socci, C. (2007). "Final demand impact on output: A macro multiplier approach," *Journal of Policy Modeling*, 29: 115–132.
32. Miller, R. E. & Blair, P. D. (2009). *Input-output analysis: Foundations and extensions* (Cambridge University Press).
33. Ciaschini, M. (1989). "Scale and structure in economic modelling," *Economic Modelling*, 6(4): 355–373.
34. Socci, C. (2004). "Distribuzione del Reddito e Analisi delle Politiche Economiche per la Regione Marche," (Dott. A. Giuffrè, Milano, Italy). pp. 81–147.

APPENDICES

Appendix A

Table A.1. Correspondences Table Between I–O Industry Classification and UNCTAD Products Classification.

International Standard Industrial Classification of All Economic Activities I–O Table		Standard International Trade Classification UNCTAD ANALYSIS	
		1. Chemicals and related products, n.e.s.	
		Division: Medicinal and pharmaceutical products	
	Chemicals and Chemical Products	**Medicinal and pharmaceutical products**	Provitamins and vitamins, natural or reproduced by synthesis (including natural concentrates), derivatives thereof used primarily as vitamins, and intermixtures of the foregoing, whether or not in any solvent
			Antibiotics
			Vegetable alkaloids, natural or reproduced by synthesis, and their salts, ethers, esters, and other derivatives
			Hormones, natural or reproduced by synthesis; derivatives thereof, used primarily as hormones; other steroids used primarily as hormones
			Glycosides; glands or other organs and their extracts; antisera, vaccines, and similar products
			Pharmaceutical goods, other than medicaments
		Medicaments (including veterinary Medicaments)	Medicaments containing antibiotics or derivatives thereof
			Medicaments containing hormones or other products of subgroup 541.5 but not containing antibiotics
			Medicaments containing alkaloids or derivatives thereof but not containing hormones, other products of subgroup 541.5, or antibiotics
			Medicaments, n.e.s.
		2. Machinery and transport equipment	
		Division: Electrical machinery, apparatus and appliances, n.e.s., and electrical parts thereof (including nonelectrical counterparts, n.e.s., of electrical household-type equipment)	

(*Continued*)

Table A.1. (*Continued*)

	Standard International Trade Classification UNCTAD ANALYSIS	
Machinery, Nec + Electrical and Optical Equipment	**Electro-diagnostic apparatus (other than radiological apparatus)**	Electrocardiographs
		Other electro-diagnostic apparatus (including apparatus for functional exploratory examination or for checking physiological parameters)
		Ultraviolet or infrared ray apparatus
	Apparatus based on the use of X-rays or of alpha, beta, or gamma radiations, whether or not for medical, surgical, dental, or veterinary uses (including radiography or radiotherapy apparatus), X-ray tubes and other X-ray generators; high-tension generators, control panels, and desks, screens, examination or treatment tables, chairs, and the like; parts and accessories	Apparatus based on the use of X-rays, whether or not for medical, surgical, dental or veterinary uses (including radiography or radiotherapy apparatus)
		Apparatus based on the use of alpha, beta, or gamma radiations, whether or not for medical, surgical, dental, or veterinary uses (including radiography or radiotherapy apparatus)
		X-ray tubes
		Other (including parts and accessories)
	3. Miscellaneous manufactured articles	
	Division: Professional, scientific, and controlling instruments and apparatus, n.e.s.	
	Instruments and appliances, n.e.s., for medical, surgical, dental, or veterinary purposes	Dental instruments and appliances, n.e.s.
		Instruments and appliances used in medical, surgical, or veterinary sciences
		Mechanotherapy appliances; massage apparatus; psychological aptitude-testing apparatus; ozone therapy, oxygen therapy, aerosol therapy, artificial respiration, or other therapeutic respiration apparatus; other breathing appliances and gas masks
		Medical, dental, surgical, or veterinary furniture; barbers' chairs and similar chairs with rotating, reclining, and elevating movements; parts of the foregoing articles

Appendix B: The Model Specification

The multisectorial model used for our analysis is described by the linear system:

$$\boldsymbol{x} + \boldsymbol{z} = \boldsymbol{A} \,.\, \boldsymbol{x} + \boldsymbol{f} \tag{B.1}$$

where $\boldsymbol{A}$ is the constant technical coefficients matrix in which the generic element indicates the *j*th intermediate good requirement, necessary for the production for a unit of the *j*th good; $\boldsymbol{x}$ is the vector of total internal production for I–O industry; $\boldsymbol{z}$ represents the vector of imports and $\boldsymbol{f}$ the vector of final demand by I–O industry.

Imports are given by

$$\mathbf{z} = \mathbf{A}^m \boldsymbol{x} + \boldsymbol{f}^m \tag{B.2}$$

where $\boldsymbol{A}^m$ is the technical coefficients matrix of intermediate goods imports and $\boldsymbol{f}^m$ the vector of imports for final demand. Substituting Eq. (B.2) into (B.1) and defining $\boldsymbol{f} = \boldsymbol{f}^0 - \boldsymbol{f}^m$, the solution of the model[30] is expressed by:

$$\boldsymbol{x} = [\boldsymbol{I} - (\boldsymbol{A} - \boldsymbol{Am})]^{-1} \,.\, \boldsymbol{f}^0 \tag{B.3}$$

The original I–O problem consists in the search of the output vector consistent with the final demand vector for the I–O industries, given the structural interrelation among industries.[31]

Model inverse matrix is defined as:

$$\boldsymbol{R} = [\boldsymbol{I} - (\boldsymbol{A} - \boldsymbol{A}^m)]^{-1} \tag{B.4}$$

and transforms each final demand in a vector of total output.

R generally exists, as in general the technology can be expected to be productive, i.e., the technology is such that a part of total output is still available for final use, after the intermediate requirements have been satisfied. In this case, the inverse matrix is usually referred to as the Leontief-multipliers matrix[30] and its elements show the direct and indirect requirements of industry output *i* per unit of final demand of product at industry *j*.[32]

The information derived from Leontief multipliers attests that the impact on production due to changes in final demand is not independent from the manner in which industries react to demand shocks.

The column sum of elements of inverse R entails the use of final demand vector taken from a set, exogenously given, of the type:

$$f^1 = \begin{bmatrix} 1 \\ 0 \\ . \\ 0 \end{bmatrix}, f^2 = \begin{bmatrix} 0 \\ 1 \\ . \\ 0 \end{bmatrix}, \ldots, f^m = \begin{bmatrix} 0 \\ 0 \\ . \\ 1 \end{bmatrix} \tag{B.5}$$

Whereas when we use indices based on the row sum of elements of R, we implicitly assume a final demand structure of the type:

$$f = \begin{bmatrix} 1 \\ 1 \\ . \\ 1 \end{bmatrix} \tag{B.6}$$

Final demand's structure produces direct and indirect effects on the level of total output that may be significantly different.[33] These differences depend on the various composition of the vector and these considerations can assume greater importance when we are interested in evaluating the impact that the final demand determines on the output level using the inverse matrix.

B.1. *Multisectorial tools*

Taking into account the model inverse matrix R, the sum of the elements in the jth column

$$r_{\cdot j} = \sum_{i=1}^{m} r_{ij}$$

detects the increase in all industries output due to an increase of one unit in the exogenous demand of the jth industry's production.

It shows the potential stimulus to the activities from investment in any industry *j*; the amount by which *j*th industry's production depends on inputs.

It is possible to take into account the average values of the column to the estimate the average stimulus imparted to other industry by a unit's worth of exogenous demand for industry *j*.

$$\frac{1}{m} r_{\cdot j} \ (j = 1, 2, \ldots, m) \tag{B.7}$$

The *i*th row sum

$$r_{i\cdot} = \sum_{j=1}^{m} r_{ij}$$

points out, however, the increase in the output of the *i*th industry required to meet an exogenous unit increase in final demand of all other industries.

Considering the average values of row

$$\frac{1}{m} r_{i\cdot} \quad (i = 1,2,\ldots,m) \tag{B.8}$$

it measures the total impact on industry *i* when final demand for all industries increases by unity. However, this only measures direct backward and forward linkages and takes no account of the indirect stimuli given to the economy if the investment goes ahead. To measure both effects we need to make a comparison between industries, however, a normalization procedure is often obtained[23] by comparing the "average" stimulus with the overall average:

$$\frac{1}{m^2} \sum_{j=1}^{m} \sum_{i=1}^{m} r_{ij}$$

So we will have for column, the averages sum of the column sum:

$$\frac{1}{m^2} \sum_{j=1}^{m} r_{\cdot j} \tag{B.9}$$

and the same for row:

$$\frac{1}{m^2}\sum_{i=1}^{m} r_i \tag{B.10}$$

From Eqs. (B.5)–(B.8), we can derive two vectors of indices:

Power of dispersion (Backward): $\pi_{\cdot j} = \dfrac{\frac{1}{m} r_{\cdot j}}{\frac{1}{m^2}\sum_{j=1}^{m} r_{\cdot j}}$

Sensitivity of dispersion (Forward): $\pi_{\cdot i} = \dfrac{\frac{1}{m} r_{\cdot i}}{\frac{1}{m^2}\sum_{i=1}^{m} r_{\cdot i}}$

Appendix C

Table C.1. Dispersion Effects Analysis Results.

		China		Germany		Italy		France	
		Backward	Forward	Backward	Forward	Backward	Forward	Backward	Forward
Agriculture, Hunting, Forestry and Fishing	c1	0.81	1.77	1.05	0.87	0.95	0.83	1.06	1.09
Mining and Quarrying	c2	0.93	1.66	1.03	0.66	0.88	0.69	1.07	0.68
Food, Beverages and Tobacco	c3	1.11	1.45	1.17	0.81	1.26	1.01	1.35	0.89
Textiles and Textile Products	c4	1.34	1.37	0.94	0.62	1.15	0.79	1.09	0.68
Leather, Leather and Footwear	c5	1.31	0.70	0.91	0.62	1.21	0.70	0.99	0.59
Wood and Products of Wood and Cork	c6	1.22	0.99	1.10	0.78	1.13	0.78	1.27	0.80
Pulp, Paper, Paper, Printing and Publishing	c7	1.20	1.16	1.04	0.83	1.12	0.91	1.14	0.94
Coke, Refined Petroleum and Nuclear Fuel	c8	0.86	1.18	1.25	1.02	0.62	0.91	0.91	1.21
Chemicals and Chemical Products	c9	1.17	2.21	0.98	0.69	1.07	0.90	1.10	0.63
Rubber and Plastics	c10	1.28	1.11	0.96	0.76	1.09	0.77	1.06	0.80
Other Non-Metallic Mineral	c11	1.14	0.77	1.07	0.77	1.12	0.83	1.17	0.78
Basic Metals and Fabricated Metal	c12	1.16	2.16	1.00	1.28	1.07	1.38	1.18	1.51
Machinery, Nec	c13	1.21	1.12	1.03	0.93	1.13	0.82	1.14	0.88
Electrical and Optical Equipment	c14	1.24	1.60	0.94	0.84	1.02	0.79	1.15	0.74
Transport Equipment	c15	1.31	1.15	1.11	0.91	1.17	0.73	1.08	0.67
Manufacturing Nec; Recycling	c16	1.08	0.49	1.06	0.69	1.13	0.73	1.14	0.66
Electricity, Gas and Water Supply	c17	1.12	1.65	1.00	1.24	0.73	1.28	1.10	1.20
Construction	c18	1.23	0.51	1.03	0.93	1.05	1.05	1.06	0.93

Sale, Maintenance and Repair of Motor Vehicles and Motorcycles; Retail Sale of Fuel	c19	0.43	0.43	0.86	0.84	1.07	0.90	0.87	0.76
Wholesale Trade and Commission Trade, Except of Motor Vehicles and Motorcycles	c20	0.79	1.13	0.96	1.36	1.10	1.99	1.05	1.73
Retail Trade, Except of Motor Vehicles and Motorcycles; Repair of Household Goods	c21	0.79	0.58	0.97	1.23	1.00	1.38	0.91	1.19
Hotels and Restaurants	c22	1.03	0.84	0.99	0.64	1.03	0.87	1.04	0.78
Inland Transport	c23	0.88	0.92	1.06	1.19	0.99	1.52	0.94	0.92
Water Transport	c24	0.94	0.63	1.28	0.69	1.24	0.59	0.82	0.73
Air Transport	c25	1.13	0.50	1.13	0.70	1.19	0.61	0.89	0.60
Other Supporting and Auxiliary Transport Activities; Activities of Travel Agencies	c26	0.97	0.58	1.16	1.77	1.16	1.24	1.04	1.27
Post and Telecommunications	c27	0.81	0.69	1.02	0.98	0.95	0.92	0.99	0.95
Financial Intermediation	c28	0.69	1.15	1.14	1.57	0.93	1.48	1.01	1.74
Real Estate Activities	c29	0.58	0.67	0.80	1.46	0.64	1.28	0.71	1.10
Renting of M&Eq and Other Business Activities	c30	1.02	1.14	0.90	3.36	0.95	2.94	0.97	4.11
Public Admin and Defence; Compulsory Social Security	c31	0.87	0.44	0.86	0.77	0.80	0.58	0.77	0.67
Education	c32	0.84	0.51	0.81	0.77	0.67	0.64	0.70	0.68
Health and Social Work	*c33*	*1.08*	*0.49*	*0.83*	*0.65*	*0.85*	*0.62*	*0.72*	*0.63*
Other Community, Social and Personal Services	c34	0.97	0.79	0.94	1.16	0.96	0.94	0.94	0.88
Private Households with Employed Persons	c35	0.43	0.43	0.62	0.62	0.57	0.57	0.59	0.59

Chapter 7

European Healthcare Industry and Chinese FDI: Where Do Chinese Firms Invest?

Ping Lv, Yu Liang and Francesca Spigarelli

1. INTRODUCTION

The 12th Five-Year Plan for Health Sector Development has set a key step in the reform of the Chinese healthcare system. The improvement of healthcare assistance for Chinese people has leveraged on the transformation of the Chinese pharmaceutical and biotech industry.[1] The Government planned to establish an innovative production and distribution system, supported by research-based companies. Cooperation of domestic firms with international companies has been encouraged to allow the development of national global players.[2] To acquire knowledge, know how, and technologies, China has been attracting, in the last years, foreign firms, supporting them to transfer in China critical business activities, core technologies, and research development.[3]

Attracted by Chinese industrial supportive policies and booming internal demand, foreign investors have been prioritizing China as the top destination for their international ventures in the last 20 years.[4] Year by year, technological spillovers from Western firms and financial and technical support from the government allowed Chinese firms to grow in size and competitiveness. Starting from early 2000, in line with the general trend of growth of Chinese investments in the world, Chinese firms in the healthcare sector have started to go global. Several cases of greenfield and Mergers and Acquisitions (M&A) in the Western markets have attracted the attention of press, media, and policy makers.

In this chapter, we investigate the internationalization patterns of Chinese companies in the healthcare sector. We analyze the main features and investment decisions of Chinese outward foreign direct investment (OFDI) in the healthcare industry in Europe.

Currently, European countries are among the preferential target destinations for Chinese investors. Europe has developed world-class companies in several healthcare subsectors. European firms can offer technology, know-how, and managerial competencies to allow the upgrading of Chinese firms capability and innovation capacity, while supporting their affirmation in the world stage.

We specifically focus on three subsectors of the healthcare industry, namely pharmaceutical, medical device and equipment, and biotechnology.

2. CHINESE HEALTHCARE REFORM AND HEALTHCARE INDUSTRY

In 2009, the Chinese government released a new plan to reform the national healthcare system.[5] The guidelines on *Deepening the Reform of Health-care System*[6] set several phases to ensure a rapid and effective transition to a universal healthcare system that could bring "safe, effective, convenient and affordable" health services to the Chinese people.[6]

The 12th Five-Year Plan (2011–2016) recognized the role of healthcare reform toward a harmonious and sustainable transition for China to the New Normal growth.[7–10] In 2012, the Pharmaceutical Industry 12th Five-Year Development Plan set the priorities in the process of development of this key industry, along with the need to promote a reinforcement and concentration of the sector, the necessity to improve managerial and quality standards of domestic firms, and the urgency of enhancing international competitiveness through export and international ventures.[11]

Table 1. 13th Five-Year Plan: Key Goals for Healthcare Reform in China.

• Improved health insurance system • Health insurance policy for workers, including coverage for serious diseases both in urban and rural areas • Specialization and diversification of medical personnel • Comprehensive reform of public hospitals • Developing the quality of health services, even at a distance	• Reform of payment systems of care, control over insurance rates • Harmonization of inter-hospitalization expenses for pensioners • Integration between the urban and rural insurance policies • Development of knowledge of "first aid," especially in rural areas • Equality of treatment for public and private hospitals	• Development of the health insurance market, with more openness and encouragement of private sector • Integration maternity insurance and basic health • Construction of harmonious relationship and trust between patients and doctors

Source: Spigarelli and Lv (2017).

In 2015, the Government released a new Plan for the healthcare sector focused on "Essential Points of the National Plan for the Health System and Healthcare (2015–2020)".[a] Later, in 2016, the 13th Five-Year Plan (2016–2020) reaffirmed the importance of the healthcare reform (see Table 1) and the relevance of healthcare industry as a strategic sector for Chinese growth.

3. CHINESE INVESTMENTS IN EUROPE

Within the landscape of deep changes in Chinese healthcare system and industry, we intend to contribute to the analysis of Chinese firms' active role in the global market. In particular, we provide a general overview of location choice and motivation of Chinese firms investing in Europe, using a very unique data set from Mofcom grounded on detailed information on Chinese investors abroad.[b]

---

[a] Available at: http://www.gov.cn/zhengce/content/2015-03/30/content_9560.htm.

[b] MofCom is the Ministry of Commerce of PR China. It releases statistics about officially approved investments (on official statistics on Chinese outward FDI, see Ref. 12).

The database covers both greenfield and non-greenfield (e.g., M&A, joint venture) investments. For each investment decision, the database provides data on the year of investment, the destination country, the entry mode, and overseas activities of the investment. We also collected parent firms' information, such as the year of foundation, the ownership structure, the number of employees, and whether it is a listed company, from the sample firms' homepages or their annual reports.

Our research target is all Chinese firms in the healthcare sector with foreign subsidiaries in EU, by the end of 2015. We identify three main subsectors of healthcare industry, namely, pharmaceutical, medical device and equipment, and biotechnology.

For each subsector included in the analysis, we provide a map of the home provinces of Chinese investors as well as of host country target locations. Thanks to the *where to where* map, we can have a clear understanding of the level of concentrations in both home and host locations and define, eventually, some pairs. Also, we define the prevailing activity performed by the European subsidiary, as declared to MofCom by Chinese firms: sales and services, production, R&D, or capital operations. Multiple choices for activity are possible. This information is quite relevant to assess the motivations behind investments.

In the pharmaceutical subsector, the dataset incorporates 38 location choices by 38 Chinese firms from 1988 (time of the first investment into Europe) to 2015. Over this period, 11 EU countries were the target destinations for Chinese firms, and investments came from 13 provinces.

As shown in Table 2, more than 30% of the sample firms invested in Germany. The next most important destinations are Netherlands, UK, and France. The concentration of investment in Germany is not surprising, in the light of long-lasting bilateral diplomatic ties with China, the country's leading position in pharmaceutical sector, and local firms' strong competitiveness, such as Bayer. Also, Germany had a very focused promotion policy to attract foreign FDI by decreasing the taxation rate in the last decade. Netherlands, UK, and France are all countries with strong healthcare systems and healthcare quality. Besides, population over 65 years old accounts for over 35%, which means huge demand markets.

We also note a strong concentration in investment sources on the Chinese side. Investing firms are based in 13 provinces, but 26.32% of

Table 2. Country Distribution of Chinese OFDI in Pharmaceutical Sector, 1988–2015.

Country	No. of Chinese Outward FDI	Percentage	Country	No. of Chinese Outward FDI	Percentage
Ireland	2	5.26%	Netherlands	5	13.16%
Czech Republic	1	2.63%	Sweden	255	5.26%
Belgium	3	7.89%	Spain	2	5.26%
Poland	1	2.63%	Italy	1	2.63%
Germany	12	31.58%	UK	5	13.16%
France	4	10.53%	Total	38	100.00%

Source: MofCom and authors' calculations.

Table 3. Source Province Distribution of Chinese OFDI in Pharmaceutical Sector, 1988–2015.

Province	No. of Chinese Outward FDI	Percentage	Province	No. of Chinese Outward FDI	Percentage
Beijing	2	5.26%	Shandong	5	13.16%
Guangdong	4	10.53%	Shanghai	1	2.63%
Hainan	2	5.26%	Sichuan	1	2.63%
Hebei	1	2.63%	Tianjin	2	5.26%
Hunan	2	5.26%	Zhejiang	10	26.32%
Jilin	2	5.26%	Chongqing	2	5.26%
Jiangsu	4	10.53%	Total	38	100.00%

Source: MofCom and authors' calculations.

them are located in Zhejiang Province (see Table 3). Zhejiang is in the Yangtze River Delta region and is one of the most active areas for the pharmaceutical sector in China, with strong R&D and powerful production capability. It is the home province, among others, of Zhejiang Pharmaceutical Holdings Limited, one of the most active firms in globalization strategies. Also Shandong, Guangdong, and Jiangsu attract a good amount of investments: they are coastal provinces and offer opening-up policies for foreign firms.

As for activities performed in Europe, 86.8% of branches/subsidiaries of the Chinese investor is in sales and services, 23.7% in R&D, and 13.2%

Table 4. Country Distribution of Chinese OFDI in the Biotech Sector, 1988–2015.

Country	No. of Chinese Outward FDI	Percentage	Country	No. of Chinese Outward FDI	Percentage
Ireland	1	1.82%	Netherlands	11	20.00%
Belgium	1	1.82%	Sweden	4	7.27%
Poland	1	1.82%	Slovakia	1	1.82%
Denmark	2	3.64%	Spain	1	1.82%
Germany	11	20.00%	Hungary	2	3.64%
France	5	9.09%	Italy	2	3.64%
Finland	2	3.64%	UK	11	20.00%
			Total	55	100.00%

Source: MofCom and authors' calculations.

in production. This shows that the firms' motivation are primarily market-seeking. A good interest in R&D is reported, but it does not seem to be a key attraction factor for Chinese firms.

For the biotech sector, the dataset incorporates 55 location choices by 47 Chinese firms from 1988 (time of the first investment into Europe) to 2015. Over this period, 14 EU countries were target destinations for Chinese firms.

As shown in Table 4, Germany, Netherlands, and UK attract 20% of OFDI, separately. The top three destination countries in biotech are the same as in the pharmaceutical sector. They all have solid position in the healthcare industry. First, there are many universities and healthcare institutions which serve strong research and development capability. A good transit from research to production helps firms take full advantage of knowledge achievements. In addition, a mature capital market provides abundant capital to conduct research, and an advanced intellectual property rights (IPR) system protects the research outcomes.

Also in this case, there is a concentration in investment sources on the Chinese side. Investing firms are based in 20 provinces, but a large number of firms are located in Beijing, Shandong, and Jiangsu (Table 5). Beijing has unique capital and policies to develop research and development capability. It offers a concentration of universities that provide

Table 5. Source Province Distribution of Chinese OFDI in Biotech Sector, 1988–2015.

Province	No. of Chinese Outward FDI	Percentage	Province	No. of Chinese Outward FDI	Percentage
Anhui	4	7.27%	Jiangsu	5	9.09%
Beijing	8	14.55%	Zhejiang	1	1.82%
Liaoning	4	7.27%	Ningxia	1	1.82%
Guangdong	3	5.45%	Qinghai	1	1.82%
Guangxi	1	1.82%	Fujian	4	7.27%
Hainan	3	5.45%	Shandong	6	10.91%
Hebei	2	3.64%	Shanxi	2	3.64%
Heilongjiang	1	1.82%	Shanghai	2	3.64%
Hunan	1	1.82%	Sichuan	1	1.82%
Jilin	3	5.45%	Tianjin	2	3.64%
			Total	55	100.00%

Source: MofCom and authors' calculations.

hundreds of thousands of talented recruits. Besides the geographic advantages mentioned earlier, Shandong and Jiangsu set a goal to prioritize the development of the biotech industry.

As for the main reasons for investing in Europe, 71% of the firms in the biotech sector are engaged in sales and services, 40% in production, and 55% in R&D. Market-seeking is still the main target of Chinese OFDI. But, in this sector, R&D accounts for a larger percentage than the other sectors. More than half of the Chinese firms invest abroad to seek advanced technology.

The last subsector to be analyzed belongs to medical devices and equipment. The dataset incorporates 67 location choices by 57 Chinese firms from 1988 (time of the first investment into Europe) to 2015. Over this period, 13 EU countries were target destinations for Chinese firms.

As shown in Table 6, more than 30% of the sample firms invested in the Germany. UK was the next most important destination for investors (with 20% of initiatives), followed by Netherlands. A strong healthcare capability is an important pull factor of Chinese OFDI.

Table 6. Country Distribution of Chinese OFDI in Medical Devices and Equipment Sector, 1988–2015.

Country	No. of Chinese Outward FDI	Percentage	Country	No. of Chinese Outward FDI	Percentage
Ireland	1	1.49%	Netherlands	8	11.94%
Austria	1	1.49%	Croatia	1	1.49%
Belgium	2	2.99%	Sweden	2	2.99%
Poland	1	1.49%	Spain	2	2.99%
Germany	22	32.84%	Italy	6	8.96%
France	5	7.46%	UK	14	20.90%
Finland	2	2.99%	Total	67	100.00%

Source: MofCom and authors' calculations.

Table 7. Source Province Distribution of Chinese OFDI in Medical Device and Equipment Sector, 1988–2015.

Province	No. of Chinese Outward FDI	Percentage	Province	No. of Chinese Outward FDI	Percentage
Beijing	10	14.93%	Ningxia	1	1.49%
Guangdong	2	2.99%	Shandong	14	20.90%
Guangxi	1	1.49%	Shanghai	8	11.94%
Hunan	2	2.99%	Zhejiang	10	14.93%
Hunan	6	8.96%	Chongqing	3	4.48%
Jilin	1	1.49%	Other	3	4.48%
Jiangsu	6	8.96%	Total	67	100.00%

Source: MofCom and authors' calculations.

As for the Chinese side, investing firms are based in 13 provinces, but 20% of them are located in Shandong Province (see Table 7), followed by Zhejiang and Beijing. Results are similar in the three subsectors of the healthcare industry. Abundant capital, advanced healthcare capability, rich research and development resources, opening-up policy, and superior geographic location are the factors that are encouraging Chinese firms invest overseas.

Table 8. Motivations of Investments in Europe, Percentage of Motivations, 2015.

Sectors	Production	Sales and Services	R&D
Pharmaceutical sector	27.27%	81.82%	36.36%
Biotech sector	20.43%	78.26%	52.17%
Medical devices and equipment sector	36.84%	68.42%	68.42%

In terms of activities performed by Chinese firms in Europe, 91% of the investment in the medical device and equipment sector involves sales and services, 31% production, and 30% R&D. This indicates that the firms' motivation is primarily market-seeking, rather than strategic-asset–seeking. Anyway, there is also a good percentage of cases where production takes place abroad.

Besides the subsector analysis described earlier, we conclude with a table of motivations of investments in Europe in 2015 (Table 8). As shown in the table, the results are similar. Sales and services explain over two-thirds of all investments in 2015, which shows that market-seeking is the top attractive factor of Chinese firms. Following sales and services, R&D is the second motivation. Since there is still a gap between China and Europe in scientific and technological strength, firms go abroad to learn advanced technology and cooperate with EU firms to improve R&D capability.

4. CONCLUSION

The main findings of our analysis can be summarized as follows.

In general, the Chinese investing provinces are mainly located in the coastal areas. This spatial allocation reflects the unbalanced industrial development of China, as well as the different level of openness to international trade and investments of Chinese provinces.[13]

Chinese investments are also spatially concentrated in key European countries: investments from more industrialized provinces tend to target leading EU countries, where they can find expertise and market.

The situations in the three healthcare sectors are almost the same, regardless of the most attractive EU countries or the most active Chinese investing provinces. Characteristics of both home and host regions seem to play a critical role in explaining the path of Chinese OFDI in Europe.

While "secondary" motivations vary over sector, there is a huge focus on Europe as an outlet market. This might reflect the fact that in all three subsectors, China has developed a good technological capacity and needs to strengthen the penetration capacity in Western markets. R&D can be also a secondary motivation, especially for biotechnology.

REFERENCES

1. Ministry of Health PRC (2013). *Healthcare in China* (People's Medical Publishing House, Beijing).
2. MofCom (2012). Catalogue for the Guidance of Foreign Investment Industries. Available at: http://english.mofcom.gov.cn/article/policyrelease/aaa/201203/20120308027837.shtml. Accessed 12 December 2015.
3. Wilsdon, T. & Fiz, E. (2013). "Encouraging pharmaceutical innovation in middle-income countries," *Wipo Magazine*, April. Available at: http://www.wipo.int/wipo_magazine/en/2013/02/article_0008.html. Accessed 12 December 2015.
4. Spigarelli, F. & Wei, H. (2014). "The Chinese pharmaceutical market: Driving forces and emerging trends," *L'industria*, 35(3): 505–530.
5. Rein, S. (2009). "Health-care reform, China style," *Bloomberg Businessweek*. Available at: http://www.businessweek.com/globalbiz/content/aug2009/gb20090821_005732.htm. Accessed 21 December 2015.
6. Freeman, C. & Lu Boynton, X. (2011). Implementing Health Care Reform Policies in China. Available at: http://csis.org/files/publication/111202_Freeman_ImplementingChinaHealthReform_Web.pdf. Accessed 8 January 2016.
7. Tung, A. (2011). "Alliances form in growing pharmaceutical market," *China Daily*. August 3.
8. Deloitte (2014). China's Pharmaceutical Market: Summary and Prospects. Available at: https://www2.deloitte.com/content/dam/Deloitte/ch/Documents/life-sciences-health-care/ch_Studie_Pharmaceutical_China_05052014.pdf. Accessed 28 September 2017.
9. WHO (2012). China. Available at: http://www.wpro.who.int/countries/chn/5CHNpro2011_finaldraft.pdf?ua=1. Accessed 19 December 2015.
10. Wong, J., Wu, C. & Xia, M. (2014). New Rules for Winning in China's Pharmaceutical Market. The Boston Consulting Group. Available at: https://www.bcg.com/publications/2014/new-rules-winning-chinas-pharmaceutical-market.aspx. Accessed 28 September 2017.

11. CCCMHPIE (2012). Pharmaceutical Industry "12th Five-Year" Development Plan. Available at: http://www.cccmhpie.org.cn/Pub/3725/48117.shtml. Accessed 12 December 2015.
12. Amighini, A., Cozza, C., Rabellotti, R. & Sanfilippo, M. (2014), An analysis of Chinese outward FDIs in Europe with firm-level data, Lund University, Circle WP 2014/02. Available at: http://www.circle.lu.se/upload/circle/workingpapers/201402_amighini_et_al.pdf.
13. Poncet, S. (2005). "A fragmented China: Measure and determinants of Chinese domestic market disintegration," *Review of International Economics,* 13(3): 409–430.

Chapter 8

Monopoly in the Chinese Healthcare Market: Norms and Practices

Lihong Zhang and Changmian Zhang

1. INTRODUCTION

The *Opinions of the Communist Party of China Central Committee and the State Council on Deepening Reform of the Health Care System* (2009, 中共中央国务院关于深化医药卫生体制改革的意见), as China's healthcare reform strategy for next decade (from 2009–2010 to 2019–2020), has determined as a principle the leading position of public-owned medical institutions. Therefore it is not occasional that in the recent policy represented by the *2016 Main tasks on Deepening Reform of the Health Care System* (深化医药卫生体制改革 2016 年重点工作任务), the experimental Public hospitals are entitled to receive financial subsidy from the central government. It is not very arbitrary to assert that, in the healthcare market, the monopoly is gradually emerging.

In Sec. 2, we will draw attention to and describe an overview of the monopoly practices in the healthcare market, evocated either by administrative discretion or by the abuse of dominant market position. The illegal monopoly occurs under the control of the legal order. So in the Sec. 3, we make the effort to illustrate the co-legal system, underlining the recent legislation, *Anti-monopoly Law of PRC*. Analyzing this Statute Law, we will individuate the completeness with regard to the abuse of the dominant position, at least from the point of view of "the law in book," and, on the contrary, the ineffectiveness in the ambit of administrative monopoly. Section 4 regards a case study with the scope to illustrate the Chinese Courts' effort to specify *Anti-monopoly Law* in the definition of vertical monopoly agreement. In Sec. 5, we conclude by providing some observations on this theme.

2. A PANORAMIC VIEW OF ILLEGAL MONOPOLY IN THE HEALTHCARE MARKET

It is not very easy to provide a panoramic view of the illegal monopoly practice in the healthcare market under the legal perspective, considering the complexity and incoherence of the legal system in this field and even the fact that, in many occasions, we cannot find the statute law as its *ratio legis*. However, in this section, we are attempting to sketch an outline of this phenomenon.

2.1. *Administrative monopolies*

The first to be demonstrated in this section is administrative regulations, which can be further categorized in several aspects.

First is the accessibility to the healthcare market. Recognized as *opinio communis*, the control of accessibility, as a governance instrument, aims to regulate the market activity to contribute to the formation of a just market order. However, despite the 1994 *Regulations on the Administration of Medical Institutions* (医疗机构管理条例), in its Article 2, advocating private investment in the medical service market, the same *Regulations*, in its Article 8, provide that its establishment shall be in line with the local regional health programs and the local regional plan for the establishment of medical institutions. Such a legal norm constitutes a legal barrier to establish a competitive medical institution, especially in a region where the public institutions, in spite of their incapacity of affording a quality service, normally have a significant influence on the local government's drafting of health programs. Actually it is not only a theoretical analysis but also a reoccurring fact as proved by the registration statistics: 90% of non-profit medical institutions are represented by small hospitals, specialized clinics, and private clinics. If one does not tend to evaluate the norm in an isolated manner without taking in consideration the cultural circumstances related to the function of the legal norm, one may accept the conclusion that Article 8 of *Regulations* presents one of the distinctive limitations to healthcare market accessibility.

The situation becomes even worse as far as foreign investment is concerned. According to the 2000 *Interim Measures for Administration of Chinese-foreign Joint Venture and Cooperative Medical Institutions* (中外合资、合作医疗机构管理暂行办法), just as this denomination implies, it is permitted to establish a wholly foreign-owned medical institution in PRC. Its Article 8 provides a restrictive condition for the foreign investment, i.e.,

> *1. It has to be an independent legal person; 2. The total amount of investment must not fall below RMB20 million yuan; 3. The equity proportion or interest the Chinese party to a Chinese-foreign joint venture medical institution or a cooperative medical institution hold therein shall not be less than 30%; 4. The period of the joint venture or the cooperative medical institution shall not be longer than 20 years; and 5. Other conditions laid down by the administrative departments of health at or above the provincial level.*

The requirements related to the establishment of Chinese–Foreign Joint Venture and co-operative medical institutions are regulated by its Articles 6, 7, and 9.[a]

---

[a]Article 6: "Chinese-foreign joint venture and cooperative medical institutions shall be established and developed in line with the local regional health programs and the local regional plan for the establishment of medical institutions, and be governed by the Basic Standards for Medical Institutions formulated by the Ministry of Health." Article 7: "The

These administrative-coercive regulations facilitate the public-owned medical institutions to occupy dominance in the healthcare market.

The second aspect on the monopoly of State-owned medical institutions consists in China's taxation policy. The 2000 *Guidances on Medical-sanitary Reform in City and Town* (关于城镇医药卫生体制改革的指导意见) has categorized the medical institutions into profit and non-profit entities and then afforded generally some taxation privileges for the latter. It is detailed by the 2000 *Notice of Taxation Policies for Medical Institutions*, formulated by the Ministry of Finance and State Administration of Taxation (财政部、国家税务总局关于医疗卫生机构有关税收政策的通知), which states that while the non-profit institutions can facilitate taxation privilege without any limitation, the for-profit institutions can make profit from the policy within three years from its establishment. In other words, once the three-year period has expired, the for-profit institutions shall pay taxes regularly, while the non-profit institutions continue to maintain their privileges. It seems, at first glance, to be reasonable. However, this policy discriminates against the private medical institutions,

---

Chinese and foreign parties that apply for the establishment of a Chinese-foreign joint venture medical institution or a Chinese-foreign cooperative medical institution shall be legal persons who can independently bear their civil liabilities. The Chinese and foreign parties to a joint venture medical institution or a cooperative medical institution shall have direct or indirect experience in medical and health investment and management, and shall answer to one of the following requirements:

(1) They are in a position to provide internationally advanced managerial experience in managing medical institutions, modes of management and modes of services;
(2) They are able to provide international cutting-edge medical technologies and equipment; and
(3) They can complement or make up for the inadequacy of local medical service capacity, medical treatment technologies, funding and medical facilities."

Article 9: " The Chinese party to a joint venture of cooperative medical institution shall obtain the approval from the corresponding competent department of its investment therein with state-owned assets (including priced investment or as a condition for cooperation). The assets shall, in accordance with the pertinent provisions on the administration of asset valuation, be appraised by an asset appraisal agency recognized by the department of administration of state-owned assets before they are used as investment therein. The appraisal result of state-owned assets which are confirmed by an administrative department of state-owned assets at or above the provincial level may be taken as the basis of pricing the state-assets to be invested in a joint venture or cooperative medical institution."

given that all of private medical institutions shall be registered as for-profit institutions with legal person status, and every public-owned medical institution is qualified as a non-profit institution.

The monopoly in the medical market also concerns medical insurance. Since the central government decided to set up nationwide "Basic Medical Insurance System" in 1998,[b] the medical insurance market in China has been largely increasing. According to this system, the patient whose medical fee is supposed to be covered by social insurance is obligated to get the drugs from the so-called designated medical institutions and drug stores. To operate this activity of medical insurance, the medical institutions and drug stores, however, shall apply *ad hoc* to the local authority for their specific licenses. As one can easily imagine, in a socialist country, priority to any public-owned institutions is always guaranteed for the issuance of this license of operation of social insurance in medical market. Therefore, the social insurance market is unavailable for the private-owned institutions without the possession of this kind of license.

With regard to the administrative power, the estimation and promotion of medical professionals is always under the domain of sanitary competence authorities. Generally speaking, the medical professionals who work for private-owned institutions can hardly obtain promotion and a fair professional esteem. This diversified treatment collaborates to preclude outstanding professionals from entering into the private profit-institutions and, consequently, decreases their competition with public non-profit institutions in terms of medical service.

2.2. *Abuse of a dominant market position*

As we have demonstrated earlier, the public-owned medical institutions, with the facility given by the legislation and the authority, are inclined to obtain a dominant market position. Statistical analysis shows that the pharmaceutical distribution by public-owned hospitals accounts for about 85% of the total distribution. The public hospitals thus occupy a dominant

[b] *The Decision of The State Council on Setting up Basic Medical Insurance System for Staff Members and Workers in Cities and Towns,* 1998 (国务院关于建立城镇职工基本医疗保险制度的决定).

position in the field of pharmaceutical distribution. Without supervision, any dominance tends to be abused. It shall be noted that there are two typical occasions, *inter alias*, with regards to the abuse of dominance in the relationship between the hospital as a purchaser and the pharmaceutical distributor. The first occasion constitutes in Exclusive Distribution Agreement, with which the distributor is compelled to make transactions exclusively with the defined hospital in a defined region. Under this agreement, the hospital shall make profit from the exclusive subdistributor in specified region, and, as a consequence, the drug's price increases. The other typical abuse can be found in tie-in purchase conduct. It means the hospital purchases one pharmaceutical product (named "A"), under the condition that the distributor shall sell the other pharmaceutical product (named "B"). In fact, the product "B" is what the hospital really desires, but from the sale of product "B," the distributor usually can hardly make profits.

On the other hand, it is easy to find an imbalance between the hospital and the patient. This kind of relationship shall be technically defined as a service contract. However, the information asymmetry breaks the equality, making the medical doctors, who always possess professional knowledge, occupy a dominant position against the patients. The abuse of this dominance commonly occurs when the medical doctors mislead the patients to undergo unnecessary medical check-up and treatment.

3. THE PRESENT LEGAL INSTITUTION ON THE REGULATION OF MONOPOLY IN THE HEALTHCARE MARKET AND ITS LIMITATION

In the current legal system, we can identify two statute laws that aim to regulate the monopoly: The 1993 *Law of PRC against Unfair Competition* and the 2008 *Anti-monopoly Law of PRC*.

3.1. *Law of PRC against unfair competition*

The 1994 *Law against Unfair Competition* determines its scope in regulating the unfair competition that infringes upon the lawful rights and interests of another business operator and disturbs the socio-economic order (Article 2). To fulfill this scope, the Articles 5–14 of this Law identifies ten types unfair competition conducts. Among these unfair conducts, it is worth mentioning that business monopoly and administrative monopoly are regulated by its Articles 6 and 7, respectively.[c] Since the recent 2008 *Anti-monopoly Law* almost redefines the monopolistic acts, we will focus on it, examining its provisions in detail.

3.2. *Anti-monopoly Law of PRC: The definition of monopolistic conducts*

The 2008 *Anti-monopoly Law* is qualified as "the constitution in business life." Pursuant to its Article 3, the monopolistic conducts are classified as follows: (1) monopoly agreements reached between undertakings; (2) abuse of dominant market position by undertakings; and (3) concentration of undertakings that lead, or may lead to, elimination or restriction of competition. As it can be easily comprehended, the last type is a "close term." This *Anti-monopoly Law* also makes efforts to clarify the monopoly agreement and the abuse of the dominant market position. In fact, while in its Capital II the monopoly agreement is further specified and individuated as horizontal[d]

---

[c] Article 6: "A public utility enterprise or any other business operator occupying monopoly status according to law shall not restrict people to purchasing commodities from the business operators designated by him, thereby precluding other business operators from fair competition."

Article 7: "Governments and their subordinate departments shall not abuse administrative powers to restrict people to purchasing commodities from the business operators designated by them and impose limitations on the rightful operation activities of other business operators."

[d] Article 13: Competing undertakings are prohibited from concluding the following monopoly agreements:

(1) On fixing or changing commodity prices;
(2) On restricting the amount of commodities manufactured or marketed;
(3) On splitting the sales market or the purchasing market for raw and semi-finished materials;
(4) On restricting the purchase of new technologies or equipment, or the development of new technologies or products;
(5) On joint boycotting of transactions; and
(6) Other monopoly agreements confirmed as such by the authority for enforcement of the *Anti-monopoly Law* under the State Council.

and vertical,[e] in its Capital III, a special attention is paid to the dominant market position. According to Article 18, the dominant market position of an undertaking can be determined by taking into account the following factors: (1) its share and competitiveness in the relevant market; (2) its ability to control the sales market or the purchasing marker for raw and semi-finished materials; (3) its financial strength and technical conditions; (4) the extent to which other business managers depend on it in transactions; (5) the difficulty that other undertakings find in entering a relevant market; and (6) other factors related to the determination of the dominant market position held by an undertaking. These determining factors become much more operable with a legal methodology: the presumed dominant market position. Under Article 19, in one of the following circumstances, the undertaking shall be presumed in possession of a dominant market: (1) the market share of one undertaking accounts for half of the total in a relevant market; (2) the joint market share of two undertakings accounts for two-thirds of the total, in a relevant market; or (3) the joint market share of three undertakings accounts for three-fourths of the total in a relevant market.

However, under the circumstance specified in points (2) or (3) of the Article, if the market share of one of the undertakings is less than one-tenths of the total, the undertaking's dominant market shall be excluded. As mentioned earlier, the 2008 *Anti-monopoly Law* uses the legal measure "presumption" in order to release the plaintiff from the burden of proof. Therefore, it is understandable that an undertaking, if there is any evidence to prove the contrary, shall not be considered to hold a dominant market position. The dominant position, *per se*, is not illegal, and only its abuse, by contrast, shall be prohibited. Article 17 clarifies the abuse conduct: (1) selling commodities at unfairly high prices or buying

---

For the purposes of this Law, monopoly agreements include agreements, decisions and other concerted conducts designed to eliminate or restrict competition.

[e]Article 14: Undertakings are prohibited from concluding the following monopoly agreements with their trading counterparts:

(1) On fixing the prices of commodities resold to a third party;
(2) On restricting the lowest prices for commodities resold to a third party; and
(3) Other monopoly agreements confirmed as such by the authority for enforcement of the *Anti-monopoly Law* under the State Council.

commodities at unfairly low prices; (2) without justifiable reasons, selling commodities at prices below cost; (3) without justifiable reasons, refusing to enter into transactions with their trading counterparts; (4) without justifiable reasons, allowing their trading counterparts to make transactions exclusively with themselves or with the undertakings designated by them; (5) without justifiable reasons, conducting tie-in sale of commodities or adding other unreasonable trading conditions to transactions; (6) without justifiable reasons, applying differential prices and other transaction terms among their trading counterparts who are on an equal footing; and (7) other acts of abuse of dominant market positions confirmed as such by the authority for enforcement of the *Anti-monopoly Law* under the State Council.

3.3. *Anti-monopoly Law of PRC: The responsibility for monopolistic conducts*

The responsibility for monopolistic conducts shall be individuated in two forms: administrative responsibility and civil responsibility.

The State council, as the exclusive authority for the enforcement of the 2008 *Anti-monopoly Law*, is equipped with the administrative power to investigate monopolistic conduct[f] and order the infringer to discontinue

[f]Article 39: When conducting investigations into a suspected monopolistic conduct, the authority for enforcement of the *Anti-monopoly Law* may take the following measures:

(1) Conducting inspection of the business places or the relevant premises of the undertakings under investigation;
(2) Making inquiries of the undertakings under investigation, the interested parties, or other units or individuals involved, and requesting them to provide relevant explanations;
(3) Consulting and duplicating the relevant documents and materials of the undertakings under investigation, the interested parties and other relevant units and individuals, such as bills, certificates, agreements, account books, business correspondence and electronic data;
(4) Sealing up or seizing relevant evidence; and
(5) Inquiring about the bank accounts of the undertakings under investigation.

the violation, confiscate its unlawful gains, and, in addition, impose a fine.[g]

On the other hand, civil responsibility is established in its Article 50, which iterates: "Where the monopolistic conduct of an undertaking has caused losses to another person, it shall bear civil liabilities according to law." Pursuant to Article 2[h] of the Supreme People's Court Interpretation on the 2008 *Anti-monopoly Law*,[i] which entered into force on January 30, 2012, the affirmative decision of the State Council on monopolistic con-

---

For taking the measures specified in the preceding paragraph, a written report shall be submitted for approval to the principal leading person of the authority for enforcement of the *Anti-monopoly Law*.

[g] Article 46: Where an undertaking, in violation of the provisions of this Law, concludes and implements a monopoly agreement, the authority for enforcement of the *Anti-monopoly Law* shall instruct it to discontinue the violation, confiscate its unlawful gains, and, in addition, impose on it a fine of not less than 1% but not more than 10% of its sales achieved in the previous year. If such monopoly agreement has not been implemented, it may be fined not more than RMB 500,000 yuan.

If the business management, on its own initiative, reports to the authority for enforcement of the *Anti-monopoly Law* about the monopoly agreement reached, and provides material evidence, the said authority may, at its discretion, mitigate, or exempt the undertaking from, punishment.

Where a trade association, in violation of the provisions of this Law, has arranged the undertaking in the trade to reach a monopoly agreement, the authority for enforcement of the Anti-monopoly Law may impose on it a fine of not more than 500,000 yuan. If the circumstances are serious, the administrative department for the registration of public organizations may cancel the registration of the trade association in accordance with law.

Article 47: Where an undertaking, in violation of the provisions of this Law, abuses its dominant market position, the authority for enforcement of the *Anti-monopoly Law* shall instruct it to discontinue such violation, confiscate its unlawful gains and, in addition, impose on it a fine of not less than 1% but not more than 10% of its sales achieved in the previous year.

[h] "Where a plaintiff directly files a civil lawsuit with the people's court or files a civil lawsuit with the people's court after a decision of the *Anti-monopoly law* enforcement authority affirming the existence of monopolistic conduct comes into force, if the lawsuit satisfies other conditions for lawsuit acceptance as prescribed by law, the people's court shall accept the lawsuit."

[i] Provisions of the Supreme People's Court on Several Issues concerning the Application of Law in the Trial of Civil Dispute Cases Arising from Monopolistic Conduct (最高人民法院关于审理因垄断行为引发的民事纠纷案件应用法律若干问题的规定).

duct does not constitute a precondition for the assumption of civil liabilities of a wrongdoer.

3.4. *The limitation: Administrative monopoly*

In our opinion, there are some serious limitations on the regulation of administrative monopoly in present legal system.

In its Capital V, the 2008 *Anti-monopoly Law,* after having enumerated several acts relating to the abuse of administrative power, offers a close-term which says: "Administrative organs may not abuse their administrative power to formulate regulations with the contents of eliminating or restricting competition" (Article 37), but the enforcement of these provision is rather less operable and effective.

In the case that a public organization abuses its administrative power to eliminate or restrict competition, under Article 15 of this law, it is not the authority for enforcement of the *Anti-monopoly Law* but the relevant administrative office at a higher level that has the power to instruct the infringer to rectify its unlawful conduct. Hence, what the authority can do is only to submit a proposal to the relevant office at a higher level. Since two administrative authorities with different levels share common interests due to their same public function and are usually characterized by nepotism, it is easy to imagine the ineffectiveness of this kind of the proposal.

Nevertheless, in the case that anyone suffers some damages from the abuse of administrative power by the relevant authorities under the 2008 *Anti-monopoly Law*, this law does not provide any administrative liabilities or sanctions for the relevant authorities for the abuse of their powers.

4. A CASE STUDY: HOW TO DEFINE A VERTICAL MONOPOLY AGREEMENT

Till now, there are few cases on monopoly of market in law practice. It is worth studying the first case on vertical monopoly agreement in China, in order to understand its definition.

The final decision on this leading litigation between *Beijing Ruibang Yonghe Technology & Trade Co., Ltd.* (hereinafter called "Ruibang") and *Johnson (Shanghai) Medical Equipment Co., Ltd/Johnson (China) Medical Equipment Co., Ltd.*, was made by the Shanghai High Court on August 1, 2012.[j]

The facts of case are as follows: *Ruibang* collaborated with *Johnson* as the latter's dealer of medical stapler and medical suture products in Beijing for more than 15 years. On January 2, 2008, the parties concluded a sale contract according to which *Ruibang* is obligated not to sell medical stapler and medical suture products in Beijing at the price lower than that established by *Johnson*. In March 2008, however, after a bid, *Ruibang* sold the products at a lower price. For this reason, *Johnson* withdrew the license of sale in several hospitals in Beijing. Thus, *Ruibang* sued *Johnson* before the court for the remedy for the losses, arguing that the sale contract constitutes a vertical monopoly agreement.

Seemingly, under the 2008 *Anti-monopoly Law,* the agreement restricting the lowest prices for commodities resold to a third party could be viewed as a vertical monopoly agreement. However, as the court of the final decision points out, in order to verify if this agreement constitutes a vertical monopoly agreement, it is necessary to take into consideration Section 2 of Article 13 on the horizontal anti-monopoly agreement, which states that "monopoly agreements include agreements, decisions and other concerted conducts designed to eliminate or restrict competition." That is to say, a vertical monopoly agreement shall bring about the unfair effect: elimination or restriction of competition.

While the courts of both instances agree on the definition of the vertical monopoly agreement, the court of the first instance, Shanghai No. 1 Intermediate Court did not hold that the sale contract led to the restriction of competition. However, the Court of the second instance, namely Shanghai High Court,

---

[j] See Shanghai No. 1 Intermediate Court's Decision (2010, the Fifth Section, decision of the first instance, N. 169) (上海市第一中级人民法院 (2010) 沪一中民五(知)初字第 169 号民事判决书), and Shanghai High Court's decision (2012, the Third Section, final decision, N. 63) (上海市高级人民法院 (2012) 沪高民三(知)终字第 63 号民事判决书).

argued that in order to demonstrate the elimination and restriction of competition, the following aspects shall be considered seriously: (1) Whether competition of relevant market is sufficient; (2) whether the defendant's market position is strong; (3) the motives of defendant to establish the minimum resale price; and (4) the effects on the competition by means of the minimum resale price. After analyzing all details of the fact, under the Article 50 of *Anti-monopoly Law*, Shanghai High Court decided that *Johnson* had restricted the competition by the conclusion of this sale contract and shall pay the losses that *Ruibang* had suffered.

This pilot case plays an important role in the understanding of the law in action on monopoly in medical market in China. The final decision of this case makes clear that, in order to verify if there is a vertical monopoly agreement, it is necessary to evaluate the effects of elimination and restriction of competition in the market. Moreover, the court of final decision lists the above-mentioned four aspects which deem to be examined to find the elimination and restriction of competition and in this way, it created the criteria for the verification of the existence of a vertical monopoly agreement in terms of the Chinese law in action.

5. CONCLUSION

Concluding this short study on the legal framework of monopoly in the Chinese healthcare market, we summarize our observations as follows:

(1) The monopoly in the healthcare market in China is an emerging issue that needs to be confronted seriously. Thanks to the Chinese legal policies and legislation, the state-owned and public medical institutions have held unreasonably and largely the monopoly position in Chinese healthcare market. Today, this situation is hindering the development of the Chinese healthcare market.
(2) Even if the 2008 *Anti-monopoly Law* has already regulated some relevant illegal monopoly, in particular, the abuse of the dominance, so far, few cases against the monopoly of healthcare market happen. As the first court decision on vertical monopoly agreement in 2012 proves, the Chinese judges are paying increasing attention to the

elimination of the monopoly for the realization of a real market-orientation economy.

(3) The rules on how to control the legal responsibility of the administrative authorities are still seriously lacking in today's Chinese law. This problem will be not easily overcome in the short term, since the Chinese government has been providing preference to the dominance of public medical institutions for a long time.

Chapter 9

The Chinese Private Hospital Sector and FDI: From Socialization to Opening Up

Federica Monti

1. INTRODUCTION

The Chinese *healthcare* and *life sciences* industry is conventionally subdivided, by government statistics, into five categories: pharmaceuticals, biotechnology, medical devices, medical services, and health administration.

With the aim to understand what the real relevance of this sector is for the Chinese government, it seems interesting to compare the current structure to those proposed at an international and European level.

For this purpose, we will consider the *International Standards Industry Classification (ISIC)*, developed by the United Nations, and the *Industry Classification Benchmark (ICB)*, operated by FTSE International Limited (London).

ISIC has organized the healthcare sector into three subsectors: hospital activities, medical & dental practice activities, and other human health activities. *ICB*, with stronger financial and management targets, is closer to the Chinese market structure. It organizes the healthcare sector (or using the classification reference "supersector") into healthcare equipment & services and pharmaceuticals & biotechnology.

In comparison, the Chinese market structure is partially correspondent with the European one, but what essentially emerges is that inside the European-proposed dual-layered market structure,[a] each layer seems to be treated more as an airtight compartment, rather than as part of a whole.

This is evidenced by the major attention paid at a European level to the pharmaceutical sector for its impressive economic significance, which makes Europe a world leader in the trade of pharmaceutical products.

On the other hand, although one cannot draw an exact comparison between the subcategories provided by the *ICB* and those conventionally referred by the Chinese government, what emerges is the greater financial and economic emphasis hidden behind each subsector. This is all conceived within the system, in which China seems to identify important areas for inbound investments.

With this in mind, consider Article 21 of the Chinese Constitution Chart, which stipulates *The state develops medical and health services, promotes modern medicine and traditional Chinese medicine, encourages and supports the setting up of various medical and health facilities [...]* with a clear aim to boost the entire healthcare industry.

Considering this as the cornerstone, over the years, China has made several efforts to develop and improve the national medical and health services sector by pursuing the policy mantra *making rural areas the focus of our work, putting disease prevention first, supporting both traditional Chinese medicine and Western medicine, relying on science, technology and education, and mobilizing the whole of society to join the efforts, improving the people's health and serving socialist modernization.*[b]

Leveraging on the government's continuous primary focus on steady economic growth and on the promotion of a national economic restructure, with particular reference to the hospital subsector, the above is confirmed

---

[a] Often used for statistical purposes by the European authorities, for examples, see the *2013 EU Industrial R&D Scoreboard* at http://iri.jrc.ec.europa.eu/scoreboard13.html.

[b] White Paper on the Medical and Health Services in China (2012). Available at: http://www.scio.gov.cn/zfbps/gqbps/Document/1435497/1435497.htm.

by a new set of rules, recently promoted by the central government. These take a new direction and break with the past to permit both domestic and foreign private investors to fully invest in the private hospital sector.

Historically, the hospital subsector has always been in the public sphere. However, since end of the 1990s, China has embraced the privatization process, which is a major step in transforming a centralized, planned economy into a market-oriented economy. In recent years, this has affected strategic sectors, such as healthcare, making the Constitutional cornerstone of "improving people's health" (as referenced in the above-mentioned Article 21) a goal with a "more economical" aim.

2. THE PRIVATIZATION OF THE CHINESE PRIVATE HOSPITAL SECTOR

Within the larger medical services category, the Chinese private hospital industry deserves particular attention because of the recent government stimulus which may involve nation-wide foreign investments in the coming years.

Nevertheless, the legal framework for the private hospital sector remains rather vague. What — at first sight — could seem like China taking a further step toward opening up to foreign investments (in this case, in the healthcare sector), could actually just be a step in China's privatization process.

This compels a consideration of the privatization phenomenon due to its deep impact on the Chinese socio-economic environment, with reference to the hospital sector.

The term *privatization* shall not be meant — simply — as a process through which government turns state sectors into private economic sectors.

This partial and incorrect association between the concept of *transfer of ownership* with the term *privatization* originated through a long history of political and ideological thought, which makes this term a taboo for the government.

Observing the background, China has known *privatization* since the end of the 1980s, when the country embraced new directions and disrupted Mao's communist policy.

The *privatization* process is better defined by the Chinese terms 私有化 (*sīyǒu huà*, literally *denationalization*), 民营化 (*mínyíng huà*, literally *managed by the people*), or 私营化 (*sīyíng huà*, literally *privatization of operations*) which all go beyond the *transfer of ownership* (from state to private). These terms emphasize the shift in control and/or management (once exclusively in the state's hands) to the market, which is one of the authentic features of *socialism with Chinese characteristics*.

Many authors[1–3] in the literature still make *privatization* (in general) a focus of their discussion due to several theoretical issues. Among them are those which see government's goals as inconsistent with efficiency, inconsistent with maximizing social welfare, or even malevolent.[4,5] This can also be observed specifically in the Chinese healthcare sector.

A better understanding of the causes and history of the Chinese healthcare sector reform and development — with particular reference to the medical market and its socio-economic environment — would shed light on the accomplishments of the healthcare reforms and, consequently, also on new regulations addressing investment in the private hospital market.

Generally, the Chinese healthcare sector's development path can be divided into three periods as elucidated in the following subsections.

2.1. *The first period (1949–1979)*

Before the foundation of the People's Republic of China (in 1949), the Chinese healthcare sector was mainly private. This was true in urban areas, but in rural areas, there were no formal healthcare facilities, private or otherwise.[c] If there were providers, they were either individual doctors or practitioners who were principally engaged in Traditional Chinese Medicine (TCM). As soon as the socialist system was established, the Chinese Communist Party began the *economic socialization* path (in the 1950s), transferring private ownership to public ownership. What happened in the Chinese healthcare sector corresponded substantially with what happened in all other Chinese economic sectors. Anything "private"

[c] A popular saying sounds like *just put up with it when you are not well, stay in bed if you get worse, and die if you are seriously sick.*

was confiscated and/or bought out by the state. The system, until then based on private ownership, was destroyed and replaced by a state ownership structure. The market share of private industry up until 1949 was 63%. By 1956, it had decreased to 0.04%.[6] The healthcare environment changed radically, and during the Mao era, the healthcare system became crude and completely supported by the state. This meant that, in urban areas, hospitals and other facilities[d] were 100% public (100% composed of state-owned enterprises) and/or mainly public (state-owned enterprises mainly controlled by the government).[7] The entire framework was completely under state control: insurers were managed and directly financed by the state and, furthermore, providers were paid on a fee-for-service (FFS) scheme for most services provided to patients.

The government was simultaneously the owner, financier, and operator of all medical structures (from the largest ones in the urban areas, to the smallest in the countryside). No private activities were allowed in this sector, and all medical professionals were considered state employees. Doctors, physicians, and nurses previously engaged in any individual private practices were gradually recruited into public healthcare facilities and paid a fixed salary.

Regarding health insurance schemes in urban areas, the state developed two different work unit-based schemes which covered the majority of the residents. On the other hand, in the countryside, village doctors (already in the medical field before 1949) continued to provide healthcare services. This practice, initially used as a stop-gap, then took the shape of a formal healthcare scheme based on the practical contributions of those so called *barefoot doctors*[e] (赤脚医生, *chìjiǎo yīshēng*). Since during the period, the

---

[d] Mainly there were hospitals, outpatient clinics, maternal and child care stations, epidemic prevention centers, and long-term care facilities under State control and management at central or local level.

[e] The epithet *barefoot doctor* originated during the 1960s in Chiangchen People's Commune in Shanghai's suburbs. In this Commune, with a population of 28,000 people, there was just one clinic. Given the need to provide healthcare services to the rural population, under Chairman Mao Tse Tung, a mobile service doctor team came from the cities and toured the villages, informing rural residents. They were people who were used to working barefoot in the paddy fields, and this is where the name originated. In fact, China's village doctors had been there long before. In 1951, the central government declared basic

majority of the Chinese population resided in rural areas (about the 80% of the population resided in the country[8]) and epidemics, infectious diseases, and poor sanitation were widespread, the government initiated a healthcare policy based on prevention. Peasants and workers started a training course, for a period not longer than two or three months, introducing themselves to a "smarter" medical education for solving more frequent health problems and diseases that might normally be dealt with by physicians or skilled doctors. The expression "barefoot doctors" came into use.

Barefoot doctors became the principal suppliers of primary healthcare in rural areas, at a low cost. The state did not focus on individual patients, but rather the whole community lagging behind in the economy[9] and aiming at prevention rather than cure.

Regarding the health insurance scheme, before the mid-1950s, in rural areas there were no assistance programs or structured services; as briefly mentioned above, rural residents had to pay for all services they might need on an FFS basis.

After economic socialization, the cornerstone of the healthcare system was the *communes* (人民公社, *rénmín gōngshè*, set up under Mao Zedong, which made up the crucial organizational structure[f] of the rural areas). Each *commune* managed the areas within its own jurisdiction, also providing healthcare services through the so-called Cooperative Medical System (CMS), which substituted the previous FFS scheme.

All services offered were paid through health insurance payments, largely for medicines, but funding was primarily channeled to public facilities.

2.2. *The second period (1980–2003)*

During the Deng Xiaoping Era (from 1979 onward), China launched its economic reform aimed at boosting its economic growth, leading to

---

healthcare should be provided by healthcare workers and epidemic prevention staff in villages. In 1957, there were already several village doctors across the nation, enabling farmers to receive basic healthcare at home and work every day. Barefoot doctors were paid on a work-point basis, permitting them to slightly increase their personal income.

[f] *Communes* were the major geographic and administrative units within a county. Their members were principally peasants, and some of them were allowed to work in state-owned enterprises or non-profit organizations. Each *commune* was divided into brigades and teams.

radical changes in the organization and the management of the Chinese healthcare framework. All medical institutions of all types and levels were made responsible for their own well-being as the consequence of a renewed profit-seeking healthcare system. They were often too expensive for patients (especially those in rural areas, where insurance programs were weak). A commonly-heard phrase, 看病难，看病贵 (*kànbìngnán, kànbìngguì*, "seeing a doctor is hard and expensive") clearly summarizes the healthcare situation during that period. But what really mattered in this period was how the government financial activity changed, because it represented the trigger for this Reform Period. Between the late 1970s and early 1980s, in parallel with the "opening up" policy, the Chinese government transformed itself from a centralized structure to a decentralized market-guided model with multiple components.[10] Before these years, as discussed, social welfare benefits and social services were paid, in urban areas by the government, and in rural areas by collectives or communes, which in turn were backed by the government. With the new decentralized management, the government dramatically changed how healthcare was financed. China started to transfer much of the responsibility for funding healthcare services to its local branches, requiring them to provide financial support through local taxation. At the same time, central government investments in healthcare sectors were reduced.[11] This meant local authorities should pay taxes to the government and simultaneously keep and make use of all the after-tax profits.

There was a consequential reduction of government subsidies to urban healthcare structures and organizations. Hospitals therefore relied on themselves to cover all expenses (including taxes, medical equipment, and salaries for all professionals involved in the structure) and were allowed to earn money from sales of services and drugs.

It is clear in these conditions that hospitals were particularly pressed to devote more attention to cost control and income maximization than the quality of provided services, often to the detriment of patients' interests and needs. Patients were seen more as a source of financial profit than as people in need.[12]

Aggravating the situation (due to changing the way professionals were remunerated), the profit-seeking goal lead to a situation where public doctors in government structures received (and, in some cases, continued to receive) bonuses over and above their base salaries based on the quantity of drug prescriptions they wrote. The more drugs doctors prescribed, the more they could earn (see Ref. 13).[g]

An interesting study[14] conducted in 2004 demonstrates that the public is commonly aware of this phenomenon. Complaints (about public doctors in public medical structures) frequently concern over-prescription cases. Those surveyed in the study (mainly coming from Guangdong, Shanxi, and Sichuan provinces) noted: "The [public] doctor prescribes more drugs for you because their bonus is related to the volume of the drugs they prescribe."

Another study by Zhang *et al.*[15] in 2003 had already reported the same situation, and additionally found during surveys that less than 1% of medicine prescriptions were actually reasonable.

Even if modern China is trying to push reforms to reduce corruption and drug sales,[16] the situation remains partially the same: on one hand, many drugs companies continue to bribe doctors to choose their pharmaceutical products; and on the other hand, hospitals encourage their doctors to prescribe the drugs which bring in the most revenue,[17] promising shady payments of 25–30% of the retail price paid by the patient.

The result has been pervasive profit-seeking: over-prescription of medications, excessive and often unnecessary drugs, testing, diagnostics, and other shocking efforts to cut corners.

A side effect of giving more freedom to local authorities in managing the healthcare sector under their respective jurisdictions was favoring wealthy coastal and urban areas over less wealthy rural ones, laying the basis for growing disparities between them.

During the Reform Period, the insurance schemes and the quality of healthcare services changed radically as well: in urban areas, hospitals remained under state ownership and government control.[18] The healthcare insurance system began to collapse when state-owned enterprises (SOEs) in the healthcare sector (managing public hospitals) closed and others lost the capacity to pay insurance premiums due to the reduced public provision and the weakening of social insurance.

Private medical facilities and small clinics were established in this period but services provided, although more accessible, were often inadequate and/or inefficient because of the lack of professionals (they were

[g]As one Chinese colorfully puts, "建设靠国家，吃饭靠自己" (literally: "The hospital relied on the government to get built, but had to rely on themselves to eat").

often staffed only by practitioners or those in the early stages of training). In most cases, these services did not include medicines covered by insurance schemes.

Many doctors and physicians moved away from the country to cities, and in the space of a decade, rural areas lost most of their qualified healthcare professionals.

The privatization process and economic reform of insurance schemes in rural areas meant the implementation of the Family Responsibility System, which quickly lead to the disappearance of communes and consequently to the collapse of the CMS.[h]

Rural administrative divisions (which replace communes in townships and villages) lost their right to appropriate a portion of land output for financing CMSs. Moreover, no organizations were willing to preserve CMSs because it would mean "welcoming an innovation" introduced during the Cultural Revolution years (the 1960s) at a time when CPC was disavowing everything that came from those years. Saving CMSs would have meant going against the Party.

With the collapse of the CMS, those who could not afford to pay for healthcare themselves were denied access to care.

The first healthcare sector reform was launched between the mid-1980s and 1990s. Facing all the social economic problems that emerged from the changed circumstances, the government started to work on a universal healthcare reform, starting with the creation of an Urban Employees Basic Medical Insurance (UE-BMI) scheme which would cover all employees in urban areas while trying to revive CMSs in rural areas.

Implementation of the reform began in 1994 when the State Council carried out a pilot reform for five selected urban areas (Zhejiang, Jiangsu, and Jiangxi Provinces and Jinjiang Prefecture) then a few years later set up the Basic Medical Insurance (BMI) for urban sector workers.

The BMI initially seemed like a good initiative because of its aim to cover employees in the private sector and small public firms. Despite

---

[h] For a better and deeper understanding to urban and rural insurance schemes promoted during these years, the reader is referred to: Barber, S. L. & Yao, L. (2011). "Development and status of health insurance system in China," *The International Journal of Health Planning and Management*, 26; and Liu, Y. (2004). "Development of the rural health insurance system in China," *Health Policy and Planning*, 19: 340–341.

these significant efforts, a lack of financial and political commitments meant the reforms were not fully implemented.

2.3. *The third period (2003–current)*

Despite the commencement of the profit-seeking method, what emerged during the Reform Period with reference to the hospital sector was the steady and the impressive presence of the state behind the market, to the detriment of citizens' healthcare. From a model completely supported by the government, China's healthcare sector effectively transformed to a profit-seeking model, launching a general call to generate profit within the newly created economic sector. The management structure and economic aims had changed, but not the complex structure of the healthcare sector, mainly under public ownership. China's private economic sector was constitutionally introduced in 1999, but China never took the "great step forward" in privatizing the healthcare sector. Since 2003, stimulated by the SARS epidemic, China has tried to launch a new healthcare reform. The New Rural Cooperative Medical System (NRCMS) for rural people was established in 2003 with the main aims of improving access to and utilization of medical services, reducing costs, and providing better risk protection. Nevertheless, the planned reforms were mostly launched as a pilot project which — like in previous years — represented the status quo and the preferred method employed by the country in running this sector. Despite the initiation of the profit-seeking method, this new initiative seemed primarily focused on increasing health insurance and coverage rather than on reforming hospitals and medical system structures to provide better services. In 2009, the Chinese government announced the largest-ever healthcare reform. One pillar of the reform was reserved for the hospital sector.

3. THE NEXT OPENING-UP PHASE AND REFORMS: NEW OPPORTUNITIES FOR HEALTHCARE OR FOR THE CHINESE ECONOMY?

The above analysis shows the hospital economy segment has been experiencing fundamental changes in recent years, thanks to the intensive demand stimulus and steady economy development, which are both expected to continue their growth momentum due to the larger healthcare reform embraced by the Chinese central government in the last 10 years.

What the analysis of this sector has shown is undoubtedly its great complexity, caused by the solid link with other economic sectors such as the pharmaceutical market, as well as social problems such as the management (and economic) mechanisms behind social insurance schemes.

Nevertheless, the hospital sector now represents one of the strategic segments in the country's path to modernization, and it is to be considered as part of the wider political plan aimed at pursuing the China's inclusive growth, passed by China's National People's Congress within the 12th Five-Year Plan (2011–2015).

The Chinese government foresees the total national healthcare expenditure will rise up to USD 1.3 trillion by the end of this decade.[i] These striking data are confirmed by the World Bank, in particular with reference to the percentage of GDP spent on healthcare — expected to take up 6.5% of GDP by 2020 (or even 10% of GDP, according to more optimistic sources.[19]

In the hospital industry, it can be seen that the number of Chinese hospitals structures grew at a Compound Annual Growth Rate (CAGR) of 6% in the 2011–2013 period. The revenue of the Chinese hospital industry jumped at a CAGR of 23.6% in the same period and it is expected to maintain a growth rate of over 20% and hit $651 billion in 2017.[20]

Analyzing the available data,[j] released by the Chinese Ministry of Health (MOH), the state presence in the hospital sector is massive.[k]

It is not by chance that all hospital sector reforms embraced by China since 2003 have been irregular and unsystematic.

Officially, China started to encourage private entrepreneurs and foreign companies to invest in a wide range of services, including healthcare, as one of the key factors for new the planned economic reform, with the

---

[i] See: http://www.forbes.com/sites/jackperkowski/2014/11/12/health-care-a-trillion-dollar-industry-in-the-making/.

[j] Data retrieved from the *China Statistical Yearbook 2012*.

[k] Public hospitals count 62% of the total hospitals with 13,450 structures. Among them, 44% are totally controlled by the State, and 18% are indirectly controlled. On the other side, private hospitals count 8,440 structures.

Third Plenum Meeting, held by the 18th Central Committee of the Communist Party of China (CPC) in 2013, in line with the 12th Five-Year Plan, issued in March 2011, which first demonstrated clear proof of the further importance the country decided to assign the hospital sector.

At this point, it is expected there will be a query: *what are the real priorities of the government?*

With specific reference to foreign investments — to be rigorous — remember that China had already begun a "tiny" opening-up policy, easing procedures and reducing legal barriers, before 2013.

In 2009, partially continuing the reform plan launched at the beginning of the Third Period, the China's State Council released the final version on the long-awaited national healthcare reform, 关于深化医 生体制改革的意 (*Guidelines on Intensifying the Reform of the Pharmaceutical and Health System*), completed the year after with the issue of 关于一步鼓励和引社会本医机的意 (*Circular on Further Encouraging and Guiding Non-governmental funding for Medical Institutions*).

After an overall view emerged, the Guidelines 2009 signaled the start of the healthcare reform, once again initially as a trial version in various provinces and cities, before gradually spreading it out nationwide.

Nationally declared priorities were speeding up the establishment of a basic medical insurance system, establishing a complete national basic medicine system to alleviate patients' cost burden, improving medical services in rural areas and urban subcommunities, guaranteeing equal basic public healthcare services, and starting public hospital reform trials to reduce reliance on drug sales as a major profit source.

Finally, after a period of 20 years, consisting of many failed or never fully implemented initiatives to better control the healthcare sector and its hospitals subsector, this ongoing reform seems to draw the outlines of a universal and omni-comprehensive reform, which gives special attention to the hospital sector as the most important and challenging area in the whole reform blueprint. The premises certainly seem virtuous.

Under the Guidelines 2009, medical institutions and hospitals must stock and use essential drugs and medicine (all included in the basic medical insurance coverage). This points to deeper changes: one of the State Council's main goals was to break the for-profit chains which have for years linked hospitals to doctors and doctors to pharmaceutical companies.

For this reason, the Guidelines prescribe that drugs shall be procured through public bidding and collective purchase, and their prices shall be set at the lower end of the range to reduce duplicated manufacturing. The Guidelines also provide a new role for the government in subsiding public hospitals for basic construction, purchasing facilities, and other policy-induced losses to change or eliminate public hospitals' profiting from drug sales. Meanwhile, China has started to encourage private investment in the hospitals sector to increase the diversification of hospitals. The ratio of public hospitals to total medical institutions will be reduced, leaving more room for both domestic and foreign private investors.

If this is so, what is evident for the first time is the nature of the reform which as well as its wider view, seems to once more make people and their wellness a central priority.

In 2011, another great sign which confirms the government effort to reform the hospital sector arrived with the amendment of the Catalogue for Foreign Investments.

With this update, the general category of "medical institutions" was removed from the restricted category and passed as a permitted activity.

Before this change, belonging to the restricted category meant foreigners could invest in the hospital sector only through a Joint Venture (JV), which required a mandatory presence of a Chinese partner as co-investor.

Despite this important sign of a new direction, no changes followed into the legal framework for foreign investment projects in the hospital sector, until the issuance of the *General Plan for China (Shanghai) Pilot Free Trade Zone* (General Plan), promulgated by the State Council in September 2013, and the *Tentative Measures for the Administration of Wholly Foreign-owned Medical Institutions in the Shanghai Free Trade Zone* (Tentative Measures), jointly notified by the Shanghai Commission of Health and Family Planning (CHFP), the Shanghai Commission of Commerce (COFCOM), and the Shanghai Administration for Industry and Commerce (AIC) on November 13, 2013.

Following the set of rules released in 2013, the hospital market appeared only partially open to foreigners. As the name of the regulations suggested, the opening-up only applied within the boundaries of the *Pilot Free Trade Zone* in *Shanghai*, so it was not a nationwide reform.

As you may have anticipated, the reform is still ongoing and further confirmation of a wider opening came in recent years.

On August 27, 2014, the National Health and Family Planning Commission and the Ministry of Commerce jointly issued the "关于开展设立外资独资医院试点工作的通知" (*Circular on the Launching of a Pilot Project for the Establishment of Wholly Foreign-owned Hospitals*).

In this way, in the space of two years, the central government made a *great leap forward* in the hospital sector, in at least three new directions:

- First, allowing the possibility for foreign investors to invest by themselves without any mandatory presence of Chinese partners (this followed the of set rules issued in 2013 in line with previous changes involving the Catalogue for Foreign Investments). With reference to the investment vehicle, in fact, the new set of rules requests the possibility to choose — as well as the still-allowed JV — the Wholly Foreign-Owned Enterprise structure, which means setting up a company for the construction and the management of hospitals and/or new medical structures, fully funded by foreign capital.
- Second, the sphere of action was enlarged geographically. While under the set of rules issued in 2013 investors could only set up JVs in Shanghai, with the Circular of 2014, the pilot project was launched in six more areas (municipalities and provinces): Beijing municipality, Tianjin municipality, Jiangsu province, Fujian province, Guangdong province, and Hainan province.
- Third, as well as the extension of the investment area, the aforesaid Circular of 2014 provided new investment methods, allowing M&A operations in addition to the Wholly Foreign-Owned Enterprises structures.

4. CONCLUSION

The Chinese hospital market is complex and its comprehension requires analysis and deep consideration of many socio-economic and collateral factors which affect the sector.

The continual development of the national economy sees China facing new important challenges: disparity between rural and urban populations, which are still enormous; and the geospatial differences reflected upon healthcare across the country. It is not a new circumstance that major cities tend to benefit from better healthcare conditions than rural areas (e.g., in the number of hospital beds and the number of available specialized doctors, specialty chain structures, advanced diagnosis machinery, etc.). Among the population, there is still a great disparity in terms of wealth: public assistance is poor and the system in some cases still leaves the population with difficulties in accessing medical care.

As discussed, China has just powered up its reform agenda for a better and more open healthcare environment, forced by all these increasing general dissatisfactions, which in turn have been propagated by all the consequences deriving from the transformation of Chinese society (urbanization, aging, emergence of new diseases, regional disparity, etc.).

On the other hand, it must not be forgotten that all planned reforms fall within the country's ongoing privatization and restructuring process, which has already been partially implemented since the beginning of Deng's era.

Furthermore, looking at the big picture, this complex situation is further exacerbated by the same historical choices made by China over the years: consider the one-child policy combined with the fast-changing economy, which have both contributed to a growing percentage of Chinese people aged over 60 years, making China an aging population and an incubator for new chronic diseases, with growing healthcare needs.

Despite China's efforts, what has emerged since the beginning of the 21st century regarding the hospital sector is a legal framework that is still immature and only partially implemented.

Moreover, the national decentralized structure will not, in the author's opinion, help the country move toward easier management of the sector, due to the great amount of autonomy renewed and gradually given to local authorities. Over the years, this has led them to claim more space and power, affirming themselves as independent powers often in contraposition to the central government. This structure will hardly guarantee to China rigid control over the country.

On the other hand, again linked to this latter outlook, it remains to be seen how the detailed implementation plans will follow the guidelines and how the interests of different groups will be balanced. There will also be differences in terms of the implementation in different provinces and cities at the stage of trial reforms.

In any case, the national healthcare reform is going to be an enormous and long-term project. And before that the CCP has a big challenge in deciding whether to put the people or economic growth first, while preserving the plebiscite consensus from the nation.

ACKNOWLEDGMENTS

The research leading to these results has received funding from the People Program (Marie Curie Actions) of the European Union's Seven Framework Program FP7/2007–2013/ under the REA Grant Agreement No. 612589. The publication does not necessarily reflect the opinion of the EU. The EU-founded project is China and Europe taking care of healthcare solutions — Chetch. See www.chetch.eu.

REFERENCES

1. Vickers, J. & Yarrow, G. (1991). "Economic perspectives on privatization," *Journal of Economic Perspectives*, 5(2): 111–132.
2. Kornai, J. (1988). "Individual freedom and reform of the socialist economy," *European Economic Review*, 32(2–3): 233–267.
3. Berglof, E. & Roland, G. (1998). "Soft budget constraints and banking in transition economies," *Journal of Comparative Economics*, 26(1): 18–40.
4. Laffont, J. J. & Tirol, J. (1993). *A Theory of Incentives in Procurement and Regulation* (MIT Press, Cambridge, MA, USA), p. 644.
5. Shleifer, A. (1993). "State versus private ownership," *Journal of Economic Perspectives*, 12(4): 133–150.
6. Bo, F. L. (1989). *The Economic History of People's Republic of China* (Heilongjiang Educational Press, Harbin, China), p. 66 [in Chinese].
7. Ramesh, M., Wu, X. & He, J. (2013). "Health governance and healthcare reforms in China," *Health Policy and Planning*, 29(6): 663–672.
8. Chi, W. (1974). "Barefoot doctors in China," *The Lancet*, p. 976.
9. Chen, Z. (1998). *Medicine in China's Rural Areas — My Recollections* (Sichuan People's Publishing House, Chengdu, China), p. 66.
10. Liu, G., Liu, X. & Meng, Q. (1994). "Privatization of the medical market in socialist China: A historical approach," *Health Policy*, 27(2): 157–174.

11. Hesketh, T. & Zhu, W. (1997). "Health in China: The healthcare market," *BMJ*, 314(7094): 1616–1618.
12. Zhong, H. (2009). "The patient-centred care and hospital marketing strategies," Manage Obs, 30, pp. 234–235 [in Chinese].
13. Cao, Y., Wei, Z. & Wang, J. (2010). "Discussion on the public hospitals' independent legal status," *Chinese Hospitals*, 14(12): 18–19 [in Chinese].
14. Meng, K. L., Yang, H., Zhang, T., Feng W. & Zhou Z. (2004). "Public perceptions of private health care in socialist China," *Health Affairs*, 23(6): 222–234.
15. Zhang, X., Feng, Z. & Zhang, L. (2003). "Analysis on quality of prescription of township hospitals in poor areas," *Journal of Rural Health Service Management*, 23(12): 33–35 [in Chinese].
16. Hui, Z., "Pharma news: China restricts hospital drug sales," Available at: http://www.fcpablog.com/blog/2015/5/28/pharma-news-china-restricts-hospital-drug-sales.html. Accessed 6 October 2017.
17. He, J. (2014). "The doctor patient relationship, defensive medicine and overprescription in Chinese public hospitals: Evidence from a cross-sectional survey in Shenzhen city," *Social Science & Medicine*, 123: 66.
18. Daemmrich, A. (2013). "The Political Economy of Healthcare Reform in China: Negotiating Public and Private," *Springer Plus*, 2: 448.
19. Li, Y. (2015). "Closer Look: How a glass door stops growth of private hospitals", *Caixin*.
20. "China Hospital Development and Investment Report, 2014–2017," *Research in China*, 2014, p. 4.

Chapter 10

Investments, Research, Education, and TCM

Paolo Sospiro

Science should not use the terms 'mainstream' and 'alternative'. Science is science.

Dr. Micozzi, the founding editor of the *Journal of CAM*[1]

1. INTRODUCTION

This chapter introduces the main private and public investment in Traditional Chinese Medicine (TCM) in accordance with the strategy outlined in the last few Five-Years Plans (FYPs) by the Chinese government. In fact, since the 12th FYP, the Chinese government emphasized its engagement on increasing the scientific reliability of TCM and investing on it. Therefore this chapter will first introduce the main theoretical approaches which may define how to develop a new economical sector, the endogenous growth model, analyze the main aspects which affect Traditional Medicine (TM) and mainly TCM. Next, the chapter analyzes the steps made in the last two decades to increase the reliability of TCM through the recognition of the TCM, the recognition of the competences and skills of the TCM doctors and practitioners, the research on TCM, and finally the promotion of TCM in a different perspective and in accordance with its scientific evidence-based effects.

Regarding the literature review methodology, the author applied the methodology of Smith.[2] Moreover, a study visit was undertaken for three months to Beijing Normal University (BNU) in China, involving several meeting with experts, scholars, and as well as practitioners.[a]

2. THE THEORETICAL FRAMEWORK

2.1. *A brief introduction to the endogenous growth model*

The relationship between Gross Domestic Product (GDP), Saving, Investment, R&D, and Capital date back to the Harrod–Domar (H–M) model, which stressed the importance to transfer the national savings to Investment and to physical capital in order to stimulate growth.[3]

$$\frac{s}{\theta} = g + \sigma \tag{1}$$

where s is the saving rate, θ is the capital rate, g is the growth rate, and finally s is the physical capital depreciation rate, and where g is the variation of the output of a plant, factory, company or country (GDP).

$$g = \frac{Y(t+1) - Y(t)}{Y(t)} \tag{2}$$

However the H–M was a classical Mechanical model based on a classical cause–effect relationship within the considered variables, and it cannot explain how to boost the economy, a sector, or a specific product.

The second model, which aimed to improve the knowledge of economic growth, was the Solow model which emphasized the role of the

[a]The author was the EU Marie Sklodowska-Curie Visiting Scholar at BNU.

productivity from the microeconomic and, in particular, from the Cobb–Douglas function point of view. Solow stressed that, in certain conditions, which means in a developed country, the economy is already in its steady-state condition (y^*, k^*) and may grow if and only if there is an increase in productivity. Productivity is denoted by efficiency ($E(t)$), which is the workers' productivity.

$$\frac{k^*}{y^*} = \frac{s}{n+\delta} \tag{3}$$

$$L(t) = E(t)P(t) \tag{4}$$

where the increase in efficiency is denoted by workers' productivity, π.

$$E(t+1) = (1+\pi)E(t) \tag{5}$$

Therefore, the endogenous growth model introduces the role of R&D on growth, following the intuition of Solow. Indeed saving becomes physical capital and human capital instead only physical capital:

$$K(t+1) - K(t) = sy(t) \tag{6}$$

and

$$h(t+1) - h(t) = qy(t) \tag{7}$$

which become

$$\frac{k(t+1) - k(t)}{k(t)} = sr^{1-\alpha} \tag{8}$$

and

$$\frac{h(t+1) - h(t)}{h(t)} = qr^{-\alpha} \tag{9}$$

Then in each company, sector, or economy we have two different production functions in which the original Cobb–Douglas production function becomes, where *P* (Population) becomes *H* (Human Capital),

$$y = k^{\alpha} h^{1-\alpha} \tag{10}$$

and

$$Y = AK^{\alpha} P^{1-\alpha} \tag{11}$$

And then

$$Y(t) = E(t)^{\gamma} K(t)^{\alpha} [uH]^{1-\alpha} \tag{12}$$

where $E(t)$ is the progress-efficiency and u is the fraction of the human capital dedicated at the production of the final goods while the role of the progress-efficiency is given by

$$\frac{E(t+1) - E(t)}{E(t)} = a(1-u)H \tag{13}$$

Where the increase in efficiency, the left side of equation, is denoted by the small portion of the human capital involved on R&D, $(1-u)H$, which means education and R&D. Taking into account that investment in education and R&D only increase the probability of innovation but cannot assure it. Of course as higher is the investment as higher will be the probability of success but there is not a guarantee of success. Therefore a, represent the probability of success. In conclusion, in our case, saving and investment in human and physical capital will increase the probability of improving TCM in terms of its reliability and practices.

2.2. *Evidence-based approach — Validity and reliability: Investment, research, and higher education and dissemination*

One of the main issues of the TM and thus of TCM is their validity and reliability which leads directly to the importance of investment, research, higher education (HE), cooperation between research centers and HE with the profit sector intellectual property ((IP) protection), and Dissemination and Implementation (D&I).[4] Choi[5] argues that TM faces some challenges, such as the varying degrees with which it is recognized by the governments, lack of evidence-based of efficacy of many of therapies, and difficulties relating to the protection of indigenous knowledge and problems in ensuring its proper use. Therefore more stringent and elaborate policies, regulations, standards, clinical practice, research, education, and information are needed.

Evidence-based approach is a practice that has been rigorously studied using experimental evaluation (i.e., Randomized Controlled Trials, RCT) and shown to have different positive statistical significances in important outcomes.[b] **Validity**[c] in epidemiology is used to assess the degree to which the information collected accurately answers the research question (i.e., the extent to which the results are accurate and the extent to which the conclusions derived can be generalized). **Reliability** is the degree to which a measurement procedure can be reproduced. Lack of reliability may arise from differences between observation, instruments of measurements, or instability of the attribute being measured.[d] In accordance with Tsang,[6] it is to be taken into account that TM and TCM are comprehensive conceptual systems that are very different from the Western mechanistic approach to diseases.[e]

---

[b]A program that has stood the test of rigorous experimental evaluations has to show that it is supported by data, not just based on theory; is repeatedly tested and is more effective than standard care or an alternative practice; and finally can be reproduced in other settings. See: http://www.ori.org/resources/what_does_it_mean_to_be_evidencebased.

[c]The term validity in epidemiological research is used in three different ways: Internal Validity (Study Validity), External Validity (Generalizability), and Measurement validity (Variable). Internal Validity is the degree to which the observed findings lead to correct inferences about phenomena taking place in the study sample. External Validity is the degree to which the inferences drawn from a study can be generalized to a broader population beyond the study population. Measurement Validity is the degree to which a test actually measures what it is designed to measure. See: http://www.jpma.org.pk/full_article_text.php?article_id=4775.

[d]Three main sources can result in errors of measurement: Observer Variability in measurement. Instrument Variability due to fluctuating environmental factors. There are several ways to enhance reliability (i.e., standardizing the measurement methods). In order to ensure a sound investigation, it is essential to consider the validity and reliability of the data and study design. Validity is essential for inference because indicate the conclusions are based on accurate information. Reliability because assures the same results would be obtained if the same methods are used again. See: http://www.jpma.org.pk/full_article_text.php?article_id=4775.

[e]TCM works around five solid organs (heart, liver, spleen, lung, and kidney) and six hollow viscera (large and small intestine, urinary bladder, stomach, gall bladder, and "triple burners"). They are connected by conduits and vessels with qi (energy) and blood. TCM is a holistic approach which analyzes whether all the structures are functioning harmoniously. The practitioner analyses the patient based on "syndrome identification" and comes up with a "pathophysiologic status" (the type of disharmony) — zheng or "syndrome." Viewpoint. See: www.nature.com/clinicalpractice/rheum.

2.3. *Education and research*

In accordance with the previous two subsections, there is a need for a systemic approach to boost a firm, an economic sector, or an economy and of an evidence-based approach to improve research, education, goods and services, and finally, especially, consumers' confidence. Therefore, in this perspective, HE becomes crucial to reach such a goal. Indeed, HE is crucial because it educates a large proportion of the population and generates knowledge. However, recently, many universities have a "third role": facilitating technology transfer.[7] Regarding the role of educating and generating knowledge, many scholars analyzed and developed a clear theoretical framework while the relationship between HE and firms remains still under scrutiny. Recently some scholars made an in-depth literature review about the academic engagement and commercialization. In fact, the authors argue there are different ways to transfer knowledge by HE, such as commercialization (patenting & licensing) and academic engagement. They define academic engagement as knowledge-related collaboration by HE researchers with non-HE organizations such as collaborative research, contract research, consulting or providing *ad hoc* advice, and networking with practitioners (i.e., informal technology transfer).[f] The main findings are that almost half of the investigators in the physical and engineering sciences are engaged in collaborative research, contract research, or consulting at least once over a two-year period. Moreover, in Germany, 20% of the academic researchers published jointly with industrial partners. Furthermore, among the engineering and medicine faculty surveyed in Sweden and Ireland, 51–68% of respondents were involved in "soft" collaboration activities. In addition, male researchers are significantly more likely to engage with industry as senior academicians and in applied disciplines and life-science/biotech fields. Finally, country-specific regulations/policy support a positive approach by the academicians to "academic engagement."

In fact, the authors argue that engagement appears to be part of the activities responsible for the "Matthew effect" in HE: i.e., individual

---

[f]They yielded 413 results and they selected 36 articles, mainly from the US (18) and UK (5) and mainly published in *Research Policy* and *Journal of Technology Transfer* (63%), out of which 33 are quantitative articles.

Figure 1. Analytical Framework of External Engagement by Academic Researchers.

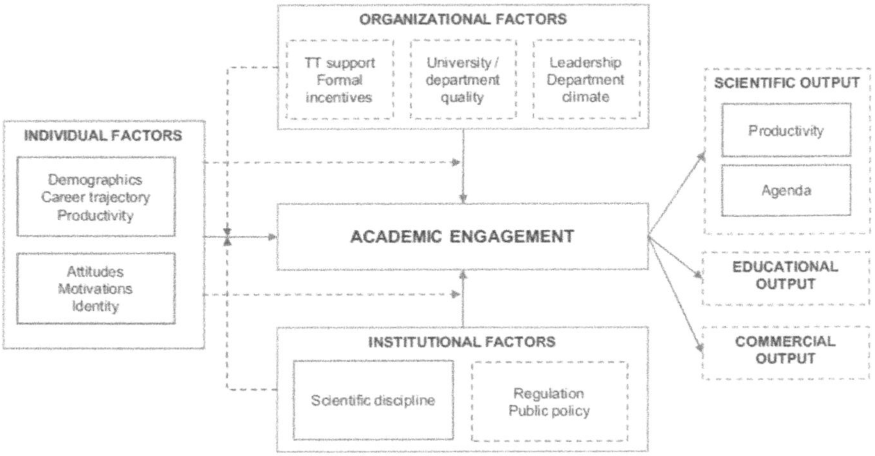

Source: From Ref. 8.

success is reinforced through a virtuous cycle of achievements and returns on those achievements. Therefore they designed an analytical framework to define HE engagement. In conclusion, it seems that, in the last decades, after the institution of the Bayh–Dole Act in 1980 in the US, and the ending of the professor's privilege in many EU and Europeans countries, HE engagement has increased in the main research areas worldwide.[g] As a consequence, there has been increased output of literature on the topic. All these aspects refer to individual, organizational, and institutional contexts which confirm the analysis made on a brief introduction to the endogenous growth model. Indeed, for instance, in order to boost TM and TCM, a systemic approach is needed which takes into account individual, organizational, and institutional approaches (see Fig. 1).

[g] Vessuri argues, there are 94.3 researchers/million in the least developed countries (LDCs), against 313 and 3.728 in the other developing countries (ODCs) and in the High-Income Countries (HICs), respectively. Enrollment in HE institutions (enrollment as a share of the corresponding age group) is 3.5% in LDCs, against 23% in ODCs and 69% in HICs. LDCs are devoting 0.3% of GDP to R&D, against 0.8% in ODCs and 2.4% in HICs. As a paradox, the brain drain hits the LDCs; therefore, LDCs have lost more than half of their HE-educated professionals.

3. R&D AND EDUCATION ON TCM

3.1. *A brief introduction*

First it is important to define TM and TCM: according to the WHO TM Strategy 2002–2005, TM[h] is "a comprehensive term used to refer both to TM systems such as TCM, Indian Ayurveda and Arabic Unani Medicine and to various forms of indigenous medicine."

The document states as well as that "in countries where the dominant healthcare system is based on allopathic medicine, or where TM has not been incorporated into the National Health Care (NHC) system, TM is often termed 'complementary,' 'alternative' or 'non-conventional' medicine."

The document refers to TM when referring to Africa, Latin America, Southeast Asia, and/or the Western Pacific, whereas "complementary and alternative medicine" refers to that practiced in Europe and/or

Table 1. Types of TM.

	CM	Ayurveda	Unani	NP	OP	HP	CP	Others
Herbal medicine	1	1	1	1	2	1		1
Acupuncture/ acupressure	1				2			2
Manual therapies	Tuina	1	1	3	1		1	Shiatsu
Spiritual therapies	1	1	1	1				Hypnosis, Healing, Meditation
Exercises	Qigong	Yoga	Relaxation					

Note: 1 — commonly uses this therapy/therapeutic technique; 2 — sometimes uses this therapy/therapeutic technique; 3 — uses therapeutic touch. *Abbreviations*: CM: Chinese Medicine, NP: Naturopathy, OP: Osteopathy, HP: Homeopathy, CP: Chiropractic.
Source: WHO TM Strategy 2002–2005.

[h]It is the first attempt to define and analyze TM by the WHO. TM therapy includes the "use of herbal medicines such as herbs, herbal materials, herbal preparations and finished herbal products, that contain as active ingredients parts of plants, or other plant material, or combinations thereof. Moreover, animal parts and/or minerals — and non medication therapies — if they are carried out primarily without the use of medication as in the case of acupuncture, manual therapies and spiritual therapies." On the other hand, TCM is a part of TM which adopts all types of therapy included as TM compared to other TM such as Ayurveda, Unani, Osteopathy, Homeopathy, Chiropractic, etc. (see Table 1).

Table 2. TCM Needs and Challenges.

National policy and regulatory framework which means	• Lack of official recognition of TM/CAM and TM/CAM providers • TM/CAM not integrated into national healthcare systems • Lack of regulatory and legal mechanism • Equitable distribution of benefits of indigenous TM knowledge and products • Inadequate allocation of resources for TM/CAM development and capacity building;
Safety, efficacy, and quality	• Lack of research methodology • Inadequate evidence-base for TM/CAM therapies and products • Lack of international/national standards for ensuring safety, efficacy & quality control of TM/CAM therapies & products • Lack of adequate regulation and registration of herbal medicines • Lack of registration of TM/CAM providers • Inadequate support for research;
Access	• Lack of data measuring access levels and affordability • Need to identify safe and effective therapies and products • Lack of official recognition of role of TM/CAM producers • Lack of cooperation between TM/CAM providers and allopathic practitioners • Unsustainable use of medicinal plant resources;
Rational use	• Lack of training for TM/CAM providers and on TM/CAM for allopathic practitioners • Lack of communication between TM/CAM & allopathic practitioners & between allopathic practitioners and consumers • Lack of information for public on rational use of TM/CAM.

Source: WHO TM Strategy 2002–2005.

North America and Australia. The reason why WHO started to include and analyze TM/CAM (Complementary/Alternative Medicine) is because over 80% of the population in Africa uses TM to help meet their healthcare needs. In Asia and Latin America, a substantial proportion of the populations continue to use TM as a result of historical circumstances and cultural beliefs. In China, TM accounts for around 40% of all healthcare delivered. On the other hand, in many developed countries, CAM is becoming increasingly popular. WHO reminds that CAM is used at least once by 48% in Australia, 70% in Canada, 42% in USA, 38% in Belgium, and 75% in France. The strategy presents TM needs and challenges (see Table 2).

On the other hand, despite allopathic medicine being based on western culture, practitioners emphasize that it is based on a scientific approach, thus it is unmarked by cultural values. On the contrary, TM/CAM therapies are influenced by the culture and historical conditions within which they first evolved. Their common basis is a holistic approach to life; equilibrium between the mind, body, and the environment; and mostly an emphasis on health rather than on disease. This more complex approach to HC makes TM/CAM very attractive but very difficult to evaluate since so many factors must be taken into account. Therefore, taking into account that TM/CAM practices have developed within different cultures in different regions, there has been no parallel development of standards and methods for undertaking evaluation. In particular, evaluation of herbal medicines is very difficult and expensive. In fact, it is RCTs are in order to analyze the benefits of each treatment.

Finally, the document highlights the importance of investment, research, and education which lead to national regulation and registration of herbal medicines; safety monitoring for herbal medicines and other TM/CAM; support for clinical research into use of TM/CAM for treating common health problems of countries; national standards, technical guidelines, and methodology for evaluating safety, efficacy, and quality of TM/CAM; and finally national pharmacopoeia and monographs of medical plants at the national level.

3.2. *TCM policies and implementation at global level*

In the last two decades, the Chinese government, in cooperation with the main TM countries such Brazil, India, Japan, and South Korea, has urged the international organizations to also take into account TM and CAM. Indeed, in the last decades, TM obtained official recognition from the WHO[i]; moreover, in 2006, Dr. Margaret Chan was appointed as the Director General of WHO and will lead WHO from 2006 to 2017. In 2008, China organized the first WHO Congress on TM in Beijing which led to the Beijing Declaration.[j] In 2009, Dr. Zhang Qi was appointed as

[i] See: http://who.int/medicines/areas/traditional/en/.

[j] See: http://who.int/medicines/areas/traditional/congress/en/.

Responsible for TM at the WHO.[k] Furthermore, three important awards honored TCM practitioners. In September 2011, the Lasker Clinical Medical Research Award honored Prof. TU You-you who discovered artemisinin and its utility for treating malaria.[l] On January 24, 2012, Dr. WANG Zhen-yi and Dr. CHEN Zhu were awarded the 7th Annual Szent–Györgyi Prize for progress in cancer research for their innovative research that led to the successful development of a new therapeutic approach to acute promyelocytic leukemia (APL).[m] Finally, in 2015, Prof. TU You-you won the Nobel prize for the same research.[n]

However, at the global level, work still needs to be done on access to existing knowledge of TM/CAM through exchange of accurate information and networking, shared results of research into the use of TM/CAM for treating common diseases and health conditions, and evidence-based research on safety, efficacy, and quality of TM/CAM products and therapies.

Therefore the main priority areas of research should be effects of each individual therapy (efficacy, safety, and cost-effectiveness); research into mechanisms of action of individual therapies, including patterns of response to treatment; research on TM/CAM genre itself, including social research on the motivation of patients seeking TM/CAM and usage patterns of TM/CAM; research on new research strategies which are sensitive to the TM/CAM paradigm; and research into the efficacy of diagnostic methods used and research into implementation and effects of TM/CAM in specific care settings. The third steps, which is very important, is education and training and as well as access to TM. Between the first and second TM strategies, two important documents updated the first TM strategy: WHO Medicines Strategies 2004–2007 and 2008–2013. The first one

[k] Dr. Zhang led the integration of TCM into the NHS of China and was the former vice-president of the China Academy of Chinese Medical Sciences. See: http://www.icihm.org/en/speakers/153-zhang-qi-md.html.

[l] She and her colleagues transformed an ancient Chinese healing method into the most powerful antimalarial medicine currently available, an artemisinin-based drug combination is now the standard regimen for malaria recommended by the WHO. See Ref. 1.

[m] By combining TCM with Western medicine (all-trans retinoic acid, ATRA), Drs. WANG and CHEN have provided dramatic improvement in the five year disease-free survival rate of APL patients (from 25% to 95%). See Ref. 1.

[n] See: https://www.nobelprize.org/nobel_prizes/medicine/laureates/2015/tu-facts.html.

Figure 2. Percentage of Population Using TM and Has at Least Once Used CAM.

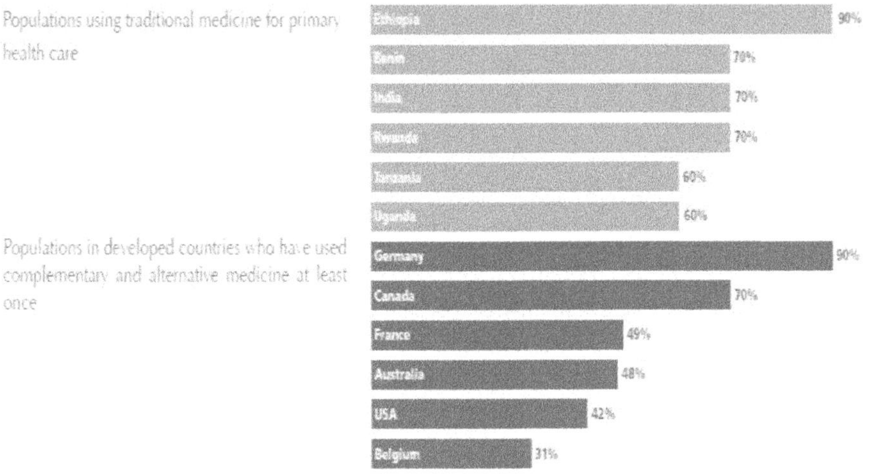

Source: WHO Medicine Strategy 2002–2005.

confirmed the importance of TM (Fig. 2) to ensure affordable access, protection of IPR, and guidance on safety, efficacy, and quality assurance.

The document confirmed the four main objectives: to integrate relevant TM and/or CAM into NHC system, as appropriate, by developing and implementing national policies and programs; promote the safety, efficacy, and quality of TM/CAM by expanding the knowledge base; and by providing guidance on regulatory and quality assurance standards and increasing the availability and affordability of TM/CAM, with emphasis on access for poor populations; and finally, to promote the therapeutically sound use of appropriate TM/CAM by both providers and consumers.

The second document confirmed the TM Strategy 2002–2005, taking into account the progress already made at the global and national levels. However, the WHO's strategic director aims to facilitate the integration of TM/CAM into the NHC systems, with a focus on better regulation of TMs and practitioners. The collection and use of better evidence on quality, safety, and efficacy will be promoted. The contribution of TM/CAM to Primary Health Care (PHC) will be explored and, where relevant and possible, promoted. Special emphasis will be placed on promoting and upgrading the knowledge and skill of the providers of TM/CAM to ensure patient safety and to build national capacity in the field of TM/CAM according to the identified needs of the country. Where needed, countries will be assisted. Once again the quality, safety, and efficacy of TM is highly correlated with the integration of the TM/CAM to the PHC system and related to the promotion of TM/CAM through the consumers. However, the document also highlights the importance of IPR protection for the first time.

In the year 2012, following the WHO Assembly resolution on TM (WHA62.13), WHO developed the new TM strategy 2014–2023 with the following goals: harnessing the potential contribution of TM to health, wellness, and people-centered healthcare and promoting the safe and effective use of TM by regulating, researching, and integrating TM products, practitioners, and practice into healthcare systems, where appropriate. Therefore the new strategy still insists on the importance of promoting the safe and effective use of TM (Fig. 3).

However, despite significant progress made in implementing the objectives of the previous strategy (see Fig. 4), the Member States continue to experience challenges related to some issues, such as development and enforcement of policy and regulations; integration, in particular, identifying and evaluating strategies and criteria for integrating TM into PHC; safety and quality, notably, assessment of products

Figure 3. Country with Education on TM/CAM.

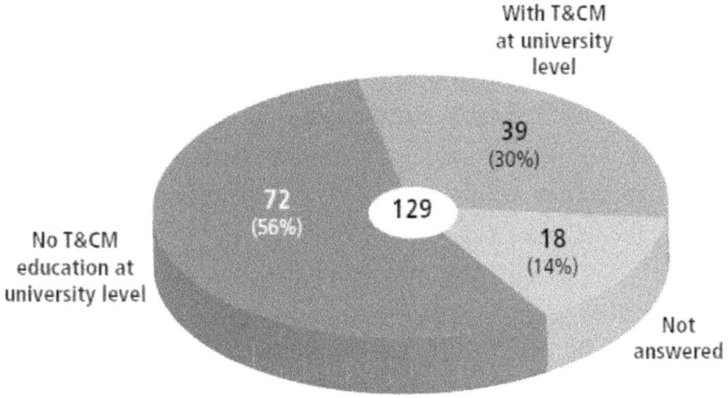

Source: WHO Medicine Strategy 2002–2005.

Figure 4. Number of Countries with National Research Institutes in TM/CAM in Different Years.

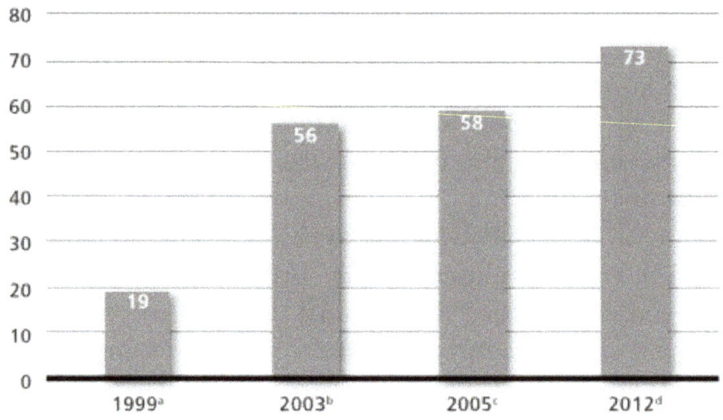

Source: WHO Medicine Strategy 2002–2005.

and services; qualification of practitioners; methodology and criteria for evaluating efficacy; ability to control and regulate TM/CAM advertising and claims; R&D, education, and training of TM/CAM practitioners; and finally, information and communication, such as sharing information about policies, regulations, service profiles, and research data, or obtaining reliable objective information resources for consumers. The strategy focuses on three main sectors: build the knowledge base that will allow TM/CAM to be managed actively through appropriate national policies that understand and recognize the role and potential of TM/CAM; strengthen the quality assurance, safety, proper use, and effectiveness of TM/CAM by regulating products, practices, and practitioners through TM/CAM education and training, skills development, services, and therapies; and finally, promote universal health coverage by integrating TM/CAM into the PHC.

New surveys state that the main benefits are the lower costs of TM/CAM and mortality rates. However, the surveys also remark on the risks associated with TM/CAM products, practitioners, and self-care, such as use of poor quality, adulterated, or counterfeit products; unqualified

Figure 5. Difficulties Faced by Countries Regarding Regulatory Issues Related to the Practices of TM/CAM.

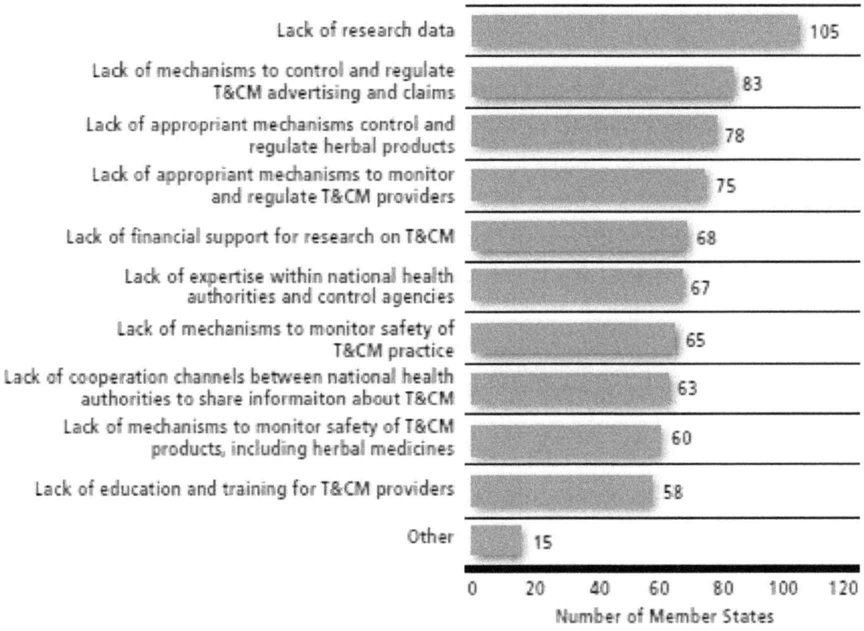

Source: WHO Medicine Strategy 2002–2005.

practitioners, misdiagnosis, delayed diagnosis, or failure to use effective conventional treatments; exposure to misleading or unreliable information; and finally, direct adverse events, side effects, or unwanted treatment interactions.

However, the integration of TM/CAM into the PHC system requires the documentation and study of the TM/CAM practice in order to categorize TM/CAM therapies or modalities that will underpin appropriate policies and regulations (see Fig. 5) such as in Sweden.[o]

[o]Where there is availability of specialist training for general practitioners, preferably computer-based documentation reflecting multi-modular management, combination of qualitative and quantitative research method, and interdisciplinary dialogue and collaboration.

A knowledge-based policy is the key to integrate Traditional and Chinese Medicine (TCM) into the national health systems. Research should be prioritized and supported in order to generate knowledge. While there is much to be learned from controlled clinical trials, other evaluation methods are also valuable. These include outcome and effectiveness studies, as well as comparative effectiveness research, patterns of use, and other qualitative methods.

There is an opportunity to take advantage of and sponsor such "real-world experiments," where different research designs and methods are important, valuable, and applicable. The importance of embracing various kinds of contributory research methods and designs in the effort to build a broad evidence base to inform national policy- and decision-making has been underlined by the National Institute for Health and Care Excellence (NICE), as well as other such institutes (Fig. 6).

Figure 6. Type of Support Required by the Countries on TM/CAM.

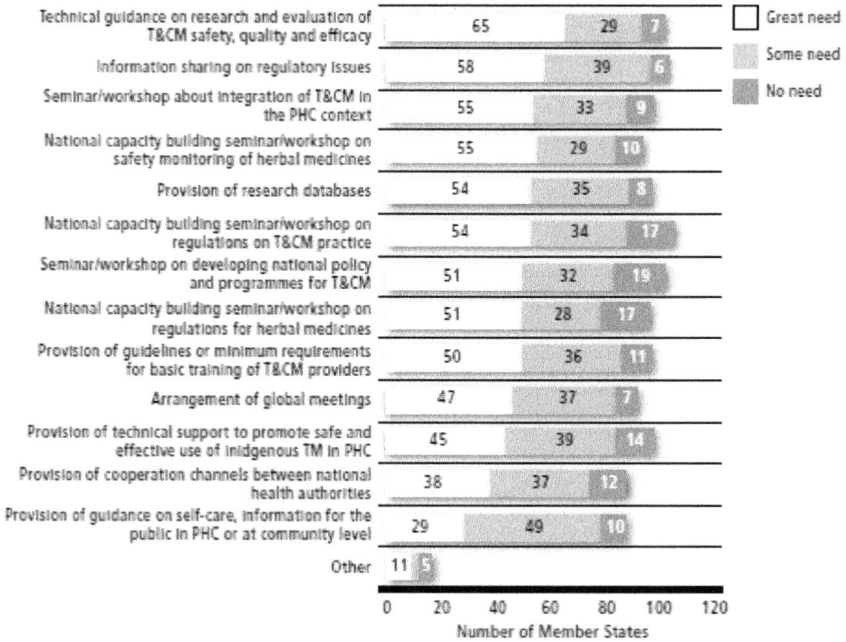

Source: WHO Medicine Strategy 2002–2005.

The surveys carried out during the last years emphasize that TM/CAM is used not only to treat diseases, especially chronic diseases, but also widely used in disease prevention, health promotion, and health maintenance and is proved to be cost-effective. Finally, the new strategy focuses on two main goals: Harnessing the potential contribution of TM/CAM to health, wellness, people-centered HC and Universal Health Care (UHC) and promoting safe and effective use of TM/CAM through the regulation, research, and integration of TM/CAM products, practices, and practitioners into the healthcare system, as appropriate. Therefore two steps are foreseen: Countries should define and better understand TM/CAM within their own national situation by identifying the forms of TM/CAM used, defining who uses them, exploring the reasons for their use, and determining both present and future needs. Moreover, countries should develop policies, regulation, and guidelines that address those forms of TM/CAM which meet the healthcare needs and choices of their people (see Table 3 and Figs. 7 and 8).

3.2.1. *Promoting the globalization of TCM*

TCM has spread to 183 countries. WHO argues that 103 Member States approved the practice of acupuncture and moxibustion, 29 enacted special statutes on TM, and 18 have included acupuncture and moxibustion treatment in their NHC. TCM medicines have been registered in Russia, Cuba, Vietnam, Singapore, and United Arab Emirates. Some 30 countries and regions have opened about 200 TCM schools to train native TCM workers. The World Federation of Acupuncture-Moxibustion Societies, headquartered in China, has 194 member organizations from 53 countries and regions, and the World Federation of Chinese Medicine Societies has 251 member organizations from 67 countries and regions. TCM becomes an important area of health and trade cooperation between China and the ASEAN, EU, Africa, and Central and Eastern Europe. China hosted the first WHO Congress on TM in Beijing in 2008. The 62nd and 67th WHO Assemblies passed two resolutions on TM, stressing its Member States to implement the WHO's TM Strategy 2014–2023. Currently, the Chinese government has signed 86 TCM cooperation agreements with other countries and international organizations and has supported the building of 10 TCM centers overseas.

Table 3. TCM Strategy at Global Level.

Strategic Objective	Strategic Direction	Expected Outcome	Critical Indicator
To build the knowledge base for active management of T&CM through appropriate national policies	Understand and recognize the role and potential of T&CM	• T&CM practices and practitioners identified and analyzed by Member State and country profile devised for T&CM. • T&CM policies and programs established by government.	• No. of countries reporting a national/provincial/state T&CM policy. • No. of countries reporting increased governmental/ public research funding for T&CM.
	Strengthen the knowledge base, build evidence, and sustain resources	• Strengthened knowledge generation, collaboration, and sustainable use of TM resources.	
To strengthen quality assurance, safety, and proper use and effectiveness of T&CM by regulating T&CM products, practices, and practitioners	Recognize the role and importance of product regulation	• Established and implemented national regulation for T&CM products, including registration. • Strengthened safety monitoring of T&CM products and other T&CM therapies. • Technical guidelines and methodology developed for evaluating safety, efficacy, and quality of T&CM.	• No. of countries reporting national regulation for T&CM products. • No. of countries reporting national/provincial/state regulation for T&CM practice. • No. of countries reporting national/provincial/state regulation/registration for T&CM practitioners.
	Recognize and develop practice and practitioner regulations for T&CM education and training, skills development, services, and therapies	• Standards for T&CM products, practices, and practitioners developed by government. • Established education/ training programs, benchmarks, and implementation capacities for T&CM practitioners. • Improved safe and effective use of T&CM.	

(*Continued*)

Table 3. (*Continued*)

Strategic Objective	Strategic Direction	Expected Outcome	Critical Indicator
To promote universal health coverage by integrating T&CM services into healthcare service delivery and self-healthcare	Capitalize on the potential contribution of T&CM to improve health services and health outcomes	• Integration of T&CM into the health system. • Improved T&CM services and accessibility. • Improved communication between conventional medicine practitioners, professional bodies and T&CM practitioners concerning the use of T&CM.	• No. of countries reporting national plan/program/ approaches for integrating T&CM service into NHC service delivery. • No. of countries reporting consumer education project/ program for self-healthcare using T&CM.
	Ensure consumers of T&CM can make informed choices about self-healthcare	• Better awareness of and access to information about the proper use of T&CM. • Improved communication between conventional medicine practitioners and their patients about T&CM use.	

Figure 7. Member States That Provide T&CM Education at University Level.

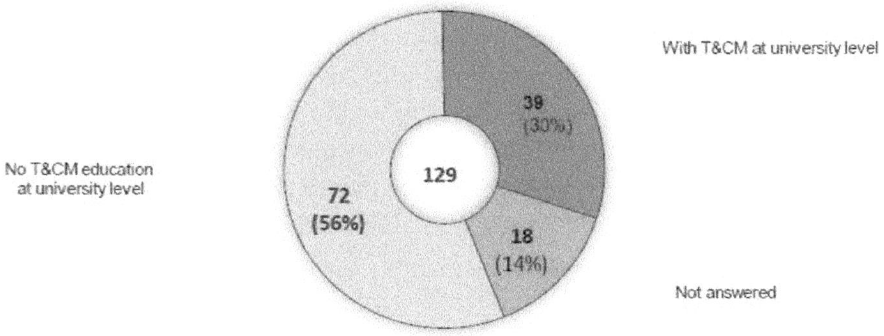

Source: Dr. Zhang Qi's Presentation: "WHO TM Strategy 2014–2023" at the *Global Health History Seminar on TM and Ayurveda*, WHO-HQ, March 19, 2015.

Figure 8. Implementation of WHO TM Strategy. Indicators for Monitoring.

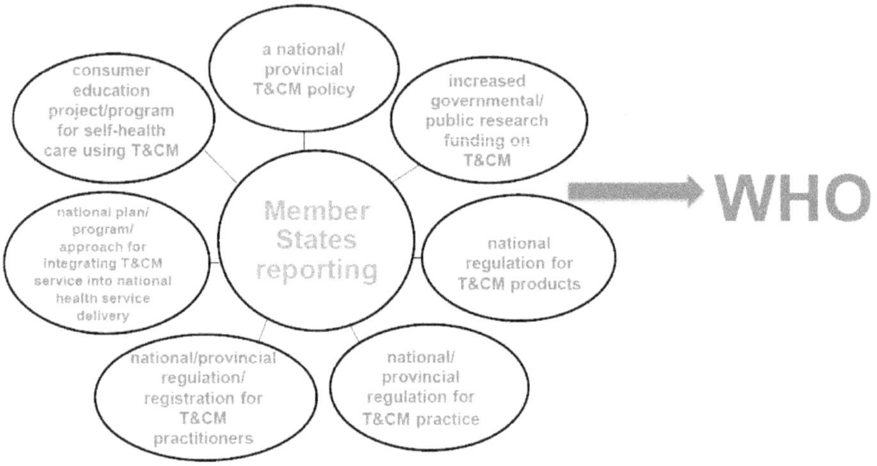

Source: Dr. Zhang Qi's Presentation: "WHO TM Strategy 2014–2023" at the *Global Health History Seminar on TM and Ayurveda*, WHO-HQ, March 19, 2015.

3.2.2. *Promoting standard management of TCM internationally*

China has facilitated the founding of the ISO/TC249 TCM in the ISO, with its secretariat in Shanghai. It has now issued a series of ISO standards on TCM. China has sent medical teams to over 70 countries in Asia, Africa, and Latin America, where about 10% are professional TCM staff. A project has been launched to build TCM centers in African countries while specialized TCM stations have opened in Kuwait, Algeria, Tunisia, Morocco, Malta, and Namibia. China sponsored 10 TCM centers overseas. In recent years, it is working on the prevention and control of AIDS and malaria in developing countries, sending a total of 400 TCM specialists to more than 40 countries.

3.3. *TCM policies and implementation in China*

At the national level, it is important to analyze the NHC System, the HE system, and the relationship between the HE system and the research on

TCM. The analysis takes into consideration the last four FYPs, the White Paper on TCM, and their implementation actions.

3.3.1. *Five-year plans analysis*

The FYP is the general or strategic plan of the Chinese government for the following five years. This section analyzes the TCM policies planned and implemented from 2000 to 2020 through the 10th FYP (2000–2005), the 11th FYP (2006–2010), the 12th FYP (2011–2015), and finally 13th FYP (2016–2020). The analysis shows that, in the first two FYPs, healthcare and TCM were not considered important areas of improvement or investment. In fact, medicine is mentioned in two areas of the program. The development of the high-tech industry includes modern medicine and development of the TCM herbal medicine. Moreover, medicine is considered in the section dedicated to the improvement of people's living and development of health and sports. In this case, in the 10th FYP, the government intends to reform the HC services and champion the vigorous development of the TCM, promoting integrative medicine. In the 11th FYP, the government plans to improve the modern TCM system and the ability to create new drugs, strengthening TCM resources survey and the development and sustainability of TCM in terms of evidence-based research, and vigorously develop the TCM industry. Moreover, protection of the TCM and construction of TCM hospitals promote its standardization and finally strengthen food and drug regulatory infrastructure. However it is with the 12th and 13th FYPs that the Chinese government, probably given the results achieved at the international level, takes an active approach on the TCM sector, for which a chapter on the plans is dedicated. Indeed, in the 12th FYP, the government emphasizes that China support the development of TCM, first, adhering to both TCM and Western medicine in the following ways: promote TCM inheritance and innovation, development of TCM education, and strengthening of TCM institutions, and TCM team-building talent; strengthen the protection of TCM resources, research, and rational use, to promote quality certification and standards; and improve HC policy and essential drugs policy to encourage the provision and use of TCM services. Finally, and most important, the government see the room to implement the export of TCM and opening at the same time the health sector to international trade and investment. The 13th FYP continues upon the previous plan, emphasizing cooperation and an open and inclusive approach toward TCM. In this case, the chapter entitled "Promote the Inheritance and Development of TCM" argues that modern TCM should become an integrated part of the NHC system, improving its basic services capabilities by: (1) strengthening clinical research base and institution-building; (2) developing medical and health services; (3) improving the TCM survey carried out to strengthen the protection of TCM resources, the establishment of TCM database, and knowledge base; (4) accelerate the standardization of TCM and the TCM medicine industry to enhance its reliability; (5) establish large, authentic, and endangered medicinal seedling breeding base and promote the development of TCM herbal medicine planting; and (6) support the development of TCM by the promotion of appropriate technology of TCM and increase its exposure in international trade. Therefore, the Chinese government, in the last 15 years, first, by timidly mentioning TC herbal medicine and then, improving its vision, started to see TCM as an important asset to improve the living conditions of the people and finally to consider TCM as an economical and industrial asset.

3.3.2. *White paper on TCM*

This approach and results leads to the release of the first White Paper on TCM in December 2016 by the Chinese government. The document tries to summarize the achievements and the next plan of action. The White Paper reminds that TCM is a combination of natural sciences and humanities and, since the founding of the country, it is mentioned into the Constitution. TCM is based on the four diagnostic methods: inspection, auscultation and olfaction, inquiry, and palpation. The government emphasizes the main interventions made on TCM since 1978 with "Report on Implementing the Party's Policies Regarding TCM and Cultivating TCM Practitioners," and in 1986, it set up a relatively independent administration of TCM. All provinces, autonomous regions, and municipalities directly under the central government have established their respective TCM administrations. In 2003 and 2009, the "Regulations of the PRC on TCM" and the "Opinions on Supporting and Promoting the

Development of TCM," were issued, gradually forming a relatively complete policy system on TCM. In 2015, the government approved the Law on TCM and, in 2016, it issued the Outline of the Healthy China 2030 Plan. It sets out a series of tasks and measures to implement the program and develop TCM. Finally, the government issued the Outline of the Strategic Plan on the Development of TCM (2016–2030), which made TCM development a national strategy, with systemic plans for TCM development in the new era. The White Paper defined the following principles and measures:

- **Putting people first,** and making achievements in TCM development accessible to everyone, supplying services, and improving community-level management, care of the elderly, and tourism.
- **Providing equal attention to TCM and Western medicine.** Equal status between TCM and Western medicine (with regard to ideological understanding, legal status, academic development and practical application).[p]
- **Upholding the dialectical unity of tradition and innovation** by establishing a series of systems.[q]
- **Making overall plans for integrated, coordinated, and sustainable development of TCM.** The state makes the overall plans for the coordinated development of TCM, integrating such areas as TCM clinical practices, healthcare, R&D, education, industry, and culture.[r]

---

[p] Improve the system of administration; increase financial input; formulate policies, laws, and regulations suited for TCM. Making TCM and Western medicine complementary creates opportunities for Western medical practitioners to learn from their TCM counterparts. Modern medicine courses are offered at TCM colleges and universities.

[q] To carry forward the theories and clinical experience of well-known veteran TCM experts and technological innovation to advance TCM progress, efforts have been made to carry out systemic research on the fundamental theories, clinical diagnosis and treatment, and therapeutic evaluation of TCM. Endeavor has been made in the R&D of new TCM medicines, and medical devices and equipment.

[r] Launching programs for training professionals necessary for TCM inheritance and innovation and improving the quality of the ranks of TCM workers. Set out to promote the green development of the entire TCM industrial chain. Further efforts have been made to upgrade the TCM industry and develop it into an emerging strategic industry.

- **Promoting TCM development.** The government has made TCM an important component of economic and social development and has included it in relevant plans and provided financial support. Moreover, it has strengthened the supervision and administration of TCM practices; initiated a market access system for TCM practitioners, TCM medical institutions, and TCM medicines; and improved the standards for the quality and safety of TCM service. Furthermore, it has developed market-driven preferential policies, encouraging social capital and private investors to support the development of TCM and to establish TCM healthcare institutions.[s]
- **Building a distinctive system of training for TCM professionals.** Thus, great efforts have been made to promote development of education in TCM with an organic link-up between college, graduate, and continuing education and run through master-apprenticeship training.[t]

In **R&D**, over 60 national TCM clinical research institutes have been built.[u] A number of laws and regulations have been enacted and

---

[s]At the end of 2015, there were 3,966 TCM hospitals in China, 446 hospitals of integrated TCM/Western medicine, 452,000 practitioners and assistant practitioners of TCM, 42,528 TCM clinics, and 7,706 for integrated medicine, which witnessed 910 million visits and treated 26.915 million patients. Moreover TCM and integrated TCM/Western medicine helped to treat SARS, influenza A HIV/AIDS and HFMD (Hand, Foot and Mouth Disease). The medical care services provided by TCM increased from 14.3% to 15.7% from 2009 to 2015. By 2020, every Chinese citizen will have access to basic TCM services, and by 2030, TCM services will cover all areas of medical care.

[t]This leads, by the end of 2015, 42 institutions of HE in TCM (including 25 TCM colleges), more than 200 Western medicine institutions of medical and non-medical HE offering programs in TCM, enrolling in total about 752,000 students. By 2015, 1,016 studios had been set up for carrying forward their expertise; 200 studios had been set up for passing on the expertise of prominent TCM experts at the grassroots level; 64 studios had been established for promoting various schools of TCM. In 2015, 124 researchers were finishing their postdoctoral studies in TCM inheritance at the CACMS. By 2015, 60 students had been awarded the title of TCM Master.

[u]A pilot program for TCM survey has been implemented, forming a dynamic information and technology system with one central platform, 28 provincial-level centers, and 65 monitoring stations. Sixty seed and seedling bases for TCM plants and two germplasm

implemented to strengthen the protection of TCM wild medicinal resources; a number of national and local nature reserves have been established; research has been conducted on the protection of rare and endangered TCM resources; and artificial production or wild tending have been carried out for certain scarce and endangered resources. A registration management system has been established for TCM pharmaceuticals.[v] In 2015, the total output value of the TCM pharmaceutical industry was RMB 786.6 billion, accounting for 28.55% of the total generated by the country's pharmaceutical industry. The export value of TCM amounted to $3.72 billion. The Outline of the Medium-Long-term Development Plan for the Standardization of TCM (2011–2020) has been issued and implemented, putting in place initially a system of TCM standards which amount to 649, with a growth of 29%. On the other hand, efforts have been reinforced to promote public awareness in TCM healthcare, including events under the campaign "TCM across China." Public talks have been organized through media and TCM education bases have been popularizing the basic knowledge and skills of TCM healthcare and prevention and treatment of illnesses.

3.3.3. *National healthcare system*

In China, there are about 440,700 healthcare institutions providing TM services, with 520,600 patient beds, including all level of TM hospitals and

---

banks have been established. The transformation and application of these research results has provided support for enhancing clinical effectiveness, ensuring the quality of TCM and fostering the development of the TCM pharmaceutical industry, resulting in the rapid development of the TCM pharmaceutical industry.

[v]Over 60,000 TCM medical drugs have been approved, and 2,088 pharmaceutical enterprises that have been approved by the Good Manufacturing Practice (GMP) of Medical Products are manufacturing TCM patents. The dosage forms of TCM medicines have increased from a traditionally limited number of forms such as pills, powders, ointments, and pellets into more than 40 (i.e., dropping pills, tablets, pods, and capsules), indicating a marked improvement in the technological level of TCM medicinal drug production. Finally, an initial establishment of a modern TCM industry based on the production of medicinal materials and industrial production and tied together by commerce has been proposed.

general hospitals, clinics, and health stations in urban and rural areas. About 90% of general hospitals include a TM department and provide TM services for both outpatients and inpatients. TM medical institutions are governed by the same national legislation on medical institutions as conventional medical institutions. TM practitioners are allowed to practice in both public and private clinics and hospitals. Government and private insurance fully cover TM, including Tibetan, Mongolian, Uygur, and Dai TM. Public or patients are free to choose TM or conventional medicine for healthcare services, or their doctors can provide advice on which therapies may be better suited to their health problems.[w]

In 2012, the Chinese government announced ambitious plans to develop the private healthcare sector, in order to relieve the strains on the public healthcare system resulting from the rapid aging of the population. It set in motion a series of reforms that aimed to raise the proportion of hospital beds funded by the private sector to around 20% by 2015. The primary way that the government sought to ease the public sector burden was by raising the attractiveness of private investment into healthcare. The plan foresees three categories: infrastructure development, cost-reduction, and expansion of insurance coverage. Also, an important step has been to remove regulatory barriers: in particular, to allow for up to 100% foreign ownership of hospitals under a Wholly Foreign-Owned Entity (WFOE) structure. Previously all investment had to be done via joint ventures with a minimum of 30% Chinese ownership. Artemed Group was the first to move, in July 2014, and the group signed an agreement to establish China's first WFOE hospital in the Shanghai Pilot Free-Trade Zone. Since 2014, domestic or foreign private investors can acquire and manage an existing public hospital.

This approach increased the interest in China's healthcare sector: mergers and acquisitions in China's healthcare sector totaled at least USD 11.3 billion in the first 11 months of 2014, continuing an upward trajectory from at least USD 10 billion in the same period in 2013.

Moreover, the government relaxed the regulation barring physicians from working at multiple sites, which made it difficult for small private

---

[w] Government of China, National Bureau of Statistics of China. *China Statistical Yearbook 2011: Chinese Medicine (1987–2010)*. The State Administration of Traditional Chinese Medicine, China (http://www.satcm.gov.cn/1987-2010/start.htm). WHO TM 2014–2023.

hospitals to offer an attractive enough salary package for skilled physicians to quit their jobs in the public healthcare sector. The barrier was particularly pronounced for elite physicians working in the largest and most famous public hospitals. Once the barrier has been lifted, private hospitals are in a better position to hire personnel staff. Finally, private hospitals are also eligible to provide reimbursable treatment for patients funded through social healthcare insurance.[x]

3.4. *TCM investment in education in China*

The earliest tertiary institution of TCM was the Nanjing University of TCM, which evolved from the Jiangsu Province Advanced School of Chinese Medicine, established in 1954. The first batch of TCM HE approved by the State Council in 1956 included four universities: Beijing University of CM, Chengdu University of TCM, Shanghai University of TCM, and Guangzhou University of CM. According to 2013 data from the SATCM, 45 TCM HE and another 215 HE provide TCM programs/majors in mainland China. TCM HE institutions in mainland China usually provide programs/majors in CM, Chinese material medica, acupuncture, moxibustion, and tuina. There are also other TCM-related or medicine-related multidisciplinary programs/majors available, such as Health Service Management, Medical English, and Nursing. For TCM education system, undergraduate programs generally take five years to complete. Master's and doctoral programs are both of three years' duration. The author takes the Beijing University of CM as an example: in 2007, it adopted a "TCM education reform experimental program." Students were admitted to this program by an independent student recruitment process that selected applicants from families of TCM practitioners instead of a college entrance examination. Once enrolled,

[x] In mid-2014, the University of Pittsburgh Medical Center (UPMC) announced a five-year consultancy deal with Xiangya Hospital in Hunan Province to establish a 200-bed international medical centre within its 3,500-bed general hospital. UPMC would provide training to medical and administrative staff in the center; make recommendations on technology, procurement, and staffing plans; as well as provide telemedicine links to its existing hospitals in Pittsburgh.[9]

students were assigned to different supervisors. This program is a combination of institutional education, master–apprentice education, and father–son education models.

In 2011, the Beijing University of CM started a nine-year TCM program called the "Qihuang Program." This is a combined undergraduate and doctoral program. During the first five years, students are trained according to an undergraduate teaching plan. In the fourth year, an entrance examination is held to enroll eligible students directly into the subsequent doctoral program. A new "cultivation model of TCM" was implemented in 2012. This includes the following programs: Doctor of TCM, Doctor of Integrative Medicine, "Doctor of TCM with Jinghua Master-apprentice Training," and "Acupuncturist and Tuina Practitioner." These programs all use an integral training model called "5+3", which comprises five years of undergraduate training with preclinical courses and three years of internship training. Graduates from these programs will obtain a Bachelor of Medicine and Master of Clinical Medicine degree. In 2015, the Beijing University of CM implemented new cultivation models of programs aimed toward non-Chinese Medicine majors. For instance, the new Chinese Materia Medica program, called the "Shizhen Guoyao Program," is an eight-year integral program comprising both domestic and international training and combining Bachelor's and Doctoral degrees. Another new Chinese Materia Medica program called the "Excellent Pharmacists of Chinese Medicine Program" is a six-year combined bachelor's and master's degree course and aims to produce highly qualified professionals who have specialized skills in Chinese Material Medica integrated pharmaceutical care. For postgraduate programs, students often attend professional courses in the first year and complete a research module. Clinical practice commences in the second and third years (Table 4).[10]

The China's University College Admissions System (CUCAS) in its website recommends Beijing, Shanghai, Guangzhou, Tianjing, and Nanjing for TCM studies in China.[y] More than 700,000 students presently study TCM in China, of which 5,510 were international students and 69% were at the bachelor level and 7% at the doctoral level. Most of the

---

[y] See: http://feature.cucas.edu.cn/Articles/Top-Places-to-Study-Medical-for-International-Students_1854.html.

Table 4. The Undergraduate Curricula for TCM Programs at the BU of TCM.

Program/Major	Curriculum Category	Examples of Courses
Chinese Medicine program	Fundamental courses of Chinese medicine	Basic Theories of CM, Chinese Materia Medica, Formulas of CM & Diagnostics of CM
	Fundamental courses of Western medicine	Anatomy of the Human Body, Physiology, and Pathology
	The classics of TCM	Selected Readings of Huangdi's *Canon of Medicine Treatise on Cold Damage* Diseases, Synopsis of Prescriptions of the Golden Chamber, and Warm Diseases
	Others	Doctrines of Different Schools in CM, Chinese Medical Classics & Acupuncture and Moxibustion
Acupuncture, moxibustion, and tuina program	Clinical practice Fundamental courses of basic theories of acupuncture & moxibustion	Meridians and Acupoints, Selective Readings of Acupuncture Classics & Acupuncture Theories of Different Schools
	Fundamental courses of acupuncture and moxibustion in clinical practice	Techniques of Acupuncture & Moxibustion, Therapeutics of Acupuncture & Moxibustion & Medical Qigong
	Fundamental courses of tuina	Massage & Tuina, Tuina techniques & Fundamentals of CM Bone-setting
	Experiment courses	Experimental Science of Acupuncture & Moxibustion, Rehabilitation of Acupuncture & Moxibustion
	Clinical practice	

Source: From Ref. 10.

international students came from other Asian countries (79%) while another 6% each came from North America and Europe (Table 5).[z] Hereafter the best university of TCM in China in the year 2014.

[z] See: http://wenr.wes.org/2016/12/traditional-chinese-medicine-surging-international-interest-shifting-educational-landscape-china.

Table 5. Best Top University of TCM in China (2014).

1	Beijing University of Chinese Medicine
2	Guangzhou University of Chinese Medicine (Guangzhou)
3	Heilongjiang University of Chinese Medicine (Harbin)
4	Shanghai University of Traditional Chinese Medicine
5	Nanjing University of Chinese Medicine (Nanjing)
6	Shandong University of Traditional Chinese Medicine (Jinan)
7	Hunan University of Chinese Medicine
8	Tianjin University of Traditional Chinese Medicine (Tianjin)
9	Chengdu University of Traditional Chinese Medicine (Chengdu)
10	Zhejiang Chinese Medical University (Hangzhou)
11	Liaoning University of Traditional Chinese Medicine (Shenyang)
12	Fujian University of Traditional Chinese Medicine (Fuzhou)
13	Yunnan University of Traditional Chinese Medicine (Kunming)
14	Anhui University of Traditional Chinese Medicine (Beijing)
15	Henan University of Traditional Chinese Medicine (Zhengzhou)
16	Capital Medical University (Beijing)
17	Gansu University of Traditional Chinese Medicine (Lanzhou)
18	GuiYang College of Traditional Chinese Medicine
19	Shaanxi College of Traditional Chinese Medicine
20	Changchun University of Chinese Medicine (Changchun)

Source: CUCAS (2014). Available at: http://www.cucas.edu.cn/studyinchina/top/2014_Top_Universities_Ranking_of_Traditional_Chinese_Medicine_Major_by_Competitiveness_3354.html.

4. CONCLUSION

In conclusion, the investment made by the Chinese government at national and global level in order to develop the TCM sector industry has been elucidated in this chapter. By analyzing the WHO policies and their implementation and the Chinese FYPs, and TCM White Papers and articles and books on TCM, it is possible to argue that China made a huge investment in terms of financial investment, reliability, and education on TCM.

Despite the international recognition of the importance of TM/CAM, the development of methodology for TM/CAM, the development of TCM educational system in China and abroad, and the promotion of TCM by the Chinese government abroad, there still remain four important aspects which need further investment and time in order to boost TM/CAM and TCM:

- Increasing and improving R&D on TCM to increase evidence-based results.
- Increasing the cooperation between HE and the pharmaceutical industry.
- Improving the IP protection on TCM.
- Finally, increasing the dissemination of the results within the consumers in China and abroad.

Further research is needed in order to analyze the academic engagement on TCM, the IP protection of TCM on a quantitative level, and finally the impact of dissemination activities.

REFERENCES

1. Xu, H. & Chen, K. (2012). "Complementary and alternative medicine: Is it possible to be mainstream?" *Chinese Journal of Integrated Traditional and Western Medicine*, 18(6): 403–404.
2. Smith, R. D. (2004). "FDI and trade in health services: A review of the literature," *Social Science and Medicine*, 59(11): 2313–2323.
3. Ray, D. (1998). *Development Economics* (New York University Press, NY).
4. Neta, G., Glasgow, R. E., Carpenter, C. R., Grimshaw, J. M., Rabin, B. A., Fernandez, M. E. & Brownson, R. C. (2015). "A framework for enhancing the value of research for dissemination and implementation," *American Journal of Public Health*, 105(1): 49–57.
5. Choi, S.-H. (2008). "WHO Traditional medicine strategy and activities 'standardization with evidence-based approaches,'" *Journal of Acupuncture and Meridian Studies*, 1(2): 153–154.
6. Tsang, I. K.-Y. (2006). "Establishing the efficacy of traditional Chinese medicine." Available at: www.nature.com/clinicalpractice/rheum. Accessed 31 May 2017.

7. Likins, P. "Corporate partnership: What's in it for the university?" Available at: http://www.columbia.edu/cu/21stC/issue-3.1/likins.html. Accessed 12 March 2013.
8. Perkmann, M., Tartari, V., McKelvey, M., Autio, E., Broström, A., D'Este, P., Fini, R., Geuna, A., Grimaldi, R., Hughes, A., Krabel, S., Kitson, M., Llerena, P., Lissoni, F., Salter, A. & Sobrero, M. (2013). "Academic engagement and commercialisation: A review of the literature on university–industry relations," *Research Policy*, 42(2): 423–442.
9. EIU (2016). "Understanding China's emerging private healthcare market," The Economist Intelligence Unit. Available at: https://perspectives.eiu.com/healthcare/understanding-chinas-emerging-private-healthcare-market-0.
10. Xue, P., Zhan, T., Yang, G., Farella, G. M., Robinson, N., Yang, A. W. & Liu, J. (2015). "Comparison of Chinese medicine higher education programs in China and five Western countries," *Journal of TC Medical Sciences*, 2(4): 227–234.

BIBLIOGRAPHY

Books and Articles

APCO (2016). "The 16th FYP: Xi Jinping Reiterates his Vision for China." It's an article by APCO, a communication consulting company, http://www.apcoworldwide.com/blog/detail/apcoforum/2015/11/13/the-13th-five-year-plan-xi-jinping-reiterates-his-vision-for-china.

Auewarakul, C., Downing, S. M., Praditsuwan, R. & Jaturatamrong, U. (2005). "Item analysis to improve reliability for an internal medicine undergraduate OSCE," *Advances in Health Sciences Education*, 10: 105–113.

BBVA Research (2016). China. The new FYP falls short of surprises on the positive side. Availabale at: https://www.bbvaresearch.com/en/publicaciones/china-the-new-five-year-plan-falls-short-of-surprises-on-the-positive-side/.

Booker, A., Johnston, D. & Heinrich, M. (2012). "Value chains of herbal medicines — Research needs and key challenges in the context of ethnopharmacology," *Journal of Ethnopharmacology*, 140: 624–633.

Cabral, A. P. (2011). "Research in HE: The role of teaching and student learning, procedia social and behavioral sciences," *29th International Conference on Education and Educational Psychology (ICEEPSY 2011).* Education and Educational Psychology, Turkey.

Cai, Y., Mao, Z., Corazzini, K., Petrini, M. A. & Wu, B. (2015). "Nursing workforce in Hubei, China. Implications for the development of traditional Chinese medicine education," *Holistic Nursing practice*, 29(6), (Wolters

Kluwer Health Inc.). Available at: http://journals.lww.com/hnpjournal/toc/2015/11000.

Clements, B., Coady, D. & Gupta, S. (2012). *The Economics of Public Health Care Reform in Advanced and Emerging Economics*, (IMF. Washington DC). Available at: https://www.imf.org/~/media/Websites/IMF/imported-flagship-issues/external/pubs/ft/books/2012/health/_healthcarepdf.ashx.

Corzo, J. (2015). "How academic institutions partner with private industry." Available at: https://www.rdmag.com/article/2015/04/how-academic-institutions-partner-private-industry. Accessed 31 May 2017.

Damsgaard, E. F. & Thursby, M. C. (2013). "University entrepreneurship and professor's privilege," *Industrial and Corporation Change*, 22(1): 183–218.

Edmondoson, G., Valigra, L., Kenward, M., Hudson, R. L. & Belfield, H. (2012). "Making industry-university partnership work: Lessons from successful collaborations." Report Prepared for Science Business Innovation Board AISBL.

Strata-Etan Expert Group on Foresight for the Development of HE/Research Relation (2002). *HE and Research for the ERA: Current Trends and Challenges for the Near Future* (European Commission, DG for Research – Unit RTD-K.2 – "Science and Technology Foresight; links with the IPTS", Brussels). Available at: https://www.google.it/url?sa=t&rct=j&q=&esrc=s&source=web&cd=1&cad=rja&uact=8&ved=0ahUKEwjXp867mNLWAhUBuRoKHbFVC8MQFggnMAA&url=http%3A%2F%2Fcordis.europa.eu%2Fdocuments%2Fdocumentlibrary%2F66638171EN6.pdf&usg=AOvVaw3iEkg8ZfrtQ-YgWTahn2ba.

Figueras, J., Robinson, R. & Jakubowki, E. (2005). *Purchasing to Improve Health Systems Performance*. European Observatory on Health Systems and Policies Series (Open University Press, Maidenhead, Berkshire, UK).

Government of China (1999). 10 FYP. Available at: http://govinfo.nlc.gov.cn/nxfz/xxgk/plxrmzfzwgkw/201204/t20120429_1433434.html. Accessed 31 May 2017.

Government of China (2004). 11 FYP. Available at: http://www.gov.cn/gongbao/content/2006/content_268766.htm. Accessed 31 May 2017.

Government of China (2009). 12 FYP. Available at: http://www.gov.cn/2011lh/content_1825838_17.htm. Accessed 31 May 2017.

Government of China (2014). 13 FYP. Available at: http://www.china-un.org/eng/zt/China123456/. Accessed 31 May 2017.

Government of China (2016). TCM White Paper. Available at: http://english.gov.cn/archive/white_paper/2016/12/06/content_281475509333700.htm. Accessed 31 May 2017.

Hong, W. & Cheung, D. (2015). "China's 13th FYP (2016–2020): Redefining China' development paradigm under new normal." PowerPoint Presentation.

Fung Business Intelligent Centre, China's Policy Think Piece Series Issue no. 3, Hong Kong (China). Available at: https://www.google.it/url?sa=t&rct=j&q=&esrc=s&source=web&cd=1&cad=rja&uact=8&ved=0ahUKEwi0nMjdmdLWAhVKahoKHZQ4AMkQFggpMAA&url=https%3A%2F%2Fwww.fbicgroup.com%2Fsites%2Fdefault%2Ffiles%2FChina%25E2%2580%2599s%252013th%2520Five-Year%2520Plan%2520%25282016-2020%2529%2520Redefining%2520China%25E2%2580%2599s%2520development%2520paradigm%2520under%2520the%2520New%2520Normal.pdf&usg=AOvVaw03IXmojRs4A5I9bcT4jJjX.

Hvide, H. K. & Jones, B. F. (2016). "University innovation and the professor's privilege." Available at: http://www.kellogg.northwestern.edu/faculty/jones-ben/htm/University%20Innovation%20and%20the%20Professors%20Privilege.pdf. Accessed 31 May 2017.

Jiang, M., Lu, C., Zhang, C., Yang, J., Tan, Y., Lu, A. & Chan, K. (2012). "Syndrome differentiation in modern research of traditional Chinese medicine," *Journal of Ethnopharmacology*, 140: 634–642.

Labontè, R. & Schrecker, T. (2007). *Towards Health-Equitable Globalization: Rights, Regulation and Redistribution. Technical report* (Institute of Population Health – University of Ottawa). Available at: https://www.google.it/url?sa=t&rct=j&q=&esrc=s&source=web&cd=1&cad=rja&uact=8&ved=0ahUKEwitpuLpnNLWAhVQSZoKHeH8BekQFggqMAA&url=http%3A%2F%2Fwww.who.int%2Fsocial_determinants%2Fresources%2Fgkn_report_06_2007.pdf&usg=AOvVaw1kSX4texBTuy-Xfr32zlfF.

Lamont, M. (2014). "How do university, HE and research contribute to societal well-being." Paper presented at the *CHER 2013 Conference*. CHER 26th annual Conference, Lausanne, Switzerland, 9–11 September 2013. The Roles of Higher Education and Research in the Fabric of Societies.

The Lancet (2012). "What can be learned from China's health system?" The Editorial.

Larkin, B. M. (2014). "Building successful partnership between academia and industry." Available at: https://www.elsevier.com/connect/building-successful-partnerships-between-academia-and-industry. Accessed 31 May 2017.

Link, A. N. & Rees, J. (1990). "Firm size, university based research, and returns to R&D," *Small Business Economics*, 2: 25-31.

Naughton, B. (2005). "The new common economic program : China's 11th FYP and what it means," *China Leadership Monitor*, fall 2005, (16).

Nolan, T., Resar, R., Haraden, C. & Griffin, F. A. (2004). *Improving the Reliability of Health Care*. Innovation Series 2004 (Institute for Healthcare Improvement, Cambridge, Ma, USA).

Park, H.-L., Lee, H.-S., Shin, B.-C., Liu, J.-P., Shang, Q., Yamashita, H. & Lim, B. (2012). "Traditional medicine in China, Korea, and Japan: A brief introduction and comparison," *Evidence-Based Complementary and Alternative Medicine*, 2012, article ID 429103, p. 9.

Peeters, M. J., Beltyukova, S. A. & Martin, B. A. (2013). "Educational testing and validity of conclusions in the scholarship of teaching and learning," *American Journal of Pharmaceutical Education*, 77(9), article 186.

Perkmann, M. & Schildt, H. (2015). "Open data partnerships between firms and universities: The role of boundary organizations," *Research Policy*, 44: 1133-1143.

Qi, Z., Liming, Z. & Van Der Lerberghe, W. (2011). "The importance of traditional Chinese medicine services in health care provision in China," *Universitas Forum*, 2(2) (2011). Available at: http://universitasforum.org/index.php/ojs/article/view/63.

Scott, P. (2015). "What is the Role of Research in HE?" PowerPoint Presentation. Available at: http://hea.ie/assets/uploads/2017/04/peter_scott_presentation_15.4.15.pdf. Accessed 4 July 2017.

Simón, L. F. R., Avilés, R. A., Botezan, I., Gastaminza, F. d. V. & Serrano, S. C. (2014). "Open data as universal service. New perspectives in the information profession," *Procedia — Social and Behavioral Sciences*, 147(2014): 126–132.

Uzuner, H., Bauer, R., Fan, T.-P., Guo, D.-A., Dias, A., El-Nezami, H., Efferth, T., Williamson, E. M., Heinrich, M., Robinson, N., Hylands, P. J., Hendry, B. M., Cheng, Y.-C. & Xu, Q. (2012). "Traditional Chinese medicine research in the post-genomic era: Good practice, priorities, challenges and opportunities," *Journal of Ethnopharmacology*, 140(2012): 458–468.

Van Dusen, V. (2013). "IP and HE: Challenges," *Administrative Issues Journal*, 3(2), article 3.

Van Rijnsoever, F. J., van den Berg, J., Koch, J. & Hekkert, M. P. (2015). "Smart innovation policy: How network position and project composition affect the diversity of an emerging technology," *Research Policy*, 44(2015): 1094–1107.

Vessuri, H. (2008). "The role of research on HE." Available at: https://upcommons.upc.edu/bitstream/handle/2099/8119/vessuri.pdf. Accessed 31 May 2017.

World Bank (2008). "Mid-term evaluation of China's 11th FYP." Available at: http://siteresources.worldbank.org/CHINAEXTN/Resources/318949-1121421890573/China_11th_Five-Year_Plan_main_report_en.pdf. Accessed 4 July 2017.

Xu, L. (2010). "The development priorities of China's 11th FYP." PowerPoint Presentation. https://www.google.it/url?sa=t&rct=j&q=&esrc=s&source=we

b&cd=1&cad=rja&uact=8&ved=0ahUKEwiK4KyspNLWAhVNK1AKHQXNApMQFggvMAA&url=http%3A%2F%2Fsiteresources.worldbank.org%2FINTEASTASIAPACIFIC%2FResources%2F226262-1143156545724%2FChina_Development_Period.ppt&usg=AOvVaw0TUhrMEDjOBAnt9mhprqyU. https://www.google.it/url?sa=t&rct=j&q=&esrc=s&source=web&cd=2&cad=rja&uact=8&ved=0ahUKEwiAvr_wyMbWAhVOY1AKHeozBOYQFggyMAE&url=http%3A%2F%2Fsiteresources.worldbank.org%2FINTEASTASIAPACIFIC%2FResources%2F226262-1143156545724%2FChina_Development_Period.ppt&usg=AFQjCNGSSvA9aYkNepWRW0Ik-MZ_ias1OA.

Websites

http://china.org.cn/top10/2012-02/22/content_24683507.htm
http://www.chinaeducenter.com/en/cedu/tcm.php
http://www.scm.hku.hk/english-school_intro_page_1.html
http://wenr.wes.org/2016/12/traditional-chinese-medicine-surging-international-interest-shifting-educational-landscape-china
http://www.satcm.gov.cn/e/action/ListInfo/?classid=143
https://www.nobelprize.org/nobel_prizes/medicine/laureates/2015/
http://www.cucas.edu.cn/studyinchina/admission/China_Academy_of_Chinese_Medical_Sciences_70_946.html
https://www.aihm.org/traditional-chinese-medicine-the-nobel-prize-and-research/
http://blog.sina.com.cn/s/blog_667242870102vqqt.html
http://www.cucas.edu.cn/server/index/2384/2384
https://nccih.nih.gov/health/whatiscam/chinesemed.htm
http://www.ontcm.com/show-36-457-1.html
http://www.sciencedirect.com/science/article/pii/S2095754816000119
https://www.google.de/webhp?sourceid=chrome-instant&ion=1&espv=2&ie=UTF-#q=investment+in+chinese+traditional+medicine
https://www.google.de/url?sa=t&rct=j&q=&esrc=s&source=web&cd=1&cad=rja&uact=8&ved=0ahUKEwjShOO98L_TAhVEPBQKHQ8eD8wQFggnMAA&url=https%3A%2F%2Fwww.takingcharge.csh.umn.edu%2Fexplore-healing-practices%2Ftraditional-chinese-medicine%2F-tcm-evidence-based-and-safe&usg=AFQjCNFgwh1-cU_LobN0MCNlGdvxh9rp9Q
https://www.google.de/webhp?sourceid=chrome-instant&ion=1&espv=2&ie=UTF-8#q=investment+in+chinese+traditional+medicine&start=10
https://www.takingcharge.csh.umn.edu/explore-healing-practices/traditional-chinese-medicine/-tcm-evidence-based-and-safe

http://www.worldsocialscience.org/activities/transformations/governance/steering-committee/vessuri/

http://www.ips.org.pk/global-issues-and-politics/996-higher-education-and-research-trends-and-challenges

https://www.aeaweb.org/econlit/jelCodes.php?view=jel

http://www.bc.edu/research/cihe/about/pga/bookchaptersandarticles.html

http://www.footnote1.com/making-scientific-research-more-reliable-by-addressing-the-%E2%80%9Creproducibility-problem%E2%80%9D/

http://www.searo.who.int/entity/traditional_medicine/en/

http://who.int/medicines/areas/traditional/en/

https://nccih.nih.gov/about

https://www.ox.ac.uk/research/innovation-and-partnership?wssl=1#

http://www.eua.be/policy-representation/research-innovation-policy/university-business-partnerships

http://www.nationalacademies.org/nasem/

http://www.nber.org/papers/w22057

WHO Publications on TM/CAM

POLICY

Policy Direction and Strategy

1. *The WHO Traditional Medicine Strategy 2014–2023* (WHO, Geneva).
2. *WHO Western Pacific Regional Strategy on Traditional Medicine: 2011–2020*, 2012.
3. *Development of TM in the South-East Asia Region: Report of a Regional Consultative Meeting*. Pyongyang, DP'sR of Korea, 22–24/6/2005, 2005.
4. *WHO Policy Perspectives on Medicines, TM – Growing Needs and Potential*, 2002.
5. *The WHO Traditional Medicine Strategy 2002–2005*, 2002.
6. *Promoting the Role of TM in Health Systems: A Strategy for the African Region*, 2001.
7. *Apia Action Plan on Traditional Medicine in the Pacific Island Countries*, 2001.
8. *Development of National Policy on Traditional Medicine*, 2000.
9. *The Promotion and Development of Traditional Medicine: Report of a WHO Meeting*, 1978.

National Policy and Regulation Monitoring

10. *National Policy and Regulation of TM: Report of the Second WHO Global Survey* (in preparation).

11. *Regulatory Situation of Manual Therapies: A Worldwide Review* (Geneva, WHO) (in preparation).
12. *National Policy on TM and Regulation of Herbal Medicines: Report of a WHO Global Survey*, 2005.
13. *Legal Status of TM/CAM: A Worldwide Review*, 2001
14. *Traditional Health Systems in Latin America and the Caribbean: Baseline Information*, 2000.
15. *Regulatory Situation of Herbal Medicines: A Worldwide Review* (Geneva, WHO, 1998)

Promotion and Preservation of Traditional Medicine Knowledge

16. *Report of the Inter-Regional Workshop on IPR in the Context of TM, Bangkok (TH), 6–8/12/2000*, 2001.

QUALITY, SAFETY, AND EFFICACY

Herbal Medicines — Quality and Safety

17. *WHO Guidelines on Good Processing Practices for Herbal Medicines.* Geneva (in preparation).
18. *WHO Guidelines on Safety Management of Toxic Medicinal Plants and Monographs on Selected Toxic Medicinal Plants* (in preparation).
19. *WHO Guidelines on Selection of Substances of Herbal Origin for Quality Control of Herbal Medicines* (in preparation).
20. *Quality Control Methods for Herbal Materials* (updated edition of 1998 publication), 2011.
21. *Safety Issues in the Preparation of Homeopathic Medicines* 2010.
22. *WHO Guidelines on Assessing Quality of Herbal Medicines with Reference to Contaminants and Residues*, 2007.
23. *WHO Guidelines on Good Manufacturing Practices (GMP) for Herbal Medicines*, 2007.
24. *WHO Good Agricultural and Collection Practices (GACP) Monograph on Artemisia Annual*, 2006.
25. *Good Manufacturing Practices: Updated Supplementary Guidelines for the Manufacture of Herbal Medicines.* Annex 3 of WHO Expert Committee on Specifications for Pharmaceutical Preparations, 40 report (WHO Technical Report Series, No. 937), 2006.
26. *WHO Guidelines on Good Agricultural and Collection Practices (GACP) for Medicinal Plants*, 2003.

27. *Basic Tests for Drugs: Pharmaceutical Substances, Medicinal Plant Materials and Dosage Forms*, 1998.
28. *Quality Control Methods for Medicinal Plant Materials*, 1998.
29. *Good Manufacturing Practices: Supplementary Guidelines for the Manufacture of Herbal Medicinal Products.* Annex 8 of WHO Expert Committee on Specifications for Pharmaceutical Preparations. Thirty-fourth Report (WHO Technical Report Series, No. 863), 1996.

Herbal Medicines — Regulation

30. *WHO Monographs on Selected Medicinal Plants Commonly Used in Newly Independent States*, 2010.
31. *WHO Monographs on Selected Medicinal Plants.* Volume 4, 2009.
32. *WHO Monographs on Selected Medicinal Plants.* Volume 3, 2007.
33. *Guidelines on Minimum Requirements for the Registration of Herbal Medicinal Products in the Eastern Mediterranean Region* (Report on the First Regional Workshop on Regulation of Herbal Medicines, Teheran, 14–17 December 2002 & Second Regional Workshop, Abu Dhabi, 7–9 June 2003), 2006.
34. *Report: Regional Meeting on Traditional Medicine and Herbal Medicines, Guatemala City, 18–20 February 2003*, 2005.
35. *WHO Guidelines on Safety Monitoring of Herbal Medicines in Pharmacovigilance Systems*, 2004.
36. *Guidelines for the Regulation of Herbal Medicines in the South-East Asia Region* [report regional workshop on the regulation of herbal medicines], 2004.
37. *Guidelines on Registration of TM in the WHO African Region* (Report on the First Regional Workshop on Regulation of TM, Johannesburg, 1–3 April 2003 & Second Regional Workshop, Madrid, 13–14 February 2004), 2004.
38. *Report of WHO Workshop on Registration of Herbal Medicines in the European Region, Yerevan, 22–24 September 2003*, 2004.
39. *WHO Monographs on Selected Medicinal Plants.* Volume 2, 2002.
40. *General Guidelines for Methodologies on Research and Evaluation of TM*, 2000
41. *WHO Monographs on Selected Medicinal Plants.* Volume 1, 1999.
42. *Guidelines for the Assessment of Herbal Medicines.* Annex 11 of WHO Expert Committee on Specifications for Pharmaceutical Preparations. 34 Report, 1996 (WHO Technical Report Series, No. 863).

Research Methodologies and Clinical Studies

43. *Key Technical Issues on Safety of Herbal Medicines with Reference to Interaction with Other Medicines* (in preparation).
44. *TM: Review and Analysis of Reports of Controlled Clinical Studies* (in preparation).
45. *Clinical Studies in Traditional Medicine: Key Technical Issues on Methodologies* (in preparation).
46. *Guidelines on Clinical Study of Traditional Medicines in WHO African Region*, 2004.
47. *SARS: Clinical Trials on Treatment using a Combination of TCM and Western Medicine*, 2004.
48. *Acupuncture: Review and Analysis of Reports on Controlled Clinical Trials*, 2002.
49. *General Guidelines for Methodologies on Research and Evaluation of TC*, 2000.
50. *Traditional and Modern Medicine: Harmonizing the Two Approaches*, 2000.
51. *Guidelines for Clinical Research on Acupuncture*, 1995.
52. *Research Guidelines for Evaluating the Safety and Efficacy of Herbal Medicines*, 1993.
53. *Clinical Evaluation of TM and Natural Products. Report of a WHO Consultation on TM and AIDS, Geneva, 26–28 September 1990*, 1990.
54. *In Vitro Screening for Anti-HIV Activities. Report of an Informal WHO Consultation on TM and AIDS, Geneva, 6–8 February 1989*, 1989.

ACCESS

Conservation and Sustainable Use of Medicinal Plants

55. *Updated Edition: WHO/IUCN/WWF/TRAFFIC Guidelines on the Conservation of Medicinal Plants* (in preparation).
56. *Medicinal Plants in Papua New Guinea*, 2009.
57. *WHO Good Agricultural and Collection Practices (GACP) Monograph on Artemisia Annual*, 2006.
58. *WHO Guidelines on Good Agricultural and Collection Practices (GACP) for Medicinal Plants*, 2003.
59. *Medicinal Plants in the Republic of Korea*, 1998.
60. *Medicinal Plants in the South Pacific*, 1998.
61. *WHO/IUCN/WWF Guidelines on the Conservation of Medicinal Plants*, 1993.

62. *Natural Resources and Human Health: Plants of Medicinal and Nutritional Value. Proceedings of the First WHO Symposium on Plants and Health for All: Scientific Advancement. Kobe, Japan, 26–28 August 1991*, 1992.
63. *Conservation of Medicinal Plants. Proceedings of an International Consultation, Chiang Mai, Thailand, 21–27 March 1988*, 1991.
64. *Medicinal Plants in Viet Nam*, 1990.
65. *Medicinal Plants in China*, 1989.

Role of Traditional Medicine in Healthcare

66. *Traditional Herbal Remedies for Primary Health Care*, 2010.
67. *Report of WHO Interregional Workshop on the use of TM in PHC*, 2009
68. *Guidelines for the Appropriate Use of Herbal Medicines*, 1998.
69. *Traditional Practitioners as PHC Workers*, 1995.
70. *WHO/DANIDA Intercountry Course on the Appropriate Methodology for the Selection and Use of Traditional Remedies in NHC Program. Report of an Intercountry Course Held in Kadoma, Zimbabwe, 26 June–6 July 1989*, 1991.
71. *Prospects for Involving Traditional Health Practitioners. Report of the Consultation on AIDS and TM, Francistown, Botswana, 23–27 July 1990*, 1990.
72. *The Role of TM in PHC in China (based on an I-R Seminar Sponsored by WHO with the MoPH of the PRC) 9–21 October 1985*, 1986.
73. *WHO/DANIDA TC: The Selection and Use of TR in PHC. Report of an I-R Workshop Held in Bangkok (Thailand), 25 November–4 December 1985*, 1986.
74. *Traditional Medicine and Health Care Coverage* (Reprinted, 1988).

RATIONAL USE

Acupuncture Nomenclature and Terminology

75. *WHO International Standard Terminologies on TM in the Western Pacific Region*, 2007.
76. *Standard Acupuncture Nomenclature*, 1993.
77. *A Proposed Standard International Acupuncture Nomenclature: Report of a WHO Scientific Group*, 1991.
78. *Report of the Working Group on Auricular Acupuncture Nomenclature*, 1991.

Consumer Information and Education

79. *WHO Guidelines on Development of Consumer Information on Proper Use of TM/CAM*, 2004.

Training and Good Practice

80. *Benchmarks for Training in Tuina.* Geneva, WHO, 2010.
81. *Benchmarks for Training in Nuad Thai.* Geneva, WHO, 2010.
82. *Benchmarks for Training in Osteopathy.* Geneva, WHO, 2010.
83. *Benchmarks for Training in Unani Medicine.* Geneva, WHO, 2010.
84. *Benchmarks for Training in Traditional Chinese Medicine.* Geneva, WHO, 2010.
85. *Benchmarks for Training in Naturopathy.* Geneva, WHO, 2010.
86. *Benchmarks for Training in Ayurveda.* Geneva, WHO, 2010.
87. *WHO Guidelines on Basic Training and Safety in Chiropractic.* Geneva, WHO, 2006.
88. *Guidelines on Basic Training and Safety in Acupuncture.* Geneva, WHO, 1999.
89. *Training Package of Practitioners of Traditional Medicine*, 1999.
90. *Guidelines for Training Traditional Health Practitioners in Primary Health Care*, 1995.

Part 2

The Integration of Western and Traditional Chinese Medicine: Challenges and Opportunities

Chapter 11

Assessing Costs, Benefits, and Cost-Effectiveness in TCM

Attilio Mucelli and Olena Liakh

1. INTRODUCTION

This chapter intends to fill the gap in evidence on the potential benefits of introducing Traditional Chinese Medicine (TCM) practices, with respect to its costs. In this regard, the different economic evaluations for the healthcare sector were described. Based on the results of the literature review, which showed a relative lack for standardized cost-benefit tools and methods examining the potential positive impact of TCM, a possible approach was structured, describing the suggested steps and necessary tools that would have to be adopted in order to run a complete appraisal of the cost-effectiveness of TCM. The steps of the evaluation include gathering cost information; identifying benefits, computing such CBA outcome measures as net benefits and benefit-cost ratios; running cost-effectiveness analyses (CEAs) for additional confirmation of the results through the cost-effectiveness, reversed cost-effectiveness, and incremental cost-effectiveness ratios; and applying additional cost-utility analysis (CUA) tools in order to obtain the cost per quality-adjusted life year (QALY) and reversed cost per QALY outcome measures. The results could also be represented visually by using the incremental cost-effectiveness plane and cost-effectiveness acceptability curve.

2. ASSESSING ECONOMIC IMPACT OF HEALTHCARE SERVICES/PRACTICES

The aim of an economic evaluation is to assess the social desirability and economic effectiveness of a certain program, usually compared with another alternative, by appraising advantages (positive consequences) and disadvantages (costs, etc.) of that particular intervention. In line with the economic theory, there are several types of economic evaluations that differ, according to the incorporated consequences and purpose of the analysis. Three of them are particularly suited for the healthcare sector and are typically used in healthcare economics:

- Cost-Benefit Analysis (CBA);
- Cost-Effectiveness Analysis (CEA);
- Cost-Utility Analysis (CUA).[1]

In the context of a CBA, a monetary value is attributed to those consequences, in this case called benefits (B), making them directly comparable with the costs (C).[2] It is thus immediately possible to understand whether a healthcare expenditure is worthwhile (under the assumption that it will improve social welfare) and should be approved. The CBA, however, requires placing a monetary value on all health outcomes.[2] For this reason, other approaches tried to express the effects in terms of non-monetary units (e.g., health status, etc.). With this regard, the most popular type of economic evaluation is the CEA, which aims at determining the treatment supplying a unit of effect at a lowest cost. Cost-effectiveness can also be calculated through an Incremental Cost-Effectiveness Ratio (ICER),[3] representing the additional cost for the additional benefit offered by the first treatment/program, which will be considered dominant if it provides better outcomes at the same, or lower, cost as the second treatment/program.[4]

When comparing completely different effects (without using prices explicitly), the CUA is the preferred approach. Interventions producing different consequences are expressed as utilities. In this case, all effects have to be converted to a common unit, called QALY,[2] which measures how much quantity of life one is willing to give up in order to achieve a higher quality of life.[5]

In order to obtain a general view of the available methodologies and results on TCM, a brief literature review was conducted. Table 1 sums up the most relevant points of these studies by considering the different topics examined throughout the review: economic evaluations (EEs), TCM, Integrative Medicine (IM), acupuncture (Acup.), and Chinese Patent and Herbal Medicine (CPM, CHM). The considerations have been divided into two columns for each topic, in order to distinguish the most important research trends from the potential gaps of knowledge that were identified.

3. POSSIBLE CBA APPROACH FOR EVALUATING THE IMPACT OF TCM, BASED ON LITERATURE REVIEW FINDINGS

Table 1 shows that the economic evaluations developed for TCM are very limited in number, and one of the possible causes is the lack of a standardized model for confirming its real cost-effectiveness in comparison with Western Medicine (WM). In order to provide a wider base for the evaluation of the TCM treatments, it might be helpful to combine some of the tools and methodologies that have already been used in research. What follows, however, is not a standardized model on its own, but only a suggestion of the most efficient steps and approaches that were gathered from reviewing the various studies on the topic.

A good initial focus could be related to the use of CBA. First of all, not many analyses of TCM have been developed through it yet, and this on its own is already a good motivation for establishing further research within this topic. Furthermore, it provides a good summary measure of multiple outcomes in a single monetary unit, which is easily comparable. The main problem though is that this analysis might not be enough on its own. Also, benefits are not easily quantifiable in monetary terms, which is why we should supplement it with other methods.

Table 1. Summary of Outcomes Obtained and Main Issues Identified.

	Summary of Outcomes Obtained so Far	Main Issues Identified so Far
EE	• CUA and CEA tools (QALY, ICER, C/E ratio): normally used in combination for optimal results; • CUAs and the related QALYs are becoming standard means for examining health outcomes (in acupuncture especially, they provide useful information in an easily comparable format for decision makers); • CUAs usually yield satisfactory results, present a low risk of bias, and are generally well-designed, high-quality studies	• Few economic evaluation researches available for TCM in general; • Very few CBAs have been performed in TCM so far: more difficult to apply as they require putting a monetary value on health; • CEAs seem less reliable: they tend to use various outcome measures and comparators, which leads to more inconsistent results
TCM	• TCM treatments present better outcomes at higher costs, compared with control; • However, they are reasonably cost-effective: ICER is below the usually recommended international threshold values; • The degree of cost-effectiveness is influenced by gender: better C/E ratio for female patients; • TCM economic evaluations could be refined by adopting specific statistical models to support them	• Inconsistent and inconclusive results of HRQL evaluations in TCM: long term effects of TCM therapies are yet unknown; • Generic instruments such as EQ-5D and SF-36, are not sensitive enough for measuring HRQL changes in patients treated with TCM (only in some cases, they managed to quantify acupuncture's effects): need for a HRQL tool that is specific for TCM; • Lack of qualitative, unbiased cost-effectiveness research in TCM: need for studies with better designs, longer duration, and right instruments to confirm the cost-effectiveness of TCM in comparison to conventional therapies
IM	• In some cases, combined WM_ TCM practices provide significant health benefits at the expense of longer length of stay, measuring time cost and higher cost per stay, measuring financial cost as total hospital expense, with better overall cost-effectiveness	• Unclear benefits of IM, since different types of economic evaluations produce different outcomes for different pathologies; • In some cases, TCM alone yields more savings than IM

(*Continued*)

Table 1. *(Continued)*

	Summary of Outcomes Obtained so Far	Main Issues Identified so Far
Acup.	• It appears to be cost-effective in the longer term: increased QALY gains tend to reduce the ICER overtime; • If £20,000 is taken as the maximum acceptable cost per QALY threshold, acupuncture normally showed to have over 90% probability of being cost-effective; • In CEAs, acupuncture is seen as dominant: cost-saving and more effective than control, with lower productivity loss and improved pain scores; • Generally, in CUAs, acupuncture is more effective but costly, yet benefits to health are obtained at a relatively minor cost	• It is challenging to generalize results: diversity of diseases and the different statuses of acupuncture in the various countries are an obstacle
CPM/ CHM	• CPM research on diabetes partially contributed to the standardization of an economic evaluation process for TCM	• Lack of cost-effectiveness research in other types of TCM practices, especially CHM: major emphasis is on acupuncture or tai chi, that are better understood by the scientific community; • Lack of a standardized cost-effectiveness evaluation model for CPM, and TCM in general

Source: Authors' own representation.

Even though CUAs present a lower risk of bias and are better designed than CEAs, CEA outcome measures are easier and faster to compute (making them useful for supporting urgent questions) and can be measured objectively. Thus a combination of CBA and CEA tools could be used for achieving better results. CUA instruments could also be added further on during the analysis, whenever a higher degree of precision is needed and sufficient data is available. In any case, when it is not possible to quantify benefits monetarily, CEAs or CUAs should be directly used, otherwise CBAs should be applied whenever possible, in order to further test the potential strengths and weaknesses of the model.

The CBA could be carried out on one of the following levels:

- National/regional/hospital level, assuming more of a societal/institutional perspective;
- Specific pathology level, assuming an individual/patient's perspective.

Depending on the choice, different types/levels of cost should be considered and identified first.

3.1. *Evaluation steps*

3.1.1. *First step: Gathering cost information*

In terms of costs, the starting point for a CBA could be the financial analysis model applied to the healthcare sector, then adapted to the specific case of TCM. With this regard, the total costs are made by the sum of the investment costs (e.g., building costs, facilities and equipment, extraordinary maintenance) and operating costs (materials/medicines, personnel cost, physician services, maintenance).

This type of information, though, could not be fully applicable to the case of a specific pathology. The investment costs in particular might not be relevant to the purpose of that kind of study. The research reviewed previously confirm that, in order to analyze the effects of a treatment on a specific pathology, one should gather data relative to the operating level (direct medical costs: consultation fees, diagnostic costs, treatment costs, drug/medication cost; and non-medical costs: transportation costs to/from the clinic, accommodation, and catering).[6]

At this point, it should already be possible to make an initial comparison in terms of costs, so as to identify which levels weight the most in either WM or TCM treatment. We can take the expenses table (simplified, to adapt it to our analysis) developed by Liao *et al.*[7] for a study on liver cancer as an example (Table 2). If we consider it from a patient's perspective, the fees represent a unit cost (NT$).

The fees for consultation, treatment, as well as drugs per visit for biomedicine were markedly higher than those for TCM: the average

Table 2. Expenditures for Outpatient Services for Liver Cancer Patients (NT$).

	Biomedicine			TCM			Biomedicine/ TCM Ratio	
	Tot.	%	Avg.	Tot.	%	Avg.	Tot.	Avg.
Unit cost for consultation/ treatment	23,205, 324,170	43.8	429.73	6,115, 161,733.80	40.02	301.93	3.79	1.42
Diagnosis cost/unit	11,725, 511,578	22.13	217.14	4,425, 149,296	28.96	218.49	2.65	0.99
Drug cost/unit	18,043, 485,487	34.06	334.14	4,738, 494,125	31.01	233.96	3.81	1.43
Total amount	52,974, 321,235	100	981.01	15,278, 805,154.80	100	754.38	3.47	1.30

Source: Authors' Own Representation Based on Ref. 7.

expenditure was NT$429.73 (USD 13.25) per biomedicine visit and NT$301.93 (USD 9.32) per TCM visit. Total average cost per visit was NT$981.01 (USD 30.28) for biomedicine and NT$754.38 (USD 23.28) for TCM. The ratio of medical expenses for all biomedicine outpatient visits relative to that for TCM was 3.47, whereas the ratio of the average medical expenses for each biomedicine outpatient visit relative to those of TCM was 1.3.[7]

3.1.2. *Second step: Identifying benefits*

Benefits can be quantified through market prices of the services (WTP) or through standard methods like QALY. It could be useful to carry out an evaluation of the benefits in terms of simple physical indicators, which are more easily quantifiable, like in CEA's case, which is more frequently used in the healthcare sector because it provides comparable results.

If we take it from an institutional perspective, we could consider the cost categories, seen in the previous example, as benefits for a healthcare institution. To clarify this concept, we shall take the data collected by Wang *et al.*[8] (extracting the year 2013 only) in the paper analyzing the development trend of TCM hospitals in China, with special reference to

Table 3. Outpatient and Inpatient Medical Fee/Person (in RMB), 2013.

	Outpatient Medical Fee		Inpatient Medical Fee	
TCM	Drug fee	118.5	Drug fee	2,519
	Treatment fee	17.4	Treatment fee	953
	Registration fee	2	Sickbed fee	267
			Surgery fee	349
WM	Examination fee	25.9	Examination fee	435
TOT		163.8		4,523

Source: Authors' own representation based on Ref. 8.

its coexistence with WM structures. The fees, within this perspective, represent the components of the revenue per unit (which should be then multiplied by the number of patients), and here they are separated in outpatient and inpatient medical fees (RMB). The WM in this case is considered as an instrumental treatment, through the examination fee.

Table 3 should be analyzed as follows. The drug fee accounted for most of the total unitary revenue in both the outpatient and medical hospital cares. Also, the proportion of the examination fee has exceeded that of the treatment fee in the outpatient case, showing an increasing usage of instrumental WM examination. The inpatient medical fee is much higher than that of the outpatient, suggesting that most of the income of TCM hospitals comes from the inpatient medical service. Of the total inpatient medical fee, the drug fee accounted for a high percentage, implying that TCM hospitals are still dependent on drugs for profit. Even though the proportion of the examination fee in this case seems lower than that of treatment, if we take a longer period of time, we can still see that it experienced a rising usage for inpatient services at TCM hospitals overtime (the study indicates an average yearly growth of 11%).

Comparing the drug revenues only, for WM and TCM, in 2013, it can be observed that WM drugs accounted for about 60% of the total drug revenue, more than TCM drugs (Table 4). The proportion of TCM outpatient drug income exceeded that of WM and reached 60.7%. Conversely, for inpatient service, WM drugs accounted for about 80% of the total inpatient drug revenue. Again, the analysis would become more complete if we analyzed a longer period of time, as done in the paper. With this

Table 4. Average Drug Revenue/Hospital (in RMB), 2013.

	Total Drug Revenue		Outpatient Drug Revenue		Inpatient Drug Revenue	
	WM	TCM	WM	TCM	WM	TCM
2013	23,500	17,115	8,151	12,608	15,349	4,507
%	57.9%	42.1%	39.3%	60.7%	77.3%	22.7

Source: Authors' own representation based on Ref. 8.

additional information, we could have added that, although the proportion of total drug revenue for TCM is lower than WM, TCM drug income has grown at a faster annual growth rate than WM, for both outpatient and inpatient services.[8]

If we assume this institutional perspective, then the revenues should be compared with the investment costs and some of the operating costs (e.g., labor, cost to the hospital of medicine drugs that are resold to patients afterward) that were presented earlier.

3.1.3. *Third step: Computing CBA outcome measure*

After having gathered all relevant information, it is possible to finalize the economic evaluation of the therapy. The following measures can be used to evaluate TCM in a CBA perspective:

- Net benefits: $(B_{TCM} - C_{TCM}) - (B_{WM} - C_{WM}) = NB_{TCM} - NB_{WM}$. Whenever the net benefits of TCM treatments exceed those of the WM intervention, expenditures in TCM are socially worthwhile.
- Benefit–cost ratio: $B_{TCM}/C_{TCM} > B_{WM}/C_{WM}$. Whenever this criterion is respected, it is sure that TCM yields more benefits per unitary cost spent compared to WM.[9]

3.1.4. *Fourth step: Running a CEA for additional confirmation of the results*

Once the CBA has been carried out, it could be integrated with some of the CEA tools suggested by the literature. Below, a list of the tools to be used for assessing the cost-effectiveness of TCM treatments through a CEA is presented:

- Reversed cost-effectiveness ratio: $E_{TCM}/C_{TCM} > E_{WM}/C_{WM}$. This is exactly the same criterion used for the B/C ratio, with the exception that benefits (P × E) have been substituted by the effects only. Here TCM achieved the most effect per cost, compared with WM.
- Cost-effectiveness ratio: $C_{TCM}/E_{TCM} < C_{WM}/E_{WM}$. When TCM's C/E ratio is smaller than that of WM, TCM is considered more cost-effective. Here TCM supplies a unit of effect a lower cost, compared with WM.
- Incremental cost-effectiveness ratio: $ICER_{TCM} = (C_{TCM} - C_{WM})/(E_{TCM} - E_{WM})$. It represents an incremental cost associated with one additional unit of effect (e.g., health/life year) gained through the TCM treatment.

One of the studies from the literature review showed how the C/E ratio and the ICER could be effectively computed by adopting the CPS as a cost measure. Figure 1 shows how the relationship between CPS and effectiveness could be graphically represented in a CEA, based on the paper developed by Li *et al.*[10]

3.1.5. *Fifth step: Including additional CUA tools*

When enough data is available from the questionnaires, QALY can be computed and included in the analysis too as a measure of the patients' utility. From QALY, we can get the different outcome measures (cost-utility ratios):

- Reversed cost per QALY, to compare competing programs (values between 1, perfect health, and 0, death or deterioration of health status): $QALY_{TCM}/C_{TCM} > QALY_{WM}/C_{WM}$. In this case we are measuring the number of additional life years gained per unit of cost spent on TCM (which, within this condition, is cost-effective).
- Cost per QALY: $C_{TCM}/QALY_{TCM} < C_{WM}/QALY_{WM}$. When the cost-utility ratio for TCM is smaller than the one for WM, then TCM produces more utility at a lower unitary cost.

Figure 1. Relation Between Adjusted CPS and Positive Effectiveness Among Four Groups (USD).

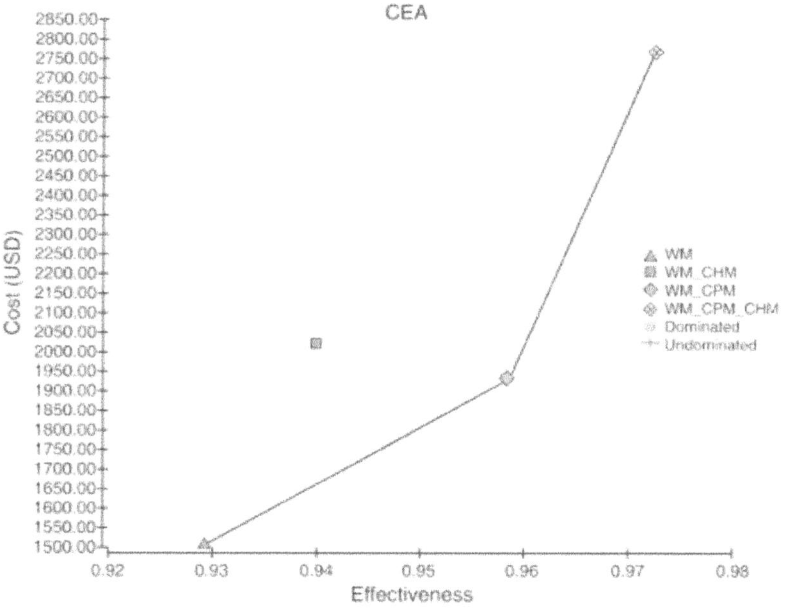

Source: From Ref. 10.

CUA and CEA tools can be combined most of the times for more accurate and broader results. The ICER, for instance, can be used for estimating utility through a single comprehensive measure of the effects, the QALY:

- Incremental cost per QALY: $(C_{TCM} - C_{WM})/(QALY_{TCM} - QALY_{WM})$. It works similarly to the ICER.
- It is useful to represent the ICER visually using the Incremental Cost-Effectiveness Plane, in which the horizontal axis represents the incremental cost (positive above, negative below) and the vertical axis shows the incremental effect (positive to the right, negative to the left), which is most commonly expressed in QALYs.
- An additional tool that supplements the analysis done through ICER is the cost-effectiveness acceptability curve (CEAC). It is a method for summarizing the uncertainty in estimates of cost-effectiveness and illustrates the probability that the data are consistent with a true

cost-effectiveness ratio falling below a specified ceiling ratio.[11] The ICER threshold value will be represented on the *x*-axis and the probability of the intervention being cost-effective on the *y*-axis. Cost per QALY could be substituted to ICER in the *x*-axis, if we want to switch to an evaluation of the utility.

3.2. *An example of a basic CEA: Integrative TCM and the risk of diabetic ketoacidosis*

In order to provide an example of a possible application of the CEA, data presented in the study designed in Taiwan by Lien *et al.*[12] (in which no explicit economic evaluation had been carried out) was taken as a reference. Diabetic ketoacidosis (DKA) is the most common complication of type 1 diabetes mellitus (T1DM), considered a catastrophic illness, leading to hospitalization. Insulin replacement is the primary WM therapy for T1DM. However, this study suggested that TCM, and CHM in particular, may have a substantial positive impact on the reduction of DKA in patients with T1DM. This study is somehow different with respect to the previous ones that compared TCM against WM in order to understand TCM's efficiency. Here, instead, the focus is on the comparison of efficacy between complete and incomplete TCM treatment sessions. With this regard, three groups of subjects have been identified:

- Non-TCM users: patients with T1DM who were TCM users for 30 days or less (1,608 control subjects).
- TCM users (416 case subjects):
    - (30–180 days): individuals diagnosed with T1DM who received TCM treatment between 30 and 180 days.
    - (> 180 days): individuals diagnosed with T1DM who received TCM treatment for over 180 days.

The costs (NT$) used in this CEA are annual medical costs of emergency room (ER) visits and hospitalizations (as taken from the paper), adjusted for the age, gender, and comorbidities factors (Table 5).

Table 5. Annual Medical Costs for ER and Hospitalization (NT$), by Users.

	Non-TCM Users	TCM Users (30–180 Days)	TCM Users (> 180 Days)
ER	2,053	2,484	1,566
Hospitalization	22,176	27,564	14,427

Source: Authors' own representation based on Ref. 12.

Table 6. Avoided DKA Events (%), by Users.

	Non-TCM Users	TCM Users (30–180 Days)	TCM Users (>180 Days)
Decreased incidence of DKA (avoided DKA events)	52.4% (N = 842)	67.1% (N = 208)	67.9% (N = 72)

Source: Authors' own representation based on Ref. 12.

The annual cost of ER visits and hospitalizations were slightly higher for TCM users who had been using TCM for less than six months, compared with non-TCM users. On the other hand, patients who used TCM for more than six months demonstrated a trend toward lower costs of ER visits and hospitalizations, with respect to both of the remaining groups.[12]

The indicator used in the study is the decreased risk of DKA events, which cannot be used as an effect in the CEA, since the decreased risk of DKA for non-TCM users was taken as a base value, zero. We are hence going to use a new effect measure instead, the avoided DKA events (which we can here interpret as the decreased incidence of DKA). This indicator has been calculated based on the number of DKA events that occurred in each group (Table 6).

The incidence of DKA in non-TCM users (48%) was higher than that of all TCM users (32.7%). Compared with non-TCM users, TCM users displayed an average of 67.3% decreased incidence of DKA events within their respective groups, among which TCM patients for less than six months displayed a 67.1% decrease, while those who received a longer period of TCM treatment (over six months) experienced a 67.9% decrease.

Table 7 represents the C/E ratios for the avoided DKA events, with respect to ER and hospitalization costs, calculated as:

$$(\text{C/E})_{\text{user group}} = \text{annual medical cost}/\%\ \text{avoided DKA events}$$

Table 7. Cost-Effectiveness Ratios for Avoided DKA Events.

	Non-TCM Users	TCM Users (30–180 Days)	TCM Users (> 180 Days)
Avoided DKA events (ER)	3,917.93	3,701.94	2,306.33
Avoided DKA events (hospitalization)	42,320.61	41,078.98	21,247.42

Source: Authors' own representation.

Table 8. Ordered Cost-Effectiveness Ratios for Avoided DKA Events by Most Preferred Group.

	Preference	1	2	3
ER	User group	TCM users (> 180 days)	TCM users (30–180 days)	Non-TCM users
	C/E ratio	2,306.33	3,701.94	3,917.93
Hospitalization	User group	TCM users (> 180 days)	TCM users (30–180 days)	Non-TCM users
	C/E ratio	21,247.42	41,078.98	42,320.61

Source: Authors' own representation.

We can now proceed to order the ratios so as to understand what interventions should be preferred first, in case the decision makers were choosing between the different alternatives, having a certain budget limit. It is true than CEAs require a budget constraint for improving the quality of the analysis; however, in this case, the budget was not imposed, as the study was not developed to provide support to any particular health policymaker decision. Still, the CEA could be carried out even without a monetary constraint, as one can also notice from the reviewed articles. And since in our case, the analysis has started from a CBA, and a CEA is a special kind of CBA, we will carry out the cost-effectiveness analysis as if it was a CBA, hence with no budget constraint (Table 8).

In this case, there are no doubts that the longer the treatment, the more TCM allows to decrease the incidence of DKA, as it helps avoid a DKA event at a much lower cost than that of the lower-period treatment group, in both the ER and the hospitalization cases. Therefore, the treatment provided to the patients who have used TCM (in particular herbal remedies) for over six months is more cost-effective than the one that lasts less than six months, and this in turn is more cost-effective than the therapy provided to the non-TCM users.

We can check the efficiency of the longer TCM treatment through ICER as well. We are going to calculate, in particular, the ICER for the longer treatment (TCM1) with respect to the less-than-six months' therapy (TCM2) on one side, and the non-TCM user group session (TCM3) on the other, through the following formulas:

- $ICER_{TCM1/TCM2} = (C_{TCM1} - C_{TCM2})/(E_{TCM1} - E_{TCM2})$
- $ICER_{TCM1/TCM3} = (C_{TCM1} - C_{TCM3})/(E_{TCM1} - E_{TCM3})$

Table 9 represents the ICER results.

Since all the incremental costs are negative and incremental effectiveness is positive, all four points fall into the SE quadrant, where they are considered cost-effective. Therefore, the TCM interventions presented in this study are all cost-effective in general, regardless of their duration (Fig. 2).

Also, $TCM_{1/3}(ER) < TCM_{1/2}(ER)$, which means that the longest TCM intervention is more cost-effective with respect to the shortest one, than it is with respect to the medium therapy in the ER case. On the other hand, $TCM_{1/2}(H) < TCM_{1/3}(H)$, meaning that the intervention lasting over six months is more cost-effective with respect to the medium term than to shortest treatment, for the hospitalization care. This result, however, might not be relevant, as the cost difference of this option is relatively larger than the effectiveness difference, meaning less cost-effectiveness.

Table 9. ICERs for ER and Hospitalization.

	$ICER_{TCM1/TCM2}$	$ICER_{TCM1/TCM3}$
ER	–114,750 ($TCM_{1/2}$–ER)	–3,141.94 ($TCM_{1/3}$–ER)
Hospitalization	–1,642,125 ($TCM_{1/2}$–H)	–49,993.5 ($TCM_{1/3}$–H)

Source: Authors' own representation.

Figure 2. Incremental Cost-Effectiveness Plane (NT$) for ER and Hospitalization.

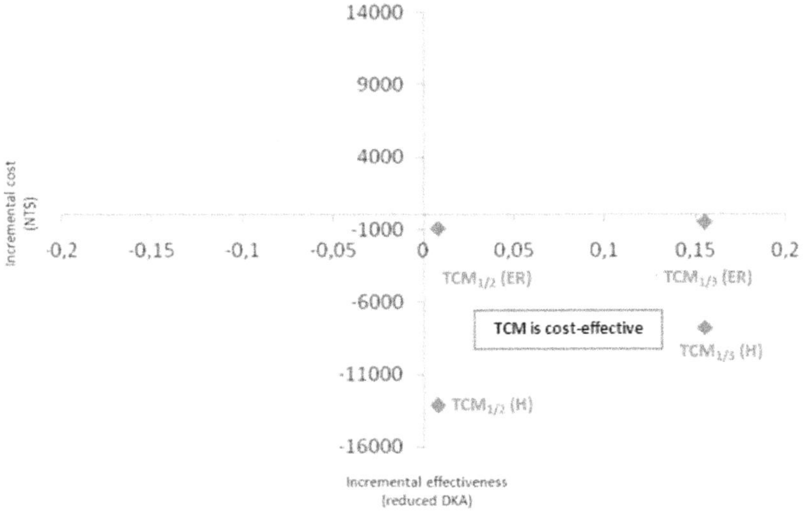

Source: Authors' own representation.

REFERENCES

1. Brent, R. J. (2003). *Cost-Benefit Analysis and Health Care Evaluations* (Edward Elgar Publishing Limited, Cheltenham, UK).
2. Kennedy, D. A., Hart, J. & Seely, D. (2009). "Cost effectiveness of natural health products: A systematic review of randomized clinical trials," *Evidence-Based Complementary and Alternative Medicine*, 6(3): 297–304.
3. EduCheer (2016). "Applying economic tools to health care setting." Available at: http://educheer.com/applying-economic-tools-to-health-care-setting/. Accessed 2 April 2017.
4. Gavura, S. (2012). "Don't call CAM "cost-effective" unless it's actually effective," *Science-Based Medicine*. Available at: https://www.science-basedmedicine.org/dont-call-cam-cost-effective-unless-its-actually-effective/. Accessed 2 April 2017.
5. Jabbour, M., Sapko, M., Miller, D., Weiss, L. & Gross, M. (2009). "Economic evaluation in acupuncture: Past and future," *The American Acupuncturist*, 49: 11–17.
6. Herman, P. M., Poindexter, B. L., Witt, C. M. *et al.* "Are complementary-therapies and integrative care cost-effective? A systematic review of

economic evaluations," *BMJ Open*, 2: e001046. doi: 10.1136/bmjopen-2012-001046.
7. Liao, Y., Lin, C., Li, T. & Lin, J. (2012). "Utilization pattern of traditional Chinese medicine for liver cancer patients in Taiwan," *BMC Complementary and Alternative Medicine*, 12.
8. Wang, L., Suo, S., Li, J., Hu, Y., Li, P., Wang, Y. & Hu, H. (2016). "An investigation Into Traditional Chinese Medicine Hospitals in China: Development trend and medical service innovation," *International Journal of Health Policy and Management*, 5.
9. Florio, M., Mafii, S., Atkinson, G., de Rus, G., Evans, D., Ponti, M., Genco, M., Parolin, R., Vignetti, S., Bollati, J., Giglio, M., Panza, G. & Sartori, D. (2008). *Guide to Cost Benefit Analysis of Investment Projects* (European Commission, Bruxelles).
10. Li, Y., Xi, H., Zhu, S., Yu, N., Wang, J., Li, Y., Yu, G., Ma, X., Zhang, J. & Zhao, L. (2014). "Cost-effectiveness analysis of combined Chinese Medicine and Western Medicine for ischemic stroke patients," *Chinese Journal of Integrative Medicine*, 20(8): 570–584.
11. Fenwick, E., Marshall, D. A., Levy, A. R. & Nichol, G. (2006). "Using and interpreting cost-effectiveness acceptability curves: An example using data from a trial of management strategies for a trial fibrillation," *BMC Health Services Research*, 6.
12. Lien, A. S., Jiang, Y., Mou, C., Sun, M., Gau, B. & Yen, H. (2016). "Integrative traditional Chinese medicine therapy reduces the risk of diabetic ketoacidosis in patients with type 1 diabetes mellitus," *Journal of Ethnopharmacology*, 191: 324–330.

Chapter 12

Evaluating the Use of TCM Through the Theory of Planned Behavior: A Consumer Survey Analysis

Olena Liakh

1. INTRODUCTION

This chapter introduces the concept of Theory of Planned Behavior (TPB) and presents the results and analysis of a consumer survey based on TPB, which is also aimed at filling the gap of knowledge with respect to the European consumer's awareness of Traditional Chinese Medicine (TCM) and the factors influencing their use of TCM. The original TPB model was extended in this case by testing three additional healthcare variables: both the health status and "having a health insurance" had an extremely weak correlation to intention, while the "presence of a local TCM practitioner" was moderately related to the frequency of use of TCM. Overall, the descriptive analysis suggests that the intention to use TCM seems to be on a transition toward a more positive attitude, despite the majority of Europeans still expected to turn to a GP in the first place. The most important limit to the diffusion of TCM among the European population appeared to be their lack of knowledge on the potential benefits of TCM, which is something that could serve as a motivation for the development of TCM knowledge diffusion national programs by decision makers.

2. THEORY OF PLANNED BEHAVIOR: AN OVERVIEW

TPB is a social cognitive framework according to which an individual's intention to perform a given behavior is a central concept in this theory. Behavioral intention (BI), a proxy of the actual behavior, is an indicator of how much of an effort people are willing to exert in order to perform the behavior in question: the stronger the intention to engage in a behavior, the higher the possibility of occurrence of that behavior, provided that the behavior in question is under volitional control (is intentional).

According to the TPB, there are three direct determinants of the strength of BI:

- Attitude Toward the Behavior (AB): It refers to the extent to which individuals view a particular behavior favorably (or unfavorably).
- Subjective Norm (SN): It measures the perceived social pressure to engage in the behavior.
- Perceived Behavioral Control (PBC): It evaluates the extent to which individuals believe that they are able to perform the behavior with ease (or difficulty), which depends on some non-motivational factors (e.g., time, money, skills, cooperation of others).

As a general rule, an individual's intention to perform a certain behavior should be stronger, the greater the PBC, and the more favorable AB and SN.[a]

3. EVALUATING THE BEHAVIOR OF EUROPEAN CONSUMERS TOWARD TCM

The present chapter contributes to the assessment of the European consumer behavior with respect to TCM and the relative treatments, by using

[a] Ajzen, I. (1991). "The theory of planned behavior," *Organizational Behavior and Human Decision Processes*, Vol. 50, 1991, pp. 179–211.

the concepts and tools provided by the TPB. In particular, the main purpose of this study is to try and understand which of the three constructs of BI are the most significant, in terms of influencing the use of TCM. Five additional variables were tested, in an attempt to give an idea of the possible extension of the original TPB model with respect to studies in TCM.

3.1. *Questionnaire*

The survey consisted of five sections related to the following aspects of TPB: Intention (6 items); Attitude (9 items) — Instrumental and experiential aspects; Perceived norm (8 items) — Injunctive and descriptive aspects; Perceived behavioral control (4 items) — Capacity and autonomy aspects; Personal information (9 items) — Collected basic demographic information of participants.

3.2. *Participants*

The questionnaire was distributed among people who have used TCM as well as those who have never tried it. The survey was conducted both online and through direct contact with the respondents, and a total of 115 questionnaires were collected. Of the participants, 67% were female and 33% male, with ages ranging from 21 to 79 years (the average age was 47 years). In terms of geographic location, most respondents were located in Italy (82%), while the others lived in Belgium, Spain, Latvia, the UK, and only one outside the EU (in China).

3.3. *Intention*

This section gathered information on the frequency and reasons for using TCM as well as the involvement with the relative treatments. First of all, in a standard situation, only a mere 7% affirmed to choose a TCM Practitioner (TCMP) over a General Medical Practitioner (GMP) when feeling sick, while those who chose the GMP accounted for a whole 63% (Fig. 1).

Most explanations for this trend, however, can be found among the reasons stated by those who chose the answer "It depends on the situation" (30%): according to most respondents, GMPs should be consulted

Figure 1. Question 1 — GP or TCMP?

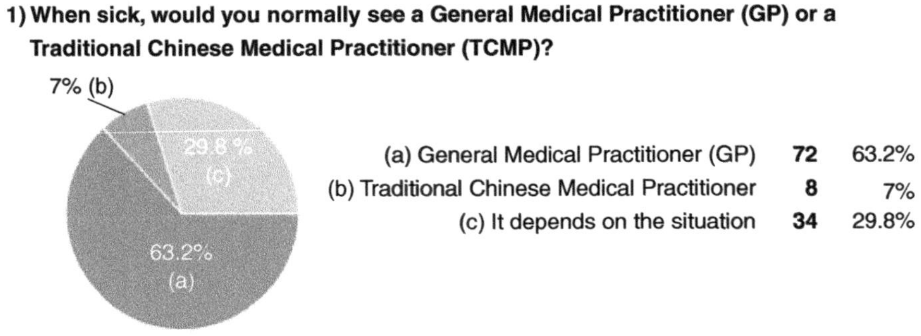

Source: Google Forms.

first as they can help deal with common diseases and general pain, then depending on the seasonal problems and only if needed, a TCMP could be consulted, for a small range of symptoms, including migraine, sciatica, and dizziness (this answer was founded on a previous experience with TCM). Also, some participants specified that they would rather see a homeopathy doctor or a phytotherapist.

Among those who tried TCM, 42% have used or are still using acupuncture. The next most popular therapy was the massage (14%) and the cupping therapy (7%). Only 5% of the respondents had experience with Chinese herbs and decoctions, and one of the participants mentioned Tai Chi (Fig. 2).

The frequency of consumption seemed to be quite varied, even though most people use it either rarely (24%) or on a non-regular basis (26%) (Fig. 3).

When enquired about the type of illness that they would apply TCM to, the majority of participants responded "both chronic and acute" (46%), only 6% of them considered acute illness while 29% would use it for chronic illnesses (Fig. 4).

The reason why people choose TCM depends on the degree of trust that they have in it (37%) and also on the fact that Western Medicine (WM) was not able to solve a particular health issue (22%). About 18% of the people surveyed followed the recommendations of somebody else in using TCM. Others mentioned that they chose it because they thought it was a good complementary medical practice to WM, it worked quite

Figure 2. Question 2 — Experience with TCM?

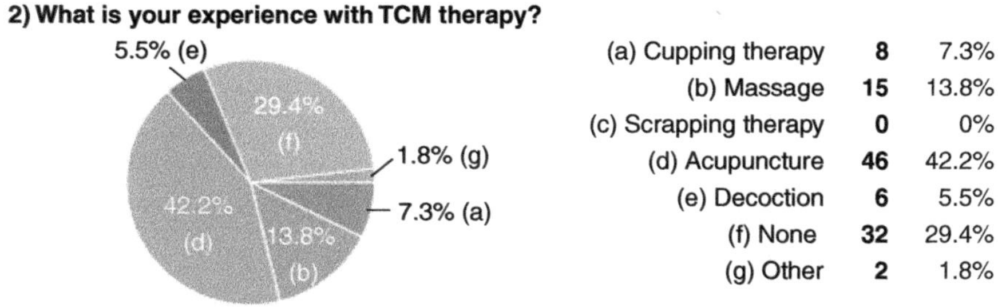

Source: Google Forms.

Figure 3. Question 3 — TCM Consumption Frequency?

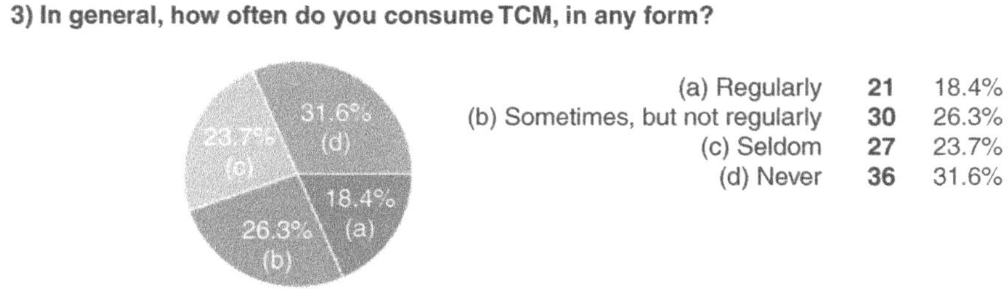

Source: Google Forms.

Figure 4. Question 4 — Type of Illness?

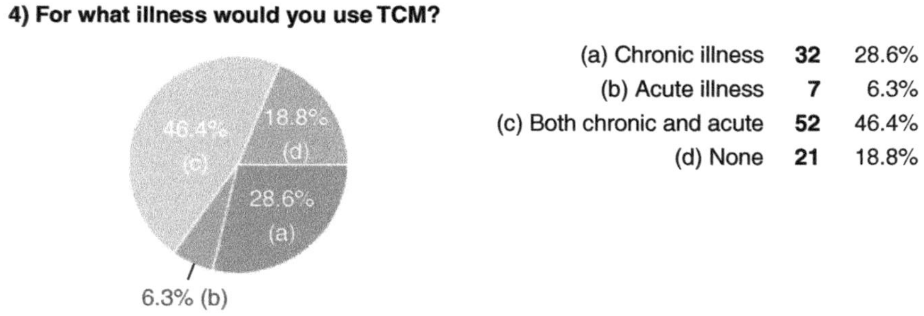

Source: Google Forms.

well according to experience, it was perceived as less invasive compared to WM, and did not harm as much (Fig. 5).

Only one person spent over €1,000 on TCM in the past years, 10 of them had expenses between €501 and €1,000, whereas 37% of participants

Figure 5. Question 5 — Reason for Choosing TCM?

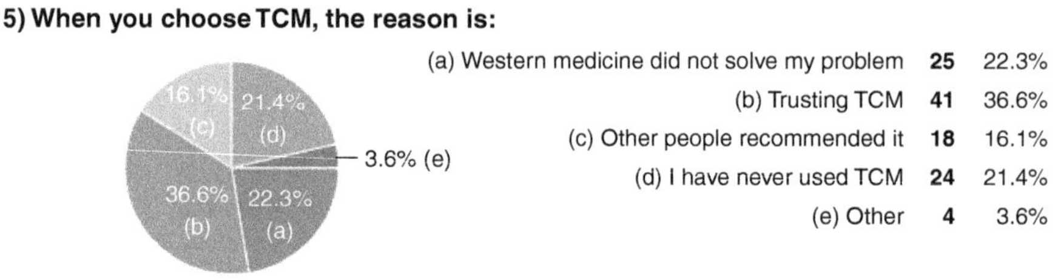

Source: Google Forms.

Figure 6. Question 6 — Average Annual Expenditure?

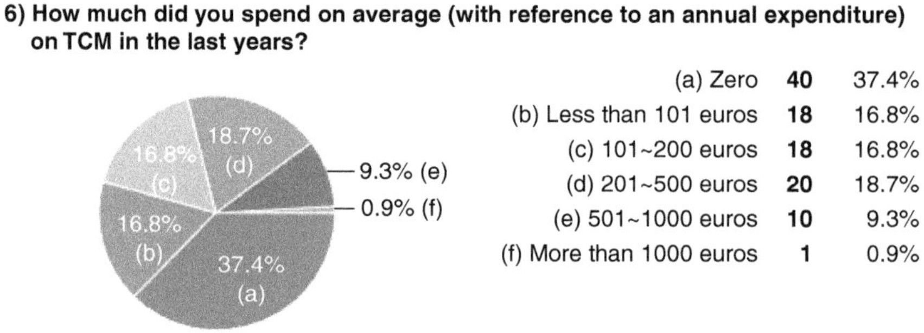

Source: Google Forms.

avoided these expenditures completely: it is to be noted that among this last category of people, not everyone was new to TCM. The null expenditure at times depended on the fact that the ones receiving the TCM treatment were either relatives or friends of the practitioners, and thus either got a very favorable discount or did not have to pay for the treatment at all (Fig. 6).

3.4. *Attitude*

Within this section, three items were measured on a 5-Likert scale ranging from 1 being "Completely ineffective" or "Slow", to 5 being "Completely effective" or "Instant" (5), with an additional option, "I do not know," in order to understand the instrumental attitudes of the respondents (null answers were not included in the computation of the mean and standard deviation, to get a more realistic result) (see Table 1).

Table 1. Mean, Standard Deviation and Percentage (Questions 7, 9, 14).

Item	Mean ± SD	Completely Ineffective (1)	(2)	(3)	(4)	Completely Effective (5)
TCM is	3.59 ± 1.01	3.6%	6.4%	30.9%	32.7%	17.3%
CHM is	3.20 ± 1.10	6.1%	11.3%	28.7%	19.1%	9.6%
1.1.1.1		**Slow (1)**	**(2)**	**(3)**	**(4)**	**Instant (5)**
Effects of CHM, compared with WM	2.51 ± 1.01	14.8%	13%	27.8%	10.4%	0%

Source: Author's own representation.

With this set of questions, participants were asked to rate the general efficacy of TCM, and Traditional Chinese Herbal Medicine (CHM) in particular, from where we could get an overall understanding of how favorably they perceived it. TCM and CHM were evaluated as a little more than neither ineffective/nor effective on average (3.59 ± 1.01 and 3.20 ± 1.10) and CHM's effects were a little slow on average, according to respondents (2.51 ± 1.01). A very small portion agreed on TCM's (17%) and CHM's (10%) complete effectiveness, and most of the respondents preferred to remain neutral, saying that TCM and CHM could be effective for some pathologies but not for others (same goes for the question on the effects of CHM). Even fewer participants stated that TCM (4%) and CHM (6%) were ineffective; however, a larger number of people said that it was somewhat effective (33% for TCM, 19% for CHM), confirming that, overall, patients tend to trust this type of medical care (as already seen in question no. 5, 37% of patients stated that their reason for choosing it was because they trusted it, thus demonstrating that their intention to use TCM depends on how much they perceive it an effective practice). Nobody rated the effects of CHM as instant, on the contrary, close to around 13–15% said they were slow or somewhat slow. Only 10% rated them as somewhat fast.

To be noted is that, for each question, there were also some people who answered "I do not know," rated as zero, which was not relevant for the computation of the mean. Nevertheless, these answers were equally relevant for the purpose of our study, as they allowed us to capture the degree of knowledge on TCM of European patients: only 9% of the respondents were not able to say whether TCM is effective or not, however, 25% of them could not evaluate how much CHM was effective (this confirms what was already noted in Chapter 2, that there is still little acceptance of CHM as an effective TCM treatment) and 33.9% of the studied population was not able to rate the speed of its effects (and among this proportion were also people who have already tried TCM in the form of other therapies).

As an explanation of the above results, we have to analyze the additional multiple-choice questions on how patients regard TCM. We can see, for example, that some people would still not completely rely on it: slightly more than 36% of participants thought than TCM should be used complementarily with WM, and this is consistent with the percentages of the neutral answers to the 5-Likert scale questions. Moreover, 9% of respondents agreed that it cures the symptoms but not the disease. Yet, nearly a quarter of them (22%) reckoned that TCM was an effective therapy (consistently with the proportions of answer 4 in the questions above) and 14% said that according to them it cures both symptoms and diseases (Fig. 7).

A series of questions then considered the advantages, disadvantages, and limits of TCM. Among the most frequently mentioned strengths of TCM were fewer side effects (43%) and the fact that it can prevent the disease and restore health (23%). Fewer people thought that WM cures symptoms while TCM cures diseases (9%), and according to a very small proportion only, TCM could cure incurable pathologies (5%) and is less expensive (2%) (Fig. 8).

Figure 7. Question 8 — Opinion on TCM?

8) You think that TCM is:

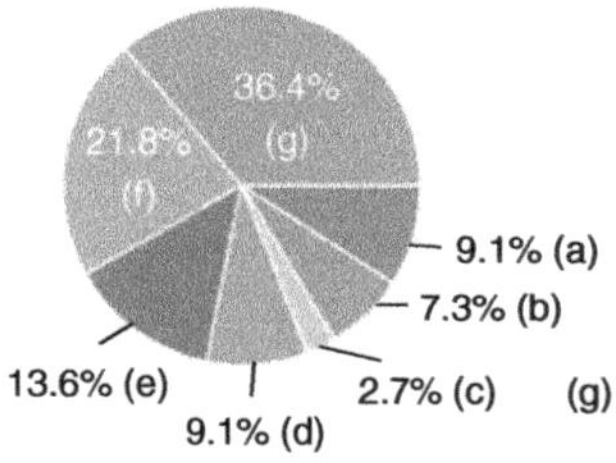

(a) Unscientific	**10**	9.1%
(b) Only an auxiliary therapy	**8**	7.3%
(c) Just a prevention of the disease	**3**	2.7%
(d) Cures the symptoms, not the disease	**10**	9.1%
(e) Cures the symptoms and cures the disease	**15**	13.6%
(f) An effective therapy	**24**	21.8%
(g) To be used complementarily with Western Medicine	**40**	36.4%

Source: Google Forms.

Figure 8. Question 13 — Main Advantage?

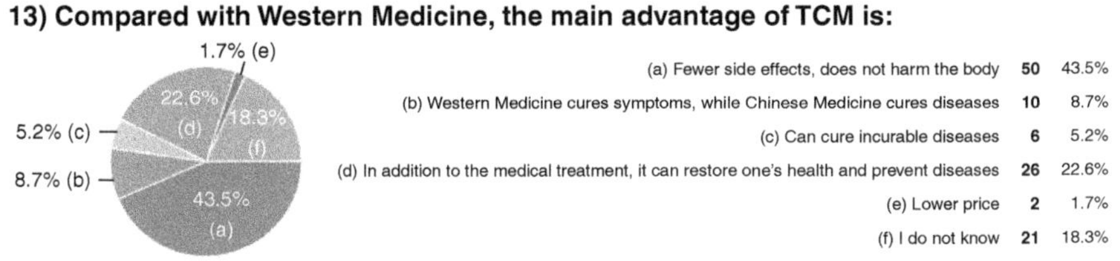

Source: Google Forms.

Figure 9. Question 12 — Main Disadvantage?

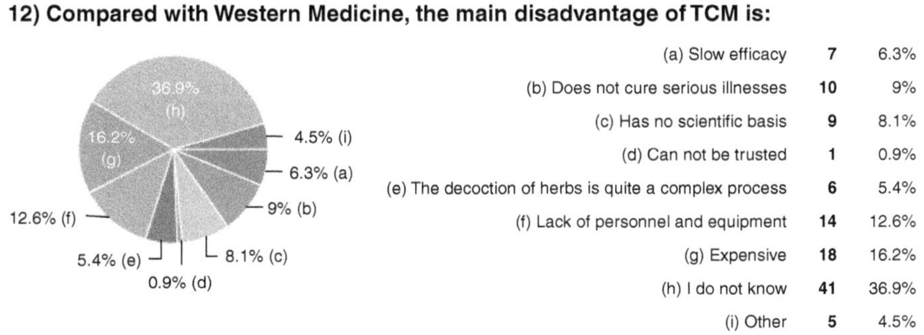

Source: Google Forms.

Regarding the main disadvantages of TCM, its cost and the lack of personnel and equipment were chosen more frequently (16% and 13%, respectively). Then around 10% of participants said that it is not able to cure serious illnesses, and about 6% of them said that the decoction of herbs is a complex process and its efficacy is slow. Only 1% of respondents states that they did not trust TCM (Fig. 9).

It was also said that the TCM lacks a scientific theory in its support, with respect to WM (24%), that its effects are slower (15%) that the decoction of herbs is not only inconvenient (7%) but the herbs themselves are not seen as having a good taste (which demonstrates how CHM products are still perceived as simple food supplements and not as part of a broader therapy).

Among other additional shortcomings that were mentioned were the current lack of diffusion of knowledge on TCM among the population,

Figure 10. Question 15 — Shortcomings?

15) What shortcomings do you see in TCM?

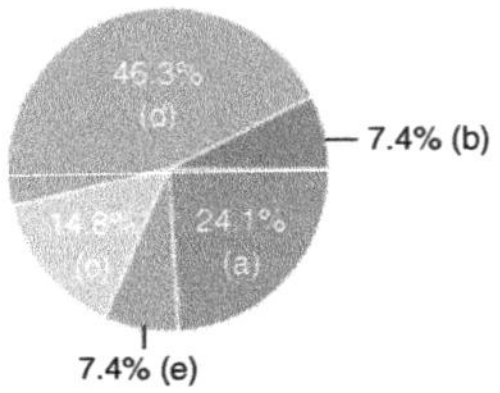

(a) Lack of a scientific theory with respect to Western Medicine	**26**	24.1%
(b) Chinese herbs have a bitter taste and it is inconvenient to boil them	**8**	7.4%
(c) Slow effects	**16**	14.8%
(d) I do not know	**50**	46.3%
(e) Other	**8**	7.4%

Source: Google Forms.

Figure 11. Question 10 — Source of Knowledge?

10) How did you learn about TCM?

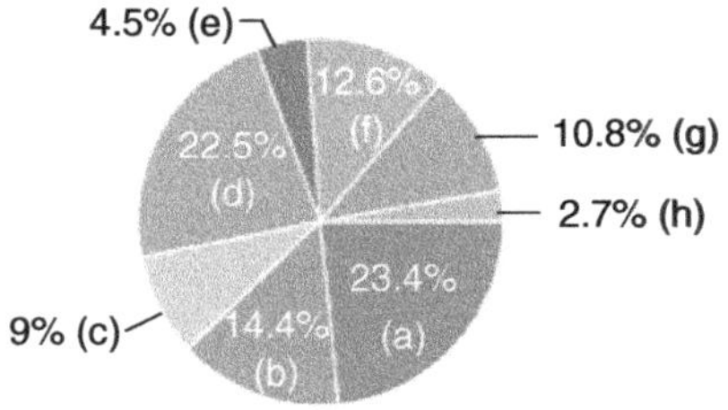

(a) Firsthand experience	**26**	23.4%
(b) Family members	**16**	14.4%
(c) Books or networks	**10**	9%
(d) Acquaintances and friends	**25**	22.5%
(e) The media	**5**	4.5%
(f) Doctors	**14**	12.6%
(g) I do not know about it	**12**	10.8%
(h) Other	**3**	2.7%

Source: Google Forms.

especially in terms of benefits that could be obtained (the reason why was said to be the idea that Western society has on Chinese medical practices). Additionally, the scarcity of TCM experts and competent Chinese patent medicine products within the national territory were seen as a limit, however, a good proportion of the "Other" answer was "None" (somebody used it regularly, even in combination with WM, and saw no shortcomings) (Fig. 10).

Concerning the experiential aspect of patients' attitude, two questions enquired on how they first came into contact with TCM and who they normally resorted to in order to receive the treatment. "Acquaintances and friends" and "Firsthand experience" were the most common cases of first-time contact with TCM (around 23%), then we find family members and doctors, accounting both for around 14%, and finally books, the Internet (9%), and the media (4%). Others mentioned work and Tai Chi/Qi Gong

Figure 12. Question 11 — Treatment Facility?

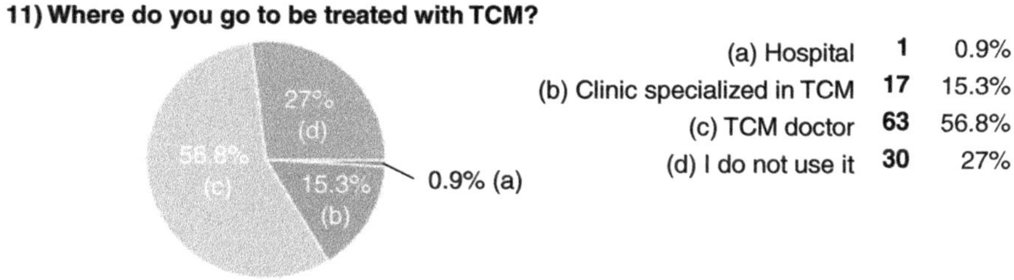

Source: Google Forms.

courses, and some responded that it is an integral part of the national culture (China) (Fig. 11).

Most patients go to a specialized TCM doctor to be treated with any of the previously mentioned TCM therapies (57%), while 15% of them prefer visiting a clinic that is specialized in TCM while only 1 respondent chose the hospital (Fig. 12).

3.5. *Perceived norm*

A 5-Likert scale measured both injunctive (I) and descriptive (D) aspects of the adoption of TCM practices (see Table 2).

The approval of Chinese herbs consumption by friends and colleagues was rated as 3.25 on average, on a scale from 1 to 5: 22% of the respondents said that they neither approved nor disapproved their consumption of CHM, while 16% of them affirmed that they somewhat approved it. However, only 5% of participants said they would be willing to comply with the advice of others, and the majority (27%) of them said it would depend on the situation. In order to understand these results, we have to analyze them in combination with the other questions in this session. So, for example, the reason why very few respondents were willing to follow somebody else's advice on their consumption of CHM was because, in almost 50% of cases, the decision on whether to purchase Chinese herbs or not depended on themselves only. When, instead, they relied on the advice of significant others, they mostly followed doctors' and friends and family's recommendations (16% and 13%, respectively). The advertising effect exerted an influence in only 3% of the cases, while pharmacists'

Table 2. Mean, Standard Deviation, and Percentage (Questions 22, 23).

Item	Mean ± SD	Completely Disagree (1)	(2)	(3)	(4)	Completely Agree (5)
(I) Your friends/ colleagues approve of your consumption of Chinese herbs	3.25 ± 1.02	2.6%	8.8%	21.9%	15.8%	6.1%
(D) You are willing to follow their advice	2.79 ± 1.20	14.2%	8.8%	27.4%	12.4%	5.3%

Source: Author's own representation.

Figure 13. Question 20 — Purchase Influencing Factors?

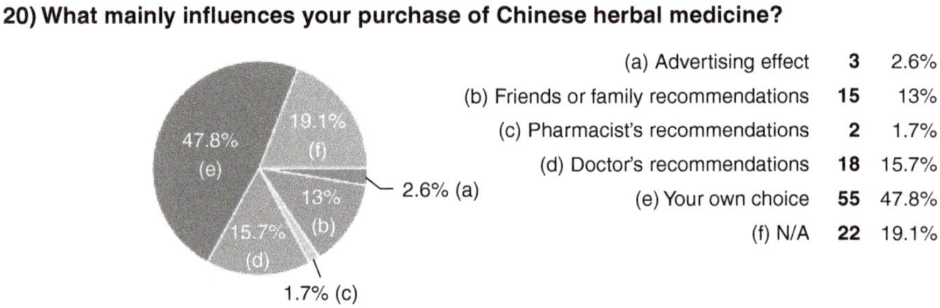

Source: Google Forms.

Figure 14. Question 21 — Friends' Experience with TCM?

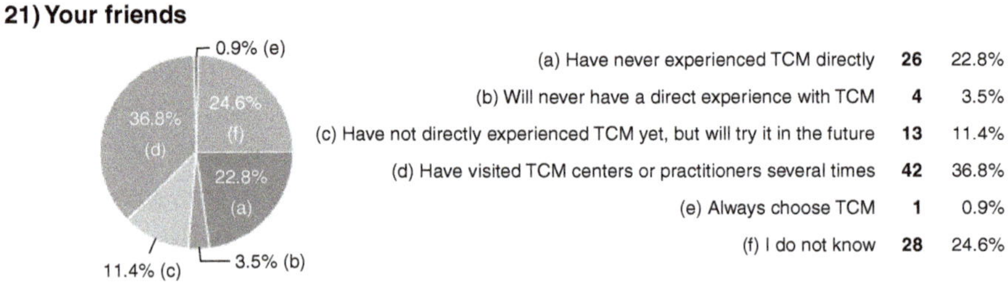

Source: Google Forms.

recommendations were followed by as little as 3% of the examined population (Fig. 13).

Among those significant others that recommend the use of TCM, 37% had visited TCM centers or practitioners several times and 1% always

Figure 15. Question 17 — People Recommending Its Use?

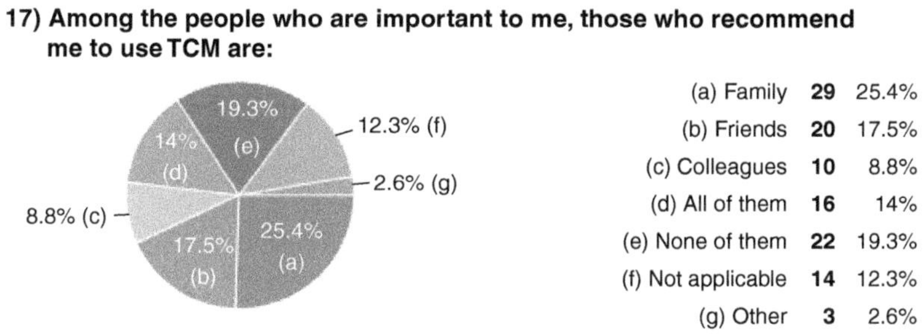

Source: Google Forms.

Figure 16. Question 16 — Most Valuable Opinions?

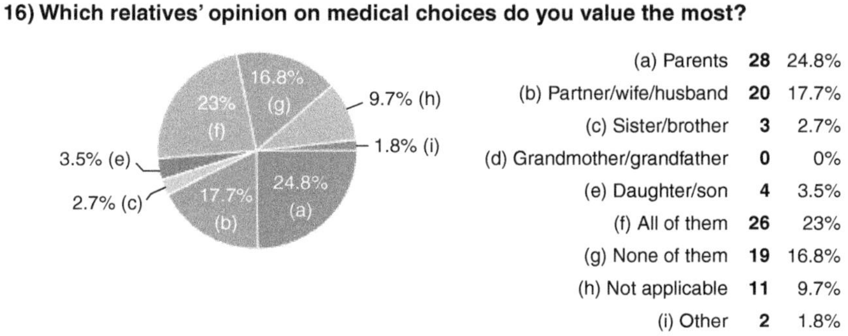

Source: Google Forms.

chose TCM. About 23% of these significant others have never experienced TCM directly, while 11% would like to try it sooner or later, and 3% do not have any intention of approaching this type of medical care (Fig. 14).

Also, significant others recommending the use of TCM were normally either family members (25%), friends (17%) or "family, friends and colleagues" altogether (14%). About 3% of the people who chose "Other" mentioned that, to them, doctors (especially the acupuncturist and neurologist) were the ones who provide the most important advice on the adoption of TCM (Fig. 15).

In terms of general medical choices, the relatives that were considered among those significant others influencing participants' decisions the most were mostly the parents (25%) and the partner (18%). In just a few cases (3%), the opinion provided by one's siblings or son/daughter was

Figure 17. Question 18 — Relatives Influencing Decisions?

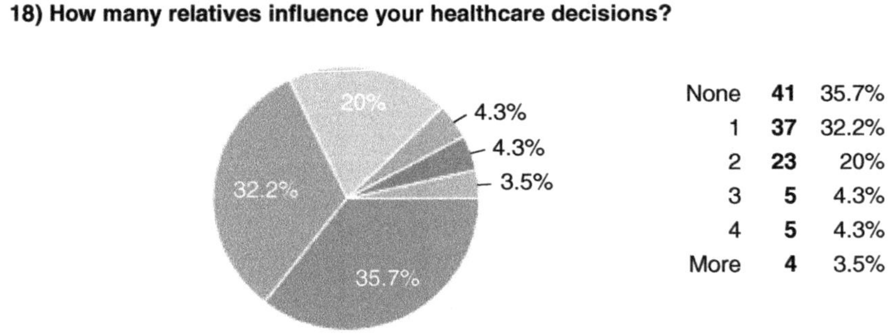

Source: Google Forms.

Figure 18. Question 19 — People Disapproving Its Use?

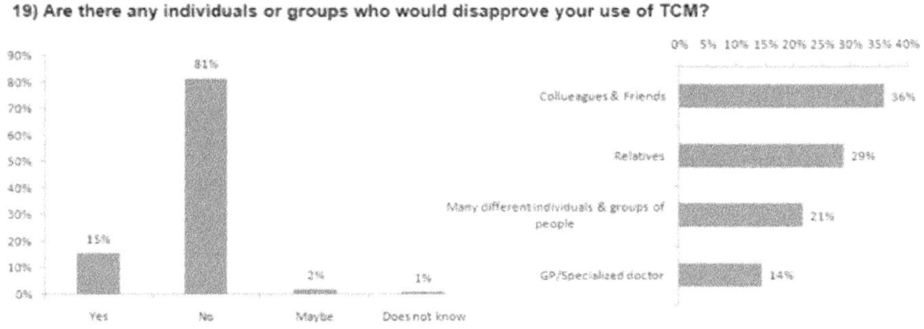

Source: Author's own representation.

considered important. There were also many respondents who affirmed to value the opinion of all of the previously mentioned relatives equally when it comes to medical decisions (Fig. 16).

Generally speaking, most participants affirmed that at least one (32%) or two (20%) relatives influenced their healthcare decisions. The majority of them (36%), however, said that those types of decisions depended on themselves only (Fig. 17).

Finally, when asked whether there were any groups of people who would not approve them using any form of TCM, a very high proportion of respondents answered "No" (somebody also added "as long as that is not the sole or major method" used). Those who replied positively (15%) stated that colleagues and friends would be against the use of TCM in the majority of cases (36%), then the relatives come at second place (29%), while 21% wrote that there would be many different people disapproving it coming from various group, and finally 14% of the population examined said it would be the general practitioner/specialized doctor (Fig. 18).

3.6. *Perceived behavioral control*

For this indicator, two items, on different Likert scales, were used to assess the perceived capacity of the respondents to evaluate their need of TCM. Since the second question had positive answers ("Definitely yes") starting from 1 in the questionnaire, all the answers had to be reversed in order to adapt it to the format of the first question (1 as negative answer) (see Table 3).

On average, respondents reckoned their capacity to identify their need for TCM, when they have some symptoms, as a little less than somewhat good (4.16 ± 2.11). Around 15% of them reported to have either a very good or somewhat good ability to assess it, while 13% of participants affirmed that their ability was very poor. Also, some of the respondents were pretty convinced of their own opinions: 18% of them were absolutely sure that they would consume Chinese herbs if they were sold in the form of beverages, also a mere 7% stated that they would never try it. Nevertheless, about 22% of the population was unsure yet and decided to

Table 3. Mean, Standard Deviation, and Percentage (Questions 24, 27).

Item	Mean ± SD	Very Poor (1)	(2)	(3)	(4)	(5)	(6)	Very Good (7)
Ability to assess the need for TCM	4.16 ± 2.11	13.2%	8.8%	7.9%	9.6%	14.9%	8.8%	14.9%
1.1.1.2		Definitely No (1)	(2)	(3)	(4)	Definitely Yes (5)		
You would use CHM if made into beverages	3.57 ± 1.20	7%	3.5%	21.9%	21.9%	18.4%		

Source: Author's own representation.

Figure 19. Question 26 — Biggest Constraint to Its Use?

26) What is the biggest constraint for you in using TCM?

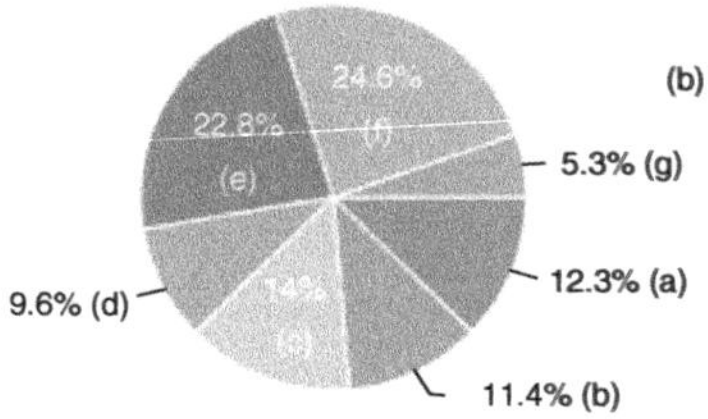

(a) Price	**14**	12.3%
(b) Being suspicious of its final effects on health	**13**	11.4%
(c) Too many fake practitioners/products	**16**	14%
(d) Lack of professional consultants	**11**	9.6%
(e) Lack of adequate knowledge	**26**	22.8%
(f) None	**28**	24.6%
(g) N/A	**6**	5.3%

Source: Google Forms.

Figure 20. Question 25 — Constraints to Its Adoption?

25) What factors or circumstances would make it difficult or impossible for you to adopt TCM?

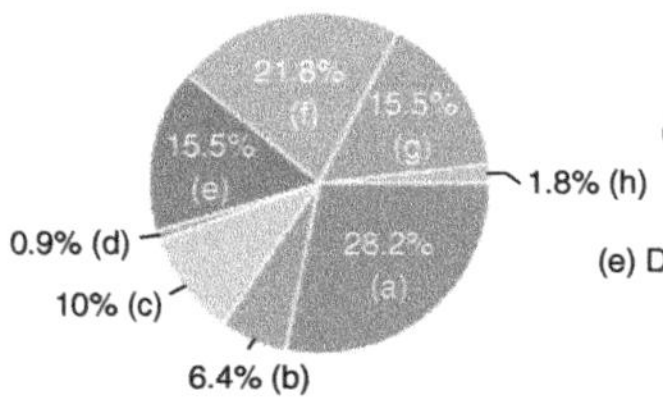

(a) Not having much knowledge about TCM	**31**	28.2%
(b) Not trusting TCM	**7**	6.4%
(c) Not trusting local practitioners who are expert in TCM	**11**	10%
(d) Bad taste of the herbs	**1**	0.9%
(e) Difficulty in identifying fake herbs or cheating practitioners	**17**	15.5%
(f) None	**24**	21.8%
(g) N/A	**17**	15.5%
(h) Other	**2**	1.8%

Source: Google Forms.

remain neutral on the matter (saying that it would depend on the recommendations of the doctor in particular, meaning that their ability to assess their need of TCM would also depend on doctors). To assess the degree of control, and thus the autonomy, over the actual usage of TCM, the participants were asked about the obstacles that currently limit, or would limit in the future, their adoption of TCM practices. Ranking the current constraints in the utilization of TCM starting from the biggest one, we find the lack of adequate knowledge (25%) as the first choice (as we assumed earlier), then comes the lack of trust toward local experts in TCM/TCM products (14%), price (12%), the distrust in the final effects on health (11%), and finally the lack of professional consultants (10%). Nevertheless, the majority affirmed to have no constraint in the use of TCM (Fig. 19).

Regarding the hypothetical factors that could prevent (in the future) a patient from adopting TCM treatments, the lack of knowledge, once again, was considered as a major cause (28%), then came the difficulty in identifying fake herbs or practitioners (15%), and the lack of trust in local TCM experts (as already seen in the previous question), followed by a general distrust in TCM (6%) and the bad taste of the herbs (1%). Other constraints mentioned were the bad quality of herbs and the economic situation of the individual (Fig. 20).

3.7. *Strength of relations between indicators*

In order to obtain a general understanding of how much the measurable direct indicators of BI, and some additional factors, influenced the intention to use TCM, we can run a rough correlation matrix analysis. It is to be taken into consideration, though, that only a few questions were selected as representative variables: a complete evaluation of the intention, attitude, subjective norm, and perceived behavioral control requires that all data available from the complete set of questions are measured through items that can be directly scored or first recoded then scored. In our case, only the 5- and 7-Likert score questions could be used to assess AB, SN, and PBC. There was no Likert score question measuring intention, so the answers to the first question regarding the choice between GP and Traditional Chinese Medicine Practitioner (TCMP) were reconverted to dummy variables indicating the choice of TCM over WM (scored as 1) or not (scored as 0) in order to generate an intention indicator. An additional measurable item was chosen to represent intention (so as to compare which one was the best approximate), that is frequency of use, which was recoded in order to provide numerical values: the correlation matrix displays a strong relationship between these two variables describing intention, which confirms the successful choice of the indicators. In addition, since the TPB researches on TCM have demonstrated the importance of "Gender" and "Age" to evaluate behavior, these two additional demographic indicators were included in the analysis. Finally, an additional set of questions related to healthcare were presented in the questionnaire, and since they are relevant to the purpose of this study, they were also incorporated to check their relevance (Fig. 21).

To begin with, general demographics such as gender and age showed a weak to extremely weak positive correlation to the intention to use

Figure 21. Correlations Among TPB Variables, Demographic, and Health Indicators.

Correlations among TPB variables, demographic and health indicators

	Intention		**Attitude**			**Norms**		**Control**		**Demographics**		**Health**		
	Freq. use	*TCM*	*Q7*	*Q9*	*Q14*	*IN-Q22*	*DN-Q23*	*Q24*	*Q27*	*Gender*	*Age*	*HS*	*Insur.*	*TCMP*
Freq. use	1,00													
TCM	0,61	1,00												
Q7	0,47	0,46	1,00											
Q9	0,07	0,28	0,22	1,00										
Q14	0,21	0,23	0,37	0,21	1,00									
Q22	0,25	0,09	0,25	-0,08	-0,11	1,00								
Q23	-0,14	-0,06	-0,06	-0,05	-0,24	0,40	1,00							
Q24	0,40	0,54	0,58	0,12	0,19	0,34	-0,09	1,00						
Q27	-0,03	0,02	-0,05	-0,17	-0,06	0,03	0,12	0,06	1,00					
Gender	0,23	0,04	0,21	-0,14	0,21	0,13	-0,17	0,29	-0,05	1,00				
Age	0,06	0,14	0,14	0,10	0,08	-0,11	0,06	0,00	-0,07	-0,10	1,00			
HS	-0,04	-0,10	-0,05	-0,09	0,08	0,09	0,00	-0,06	0,04	-0,08	-0,32	1,00		
Insur.	0,08	0,07	-0,03	0,00	-0,04	0,13	0,18	0,05	0,21	-0,12	-0,14	0,08	1,00	
TCMP	0,43	0,28	0,42	-0,03	0,19	0,26	0,04	0,39	0,11	0,28	-0,02	-0,21	0,03	1,00

Source: Author's own representation.

TCM, meaning that, in very rare cases, being a woman (also scored as 1) in her 50s (the majority of respondents) was a highly possible characteristic prompting the adoption of TCM practices. For what concerns the healthcare variables, both the health status (HS) and "having a health insurance" (Insur.) had an extremely weak correlation to intention. Only the "presence of a local TCMP" had better results: it was weakly related to the "use of TCM over WM" (TCM) but seemed to have a moderate influence on the frequency of use of TCM (Freq. use), therefore, the closer the TCM doctor or clinic, the more frequent the visits to that clinic or doctor. The next block of variables examined are the TPB indicators, hence "Attitude" measured by questions 7, 9, and 14 on instrumental attitudes; "Norms" measured both though injunctive (IN-Q22) and descriptive (DN-Q23) aspects; and "Control" described by capacity-related aspects. Within attitude, question 7 seemed to have an almost moderate degree of correlation to question 14, so the people who perceived a high TCM efficacy were somewhat likely to judge the effects of CHM as almost instant. The same variable seemed to have an even better correlation to the "presence of a local TCMP" variable (so, the closer the TCM healthcare structure/practitioner, the more occasions for trying TCM therapies out and build an acceptable perception of its efficiency). What is also interesting to notice is that this question was almost strongly related to a question from the PBC section: it appears that people who rate TCM as efficient are also able to identify their own need for TCM in many occasions. Question 7 was the only question of its group (attitude) to be moderately related to both indicators of intention: people choosing TCM over WM, and especially those who use it on a regular basis (with an even stronger coefficient) are more likely to perceive TCM's usefulness. The other two questions had a weak correlation to intention, and this could be due to the fact that CHM resulted as a relatively unknown and distrusted practice to the majority of respondents, according to the descriptive results of this study. For what concerns the questions on subjective norms, even though they showed a relatively weak degree of correlation to intention, they were moderately dependent on each other: when significant others approve the patient's use of Chinese herbs, the latter are more likely to follow their advice and imitate their behavior relatively to TCM. The last set of questions regarding perceived behavioral control had an extremely weak relation to one another, and only the question regarding the capacity to identify one's need of TCM seemed to have a moderate influence on BI: the more people are able to identify their need for TCM, the more frequently they choose it over WM. But since the evaluation is limited and provides just an approximated general evaluation of the influence of each variable on the intention to use TCM over WM, it should be combined with the descriptive analysis presented above.

4. DISCUSSION

From the descriptive analysis, we can sum up that, even though a big majority of Europeans still prefers going to a GP first (and most of them does not use TCM at all), the intention of these patients to use TCM seems to be on a transition toward a more positive attitude: they affirmed that they have such a degree of trust in TCM to be prone to reckon that it could be equally effective in solving both chronic and acute pathologies. Also, the ones that have already tried it, have done so on a regular basis (even if not so often) and affirmed to be more familiar with acupuncture, which, as was already examined in Chapter 2, is due to the fact that this therapy is the one that has been somewhat accepted by the scientific community, and therefore by the population itself. As for the instrumental aspects within attitude toward behavior, most people ranked TCM and CHM as somewhat effective procedures and expressed the opinion that TCM cures both symptoms and diseases, confirming patients' overall trust in this medical care. The ones who did not express an opinion on TCM claimed that it was due to the limited diffusion of TCM knowledge across the national territory, leading to distrust of local TCM experts and to not being able to identify qualitative herbs and TCM services. As an advantage, TCM has fewer side effects compared with WM and is both able to prevent and restore health. The main disadvantage according to the respondents is the cost, the lack of qualified personnel and equipment, and the lack of a scientific theory in its support. When it came to describing the experiential aspect, the majority of respondents affirmed that they first came to know about TCM either through friends and acquaintances or firsthand experience. For the subjective norms, many respondents claimed that they usually took their own healthcare decisions autonomously and were, therefore, not so willing to comply with others. When they accepted the opinion of significant others, these people were mostly represented by doctors, friends, and family (parents and partners especially). With respect to TCM, they stated that no significant other would disapprove their use of TCM in most of the cases, while those significant others who recommend it have had several experiences with TCM treatments already. Within the perceived behavioral control as well, people mentioned the lack of knowledge as their main limit in adopting TCM: this obstacle appeared to be the main reason why only a very small portion of the population under examination was able to assess their need of TCM. The degree of control over TCM choices that people had seemed to be quite connected to their behavior and intention to adopt TCM, and since we have just seen that their capacity and autonomy in using and controlling the use of TCM were strongly limited by the knowledge that they had on the matter, in the future, decision makers could try to develop some governmental nation-wide programs/campaigns to promote the diffusion of knowledge related to the benefits of TCM. This is also confirmed by the positive correlation between the attitude toward TCM and the actual intention to adopt it: we have seen that since attitude is moderately related to the intention and frequency of TCM use, the more effectively TCM is perceived by patients, the more they will choose it over WM. For further knowledge to be spread, new knowledge on the topic has to be gathered. In this respect, further studies could be developed to justify the need for the diffusion of such type of TCM-related knowledge: future studies could focus, for example, on the benefits to health of TCM, measuring such variables as perceived and effective improvement in patients' health status compared with WM, or the number of side effects that appeared while going through a WM treatment compared to TCM.

BIBLIOGRAPHY

Ajzen, I. (1991). "The theory of planned behavior," *Organizational Behavior and Human Decision Processes*, 50: 179–211.

Choi, Y. (2003). "The influence of patient's satisfaction and health locus-of-control belief to the use of Chinese medical treatment in Hong Kong," Hong Kong Polytechnic University.

Lee, J., Cerreto, F. A. & Lee, J. H. (2010). "Theory of planned behavior and teachers' decisions regarding use of educational technology," *Educational Technology & Society*, 13(1): 152–164.

Mou, Y. (2016). "Predicting the use of traditional Chinese medicine health maintenance approach from cultural and spiritual perspectives," *Journal of Religion and Health*.

Rochelle, T. L., Shardlow, S. M. & Ng, S. H. (2015). "Using the Theory of Planned Behaviour to explain use of Traditional Chinese Medicine among Hong Kong Chinese in Britain," *Evidence-Based Complementary and Alternative Medicine*, (Article ID 564648): 6.

Tang, S. *et al.* (2012). "The research on knowledge inheritance behavior of old TCM experts based on the Theory of Planned Behavior," *Medicine and Society*, 25(5).

Chapter 13

Legal Framework on Health Foods in China and Food Supplements in the EU: A Comparison Study in the Perspective of TCM*

Pamela Lattanzi and Qingle Hu

1. INTRODUCTION

Foodstuffs providing health and well-being benefits due to components either naturally present or added or reduced/removed are increasing popular among Chinese and EU consumers.

The search for "natural" products, the increasing cost of many pharmaceuticals and their negative effects, as well as the growing need for a healthier life feed both Chinese and EU consumer demand for

*Albeit the chapter's unitary conception, Pamela Lattanzi drafted Sections 1, 3, 5, 5.1, 6, 6.2, 7, 7.2, 8, 8.2 and 9 while Qingle Hu drafted Sections 2, 4, 6.1, 7.1 and 8.

foodstuffs having health-enhancing properties,[1] thus going beyond the main role of food that is, since the dawn of time, the satisfaction of hunger and the provision of necessary nutrients. The rise in lifestyle- and diet-related diseases and the aging population exacerbates this trend.[2]

In 1995, the Chinese Ministry of Health designed an *ad hoc* category of food having functional and nutritional properties, named *health food.* This food category includes foodstuffs having both conventional food forms and pharmaceutical oral delivery forms (such as pills, capsules, oral solutions, etc.), the latter being the most common forms marketed.[3]

Since the first health food was approved in 1996, the Chinese health market has expanded dramatically. In 2012, the health food category counted about 12,061 domestic products and 672 imported health foods.[4]

According to the data analysis, the total amount of health food sales in Chinese market was 16.10 billion, in 2014, and RMB 18.51 billion, in 2015.[a] It is expected that the total amount of health food sales would boost to RMB 20 billion in 2020.[b]

In order to keep up with this burgeoning business, the legal framework on health food has been amended several times. The latest revision occurred in 2015, aimed at simplifying the market entry procedures and introducing more stringent safety requirements.

By contrast, the EU legal framework lacks a similar category, even if several correspondences can be found in the category of food supplements (regulated by Directive 2002/46/EC, *Food Supplements Directive*), which have pharmaceutical oral delivery forms. However, the Chinese health food category is wider than that of EU food supplements because it also embraces food with special healthcare functions having traditional food forms. In the EU, such type of food is commonly considered as "functional food." Nevertheless, there is neither a legal definition nor a specific regulation of such category, except those specific rules

---

[a] See: http://www.instrument.com.cn/news/20160627/194571.shtml, updated June 2016. Accessed May 2017.

[b] See: http://www.chyxx.com/industry/201602/389194.html, updated February 2016. Accessed May 2017.

concerning nutritional and health claims which are also applicable to food and those rules on enriched food.

The EU food supplements market also presents impressive data about its development; it is projected to grow by around 9.5% in the next few years, reaching a EUR 9 billion market value by 2020.[c]

The first aim of this chapter is to compare the Chinese legislation on health food with the EU legislation on food supplements. In order to achieve this goal, the chapter will take into consideration four main topics: the legal definitions of food, health food and food supplement, the market entry procedures, the labeling rules, and the import and export rules.

Another aim of the chapter is to detect connections between such food with health-enhancing properties and Traditional Chinese Medicine (TCM).

2. THE DEFINITION OF "FOOD" IN THE CHINESE LEGAL FRAMEWORK

Linkages between food and TCM are clearly expressed in the definition of food as laid down by the main Chinese legislation on food: the *Food Safety Law* (2015).[d] According to this law, food is defined as "any substance that has been processed or not processed that is suitable for eating and/or drinking, including substances traditionally used as food and Chinese herb medicine, excluding substances solely used for disease treatment" (Article 150). This definition is strongly linked to the Chinese cultural background, where botanical (herbal) ingredients are almost equal to TCM. This could be reasoned in two points:

(1) Chinese medicinal herbs are perceived as one kind of crop (agricultural products) even under the *Food Safety Law* (2015) (Article 49).

---

[c]Euromonitor International for Nutraingredients special edition series "Inside Europe's Food Supplements Markets," 2015.

[d]The *Food Safety Law* was enacted in 2009. In 2015, the new amendment of *Food Safety Law* was promulgated by the Chinese Food and Drug Administration (CFDA), it went into effect from October 1, 2015. This new amendment has been called the strictest *Food Safety Law* in history.

(2) There is an idea held by the Chinese, especially TCM doctors, believing that medicine and food are affine, and many Chinese have knowledge of Chinese medicinal herbs function, inheriting the ability to preparing food using herbal medicine (products). Indeed, "many herbal medicinal materials are integrated into culinary and medicinal food practice with high consumer acceptance" (Ref. 4, p. 369).

According to Article 102 of *Drugs Administration Law*, which is the basic law for drug (including TCM) regulation in China, enacted by the People's Congress in 2001, TCM includes Chinese crude drugs, prepared slices of Chinese crude drugs, and traditional Chinese medicine preparations.[e]

Among these three types of TCM, medicine preparation is truly one kind of medicine, while some kinds of crude drugs and prepared slices could be used as food in the daily life of the Chinese.

This could also explain why, in 2002, the Minister of Health, the responsible regulatory department at that time, had to attach three catalogues when it issued the *Notice on Further Standardizing Management of the Raw Materials of Health Food*, named: "Catalogue of Raw Materials for Health Food," "Catalogue of Raw Materials for Both Food and TCM," and "Catalogue of Forbidden Raw Materials for Health Food," since these catalogues make the demarcation line between food and medicine (precisely herbal medicine) more clear and set a convenient structure for better regulation of food, especially health food.[f]

---

[e] Chinese crude drugs (*zhongyaocai*) are defined by *Good Agricultural Practice for Chinese Crude Drugs* (Interim) (Article 55), as: "the raw medicinal materials from the medicinal parts of plants or animals, which are collected and primarily processed." They are the original raw materials, used for prepared slices of Chinese crude drugs.

Prepared slices of Chinese crude drugs (*zhongyaoyinpian*) are firstly defined in Chinese Pharmacopeia 2010 as "prescription medicines which are used for clinic prescription and medicine preparations directly after the processing of crude medicines."

Traditional Chinese medicine preparations (*zhongchengyao*) are only used for curing illnesses, which could only be made by prepared slices.

[f] When the regulatory power of food was transferred from Ministry of Health to CFDA in 2003, the latter continues to use these three Catalogues, even until now. However, after the implementation of the Food Safety Law 2015, new Catalogues would be issued in the not-far future.

The raw materials in the first catalogue could only be used for health food production while they are banned for food production (Article 75, Food Safety Law). Moreover, these raw materials could also be used for food production while they get the permission according to the *Administrative Rules for the Safety Examination of New Food Materials*, enacted by National Health and Family Planning Commission (NHFPC) in 2013. The raw materials listed in this catalogue are mainly Chinese medicinal herbs.

The raw materials listed in the second catalogue could be used for producing both food and TCM. As mentioned earlier, health food is one kind of food in the Chinese food safety regulatory system. Therefore, the raw materials here could be used for both food (health food) and TCM production. Similarly, the raw materials listed in this catalogue are principally Chinese medicinal herbs.

The raw materials listed in the third catalogues are forbidden for use in producing health food. They again comprise principally of Chinese medicinal herbs. The reason for banning these raw materials is also based on the TCM theory: the function of some Chinese medicinal herbs is not easy to control in the absence of professional advice, so it is not suitable for daily use as food (health food).

Thus, it could be seen that, there is a strong linkage between food (health food) and TCM in China. According to statistics, the formulae of the health food containing the TCM raw materials account for more 50% of all the approved health foods in China.[5] Specifically, the approved health foods containing the TCM raw materials from 2013 to 2015, respectively, took up 60.6%, 55.1%, and 52.6% of the entire amount of the approved health foods.[6]

3. THE DEFINITION OF "FOOD" IN THE EU LEGAL FRAMEWORK

Understandably, the EU's legal definition of food does not take TCM into consideration. Actually, it does not even take into consideration botanicals (e.g., plants and preparations made from plants, algae, fungi, or lichens) commonly used in traditional western herbal medicines as well as in food production. According to Article 2, Regulation (EC) No. 178/2002,[g] known as the *General Food Law*, food is defined as: "any substance or product, whether processed, partially processed or unprocessed, intended to be, or reasonably expected to be ingested by humans." Moreover, this provision explicitly excludes medicinal products from the category of foodstuffs.[h]

However, the demarcation line between food and medicinal products is not always clear, especially in the case of food supplements, in particular when they are produced from plants and their preparations (such as garlic or ginger) used in both food supplements and medicinal products.[7] The Court of Justice of the European Union has had several occasions to define such demarcation line and it has identified some classification criteria.[8,9]

---

[g] Regulation (EC) No. 178/2002 lays down the general principles and requirements of food law as well as the procedures in matters of food safety and establishing the European Food Safety Authority.

[h] Medicinal products are defined by Directive 2001/83/EC (the Community Code relating to medicinal products for human use) as "any substance or combination of substances advertised as having properties for treating or preventing disease in human beings; or any substance or combination of substances which may be used in or administered to human beings either with a view to restoring, correcting or modifying physiological functions by exerting a pharmacological, immunological or metabolic action, or to making a medical diagnosis." Moreover, Article 2.2 of Directive 2081/83/EC states that, in cases of doubt, where, taking into account all its characteristics, a product may fall within the definition of a "medicinal product" and within the definition of a product covered by other Community legislation, the provisions of the Directive 2001/83/EC will prevail and apply (namely "the rule of doubt").

Directive 2001/83/EC, as emended by Directive 2004/24, also defines 'traditional herbal medicinal product' ("herbal medicinal product that fulfils the condition laid down in Article 16a"), "herbal medicinal product" ("any medicinal product, exclusively containing as active ingredients one or more herbal substances or one or more herbal preparations, or one or more such herbal preparations, or one or more such herbal substances in combination with one or more such herbal preparations"), and "herbal preparations" ("preparations obtained by subjecting herbal substances to treatments such as extraction, distillation, expression, fractionation, purification, concentration or fermentation. These include comminuted or powdered herbal substances, tinctures, extracts, essential oils, expressed juices and processed exudates").

4. THE DEFINITION OF "HEALTH FOOD" IN CHINA

In China, according to the *Food Safety Law* (2015), health food is considered as a kind of special food as well as formula for special medicine purposes and formula food for infants and young children.[i]

However, there is no definition for health food in *Food Safety Law*, and the same appears in the *Administrative Rules for Health Food Registration and Filing*, enacted by CFDA and went into effect on July 1, 2016. The reason for this situation may be that health food is now considered as one kind of food and a special type of food. However, the *Administrative Rules for Health Food Registration* (2005), which was repealed by the *Administrative Rules for Registration and Filing to Health Food* in 2016, defined health food as food with special healthcare functions or for providing supplements of vitamins and minerals, which means that it is suitable for a special group of people, assisting in physiology regulation but not curing illnesses, with no acute, subacute, and chronic harm to the human body.

Nutrient supplements (vitamin and mineral supplements) are considered as health food under the *Food Safety Law* (2015). Similarly, no definition is provided for them. They once were defined in the *Rules of Application and Examination for Nutrient Supplements* (*trial*), enacted by CFDA in 2005, as: "Nutritious supplements are products which aim at supplying vitamin supplements and mineral supplements but not energy. Its effect is to replenish the insufficiency of diet, preventing from alimentary deficiency and reducing the risk of suffering chronic deseases" (Article 2). However, at that time, it shall be noted that nutrient supplements were not considered as health food. Then in 2011, when *Rules for Technical Examine*

---

[i] In 2016, CFDA enacted the *Administration Rules for Registration of Formula for Special Medicine Purpose* and the *Administration Rules for Registration of the Formula to Infant and Young Children Formula Food*. The first administrative rules defines (Article 48) "Formula for Special Medicine Purpose" as "formula food which is prepared or processed specially to meet the special requirements of nutrients and meals to the groups of people who is suffering restricted eating, disorder of digestion and absorption, metabolic disorders or particular illnesses, including formula food for special medicine purpose of infant, and formula food for special medicine purpose of people above one year." For infant and young children formula food, the legislation lacks a legal definition.

Priorities of Health Food (*trial*) were published by CFDA, nutrient supplements were subject to the regulation for health food. Recently, the "Catalogue of Raw Materials Used for Nutritious Substances" as the first batch of the "Catalogue of Raw Materials for Health Food" has been published. All the raw materials listed in the aforementioned catalogue could be used for producing nutrient supplements.

Health foods may have different forms: traditional food forms and pharmaceutical oral delivery forms. For both food with special healthcare functions and nutrient supplements, primary forms marketed are pills, capsules, oral solutions, particles, tablets, and so on.[j]

5. THE DEFINITION OF "FOOD SUPPLEMENT" IN THE EU

At the EU level, a health food category as designed in China does not exist. However, among the typologies of food with health benefits regulated by the EU legislator, one that is most comparable to the Chinese health food category is that of "Food Supplements".[k] According to the *Food Supplements Directive*, food supplements are defined as "foodstuffs the purpose of which is to supplement the normal diet and which are concentrated sources of nutrients or other substances with a nutritional or physiological effect, alone

[j] Pharmaceutical oral delivery forms are the primary forms all-time for health foods approved by CFDA, representing about two-thirds to three-fourths of total approvals in the period 2003–2014. More particularly, of these approved products 41% were hard-shell capsules, 17% soft gels, 14% tablets, 13% liquid, 5% granule or powder drink forms, and 4% tea (see Ref. 3, p. 376).

[k] Other categories of food with explicitly health functions, regulated by EU Law, are: fortified or enriched food (Regulation (EC) No. 1925/2006 on *the addition of vitamins, mineral and other substances to foods*); and "Foods for specific groups" (Regulation (EU) No. 609/2013). The latter Regulation considers "special" food products: infant formulae and follow-on formulae; processed cereal-based foods and baby foods; food for special medical purposes; and total diet replacement for weight control. Regulation (EC) No. 1925/2006 does not lay down a definition of "enriched food," which is food enriched with vitamins, minerals, and other substances (such as plants and herbal extracts). In China, nutritional fortification substances are considered as food additives by *Food Safety Law* (2015) (Article 150) and consequently regulated by food additives legislation.

or in combination, marketed in dose form, namely forms such as capsules, pastilles, tablets, pills and other similar forms, sachets of powder, ampoules of liquids, drops, dispensing bottles and other similar forms of liquids and powders designed to be taken in measured small unit quantities."

Nevertheless, the Chinese health food category is wider than that of EU food supplements because it also embraces food with special healthcare functions having traditional food forms. In the EU, such type of food is commonly considered as "functional food." However, there is neither a legal definition nor a specific regulation of such category, except specific rules concerning nutritional and health claims which are also applicable to food supplements, as below better explained, and concerning fortified food as determined by Regulation (EC) No. 1925/2006. The "European Commission Concerted Action on Functional Food Science in Europe" (Fufose), launched in 1995, proposed this working definition of functional food: "a food that beneficially affects one or more target functions in the body beyond adequate nutritional effects in a way that is relevant to either an improved state of health and well-being and/or reduction of risk of disease. It is consumed as part of a normal food pattern. It is not a pill, a capsule or any form of dietary supplement."

It is worth noting that the *Food Supplements Directive* provides a harmonized list of vitamins and minerals that may be added for nutritional purposes in food supplements (Annex I to the Directive) and a list of permitted sources (vitamin and mineral substances) from which those vitamins and minerals may be manufactured (Annex II of the Directive). However, the maximum levels of vitamins and minerals used in food supplements have not been harmonized until now, so it is necessary to consider national rules established by each Member State for maximum levels permitted in its territory.

A similar situation occurs in the case of botanical-based food supplements: the *Food Supplements Directive* has not yet extended the harmonization to the use of ingredients other than vitamins and minerals (including botanicals) for nutritional/physiological purposes. Even if the European Food Safety Authority (EFSA) published in 2012 a "Compendium of Botanicals"[10] listing those plants reported to contain toxic substances or components that might otherwise be of concern, that could be considered as a EU negative botanical list (see Ref. 11, p. 284), many EU Member States have adopted their own positive and/or negative lists. This means, for example, that the use of the same herbal substance in one State could be unrestricted while in another it could be subject to authorization or prohibited on the basis of a non-harmonized national list of substances. Moreover, in some countries, product status for some botanicals is automatically linked to pharmacy-only status. Obviously, this generates a heterogeneous situation that could give rise to several problems[12] such as those relating to the effectiveness of controls on food supplements carried out by national competent Authorities and relating to trade barriers between Member States.[13]

5.1. *The linkages between EU food supplements and TCM*

It is well known that TCM comprises a wide range of practices, but herbal medicine is a core part. Medicinal herbal products pertaining to TCM manufactured in China can be sold in the EU market as medicinal products only after they have obtained a pre-market approval. This is established by Directive 2001/83/EC, which sets out the general requirements for the marketing authorization or registration of medicines, industrially made and sold without medical prescription (i.e., over-the-counter pharmaceuticals).[1]

In particular, with regard to herbal medicines, the *Traditional Herbal Medicinal Products Directive* (Directive 2004/24/EC amending Directive 2001/83/EC) introduced a simplified registration based on "traditional use" (the so-called "traditional use registration"). According to the *Traditional Herbal Medicinal Products Directive*, "the long tradition of the medicinal product makes it possible to reduce the need for clinical trials, in so far as the efficacy of the medicinal product is plausible on the basis of long-standing use and experience." Thus, for registration as traditional herbal medicine, the product is required to show a history of use of 30 years, including at least 15 years in the EU. Nevertheless, all registered herbal medicines must comply with general provisions applying to all

---

[1]Herbs and granules of single herbs, used as raw materials for the production of individual Traditional Chinese Medicine formulations in pharmacies, are not affected by Directive 2004/24/EC.

medicinal products (such as pharmacovigilance, good manufacturing practices, manufacturing licence, etc.).[m]

Despite the simplified registration introduced by the *Traditional Herbal Medicinal Products Directive*, this "has had an inhibitory effect on the registrations, as a large number of products have not been able to demonstrate the requirement of 15 years on the market in the EU. Even for products that can meet this requirement, significant change may have taken place to the product composition. Consequently, relatively few Traditional Herbal registrations have been authorized. In parallel, a large number of botanical materials are being used as ingredients in food supplements" (see Ref. 14, pp. 228–229). This is the case with several imported Chinese herbal products pertaining to TCM, which do not satisfy the European pharmaceutical legislation conditions. If very few Traditional Chinese herbal medicines have been authorized up until now, in parallel, a large number of Chinese herbal products are in common use as food supplements.[n]

This is, yet, possible since many TCM raw materials are enclosed in the national lists of permitted ingredients for food supplements.

6. MARKET ENTRY PROCEDURES

The first entry into market of a health food and a food supplement, in China and in the EU, respectively, has to follow specific market entry procedures. The EU has opted for a notification-based system (see Ref.

---

[m] The rules on labeling of traditional herbal medicinal products require that labels must claim their therapeutic effect in a specific way: "Traditional Herbal Medicinal Product used…"; moreover, they must state: "The product is a traditional herbal medicinal product for use in specified indications exclusively based upon long-standing use."

[n] The first marketing registration for a Chinese herbal medicine product was only granted on March 14, 2012 by the Dutch Medicines Evaluation Board. As reported by the China Chamber of Commerce for Import & Export of Medicine and Health Products (CCCMHPIE), in its "Analysis in the First Half and Outlook in the Second Half of 2011 of Import and Export of Pharmaceutical Products," the Traditional Chinese Medicine exports to the EU in June 2011, after the transitional period established by the Traditional Herbal Medicinal Products Directive, dropped by almost 50% compared with June 2010.

11, p. 285), while China, originally, chose a registration-based approach and, recently, it has turned to a "double way system," hence mixing the two approaches (see Ref. 11, p. 280).

6.1. *Market entry procedures for health food in China*

The new amendment of *Food Safety Law* makes a notable change for health food regulation. The single register system for health food has turned into a so-called Double Way System that integrates both registration and filing. Such Double Way System is provided in Article 76 as follows: "Health foods that use raw materials outside the catalogue of raw materials for health food or health food that is imported for the first time shall get registered with the CFDA; however, first time import of health foods that are nutritious substances, such as vitamin supplements or mineral supplements, shall be filed for record with CFDA. Other health foods shall be filed for record with the food and drug regulatory department of the provincial government."

Furthermore, the *Administrative Rules for Health Food Registration and Filing* provides details rules and procedures for health food registration and filing. To be noted, it provides that the first time import of health foods that are nutritious substances refer to those that use raw materials listed in the "Catalogue of Raw Materials for Health Food." This requirement makes a consistent supplement for the provision in the new *Food Safety Law* by emphasizing that only the health foods that use raw materials inside the catalogue of raw materials could be filed for record. With this supplement detail, the Double Way System could be explained as follows: health foods that use raw materials inside the "Catalogue of Raw Materials for Health Food" only need to be filed for record with the regulatory department, while health foods that use raw materials outside the "Catalogue of Raw Materials for Health Food" shall get registered with the regulatory department.

6.2. *Market entry procedures for food supplements in the EU*

According to Article 10 of the *Food Supplements Directive*, EU Member States have the choice as to whether or not to set up a mandatory notification procedure for the first marketing of food supplement products in their country. All EU Member States, with the exception of Austria, Lithuania, the Netherlands, Sweden, and the UK, decided to introduce a mandatory notification procedure, while in the aforementioned five States, notification for new products is optional (see Ref. 11, p. 285). The requirements of the notification procedures vary from country to country (see Ref. 14, pp. 226–227).

7. LABELING REQUIREMENTS

Both China and the EU lay down mandatory labeling requirements for health food and food supplements, respectively. Moreover, they provide rules for the use of health claims, namely assertions about a relationship between a food (or its constituents) and health.

7.1. *The labeling of health food in China*

A stricter regulation for health food in the *Food Safety Law* (2015) is reflected in the supervision on label and advertisement. Articles 78 and 79 of the new *Food Safety Law* require declarations on label and advertisement to be made explicitly that "this product couldn't replace drugs." Article 78 further states: "the label and instructions of health food shall not involve prevention or treatment of diseases; content of label and instruction shall be true and be consistent with the registered or recorded content." This amendment expressly indicates that one would violate the *Food Safety Law*, which would ensue legal liability, if the labeling and instructive contents of health food were inconsistent with those information provided in the registration or filing progress. Another change that should be noticed in Article 79 is the accountability to review and approve the content of advertisements is assigned to the provincial food and drug regulatory departments but no longer the business administration departments.

On July 28, 2015, about three months after passage of the amendment by the Standing Committee of People's Congress, CFDA published the consultative drafts of *Administrative Rules for Health Food Labelling*, which should have been published by now. However, it is worth to be noticed. With the aim to establish the rules for regulating all the health food labeling, in this consultative draft, health food labeling is classified into three classes as follows: health food label; health food instruction; and health food mark. It also imposes a requirement on the contents of health food labeling: for example, the manufacturer has to label the information of the producer, products, usage, and storage on the concerned food product. To be noticed, the provisions for health food labeling were provided in Chapter 4 of the *Administrative Rules for Health Food Registration* (2005) which is now repealed. An independent administrative rule for health food labeling would be a huge step for its regulation.

As for the labeling of health claims, there are 27 types of permitted health claims for health food. A consultative draft named *Administrative Rules for Health Food's Catalogues of Health Claims and Raw Materials* was published on July 8, 2015, with the *Administrative Rules for Health Food Registration and Filing*, already implemented. This consultative draft creatively provides for the rules and progress to adopt, re-examine, and exclude the health claims and raw materials into the health food's Catalogues of health claims and raw materials, which means these two catalogues would be controlled in a dynamic way, as stipulated in Article 7 thereof. Also, as a response to the different manners of registration or filing for different types of health food provided in the new *Food Safety Law*, the consultative draft divides the health food's catalogue of raw materials into two sub-catalogues known as the "Catalogue for Vitamin Supplements and Mineral Supplements" and the "Catalogue for Other Types of Raw Materials for Health Food." As discussed earlier, the "Catalogue of Raw Materials used for Nutritious Substances" as the first batch of the "Catalogue of Raw Materials for Health Food" was published, and at the same time, the "Catalogue of Health Claims for Nutritious Substances" as the first batch of "Catalogue of Health Claims" was published. The health claims in this published catalogue is to supplement vitamins and minerals, which is a kind of health claim not listed in the "Catalogue of Permitted Health Claims for Health Food" published by CFDA in 2012.

7.2. *The labeling of food supplements in the EU*

The labeling of food supplements has to comply with the general rules applying to all foodstuffs established by Regulation (EU) No. 1169/2011 *on the provision of food information to consumers* as well as with the specific rules established by the *Food Supplements Directive*.[o] It is also covered by the *Nutrition and Health Claims Regulation* (EU Regulation 1924/2006), in case labels bear nutritional and/or health claims.[p]

According to the *Food Supplements Directive*, presentation and advertising must not attribute to food supplements the property of preventing, treating or curing a human disease, or refer to such properties. The same rule is established by EU Regulation no. 1169/2011 for all foodstuffs, consequently, it also concerns the labeling of "functional food." However, labels on foodstuffs (including food supplements and "functional food") may refer to properties having positive effects on health and well-being, provided they respect the requirements laid down by the *Nutrition and Health Claims Regulation*. This Regulation requires that all nutrition and health claims made voluntarily on foods (including food supplements) can only be used when they have been approved by the European Commission following an assessment of the scientific data available by EFSA. Once approved, the claim are include in a specific EU register and can be used by any food business operator, except in the case of health claims for which protection of proprietary data is granted and the right of use of the claim is restricted to the benefit of the applicant.

As for health claims, the scientific assessment must demonstrate the cause-and-effect relationship between intake of a compound and a health benefit. EFSA's scientific assessment methodology is centered on

---

[o]According to the *Food Supplements Directive*, the labeling of food supplements shall bear: (a) the names of the categories of nutrients or substances that characterize the product or an indication of the nature of those nutrients or substances; (b) the portion of the product recommended for daily consumption; (c) a warning not to exceed the stated recommended daily dose; (d) a statement to the effect that food supplements should not be used as a substitute for a varied diet; and (e) a statement to the effect that the products should be stored out of the reach of young children. Moreover, the labeling shall not include any mention stating or implying that a balanced and varied diet cannot provide appropriate quantities of nutrients in general.

[p]According to Regulation (EU) No. 1924/2006, health claims are divided into three types: function health claim (relating to the growth, development, and functions of the body; referring to psychological and behavioral functions; on slimming or weight-control); risk reduction claim (on reducing a risk factor in the development of a disease) and health claims referring to children's development.

evidence at the "highest possible standard." Human studies are considered a fundamental part for achieving such evidence. Similarly, in China, data from human trials are required for most of the health claims approved (see Ref. 3 and Ref. 5, p. 3).[q]

To date, 261 health claims have been approved.[r] Of all approved health claims, very few are associated with botanicals, moreover, they only refer to active ingredients or class of active ingredients in well-defined dosages (such as olive oil polyphenols, cocoa flavanols, B-glucans from oats or barley) and not directly to botanical ingredients.[15,16]

The scientific assessment of health claims on botanicals is a controversial issue in the EU.[9] When EFSA started its assessment of the scientific evidence for the registration of health claims, more than 500 claims for botanicals failed because their dossiers were only based on the notion of "traditional use," namely evidence based solely on use and experience over time.[s] In May 2012, the European Commission adopted EU Regulation no. 432/2012, establishing a list of 222 permitted health claims ("function health claims"). Simultaneously, the Commission identified a list of more than 2,000 claims, also concerning the effects of botanical substances, not yet assessed by EFSA and the European Commission and not yet listed on its webpage in the "list of health claims on hold." According to the Commission, such health claims could continue to be used in accordance with transitional measures (Article 28, par. 5 and 6 of Regulation n. 1924/2006) provided they comply with the applicable EU and national legislation.[t]

Since then, health claims on botanicals have been on hold (in a transitional period with no defined endpoint). A contribution towards overcoming the pending situation will derive from the revision of the

---

[q]Depending on the health claim, only human studies or only animal tests or both are required.

[r]Precisely, 335 function health claims, 14 risk reduction claims, and 12 health claims referring to children's development. Moreover, 28 nutritional claims have been approved until now.

[s]On the contrary, such evidence is at the basis of the registration process for Traditional herbal medicinal products.

[t]In August 2012, the European Commission published a discussion document addressed to the Member States, asking solutions to overcome such complex situation.

Nutrition and Health Claims Regulation recently started by the EU Commission.

8. IMPORT AND EXPORT RULES

Chinese legislation on health food provides specific rules for importing and exporting health foods, by contrast, the *Food Supplements Directive* does not provide similar rules.

8.1. *Rules for imported and exported health food*

In respect of the safety of imported health food, China requires that "The imported health food shall have obtained sales permission by the competent authority of the exporting country" (Article 76, *Food Safety Law*), and they should be marketed legally at least for one year or with the food consuming safety report in the exporting country (Article 13, *Administrative Rules for Health Food Registration and Filing*).

Responsibilities are assumed by the traders. First, overseas exporters and producers shall guarantee that the imported food complies with all the requirements set by all Chinese related laws (Article 96, *Food Safety Law*). Second, they should build the pre-supervision and recall system. And in order to promote the traceability system for imported food, the importers are required to establish a food and food additive import and sale record constituted with "names and addresses of overseas exporter and buyers," and "keep the related certificates" (Article 98).

While there is no national safety standard set in China for imported food, "the overseas exporter/producer, or its entrusted importers shall submit the relevant executive national (regional) standard or international standard to the NHFPC. NHFPC shall review the relevant standard and may decide that the executive standard applies temporarily if deems it can meet the food safety requirements and develop corresponding national food safety standards in a timely manner" (Article 93). Presently, the most important standard in China is the National Standard for Health Foods GB16740-2014, which was published by NHFPC in 2014. There are 23 national standards documents concerning health food safety in total.[17]

In addition, exported foods are required to comply with standards of the exporting country (region) or meet contract requirements (Article 99).

8.2. *Rules for imported and exported food supplements*

The *Food Supplements Directive* does not provide specific rules on importing and exporting food supplements. Therefore, according to Article 11 of the *General Food Law*, which requires that imported food must comply with the relevant requirements of EU food law, all imported food supplements must follow: (a) the specific rules applying exclusively to food supplements (as laid down by the Food Supplements Directive and by national legislations on the maximum levels of vitamins and minerals and on the use of botanicals ingredients in food supplements) and (b) all the requirements established by horizontal rules applicable to all foods (such as legislation on additives, labeling, claims, hygiene, contaminants, GMOs, etc.). As for exported food supplements, Article 12 of the *General Food Law* requires that these shall comply with the relevant requirements of food law in force in the importing country.

9. SOME FINAL REMARKS

The analysis carried out has put in evidence some similarities between the Chinese health food legal framework and the EU food supplements legislation. However, several differences exist, and this aspect must be carefully considered by Chinese and EU companies aiming at exploiting the flourishing market of food with health-enhancing properties in the EU and in China, respectively.

As for the connections with TCM, these are easily distinguishable in the Chinese food legislation on health food. Coherently with the Chinese culture of considering food and medicine to be strictly linked, the use of TCM raw materials in the health food production is explicitly taken into consideration. In the case of EU Food Law, the EU food supplements category could be considered as a sort of "Trojan Horse" for the import of TCM products in Europe, which fail to comply with the strict requirements for obtaining pre-market authorizations as established by the EU legislation on medicinal products.[18] This is, yet, possible since TCM raw materials are enclosed in the national lists of permitted ingredients for food supplements.

REFERENCES

1. Nicoletti, M. (2012). "Nutraceuticals and botanicals: Overview and perspectives," *International Journal of Food Sciences and Nutrition*, 63: 2–6.
2. Malla, S., Hobbs, J., Sogah, E. K. & Yeung, M. T. (eds.) (2014). *Regulating Health Foods: Policy Challenges and Consumer Conundrums* (Edward Elgar Publishing, Cheltenham, UK).
3. Hu, C. (2017). "Developing new functional food and nutraceutical products." In *Nutraceutical Innovation and Health Claims in China*, Bagchi, D. (ed.) Chapter 19 (Elsevier, London, Waltham, San Diego), pp. 369–389.
4. Hu, C. (2014), "Nutraceutical innovation and health claims in China." In *Nutraceutical and Functional Food Regulations in the United States and Around the World,* Bagchi, D. (ed.) Chapter 21 (Elsevier, London, Waltham, San Diego), pp. 363–388.
5. Hou, H., Li, S. & Ye, Z. (2016). "Health food and traditional Chinese medicine in China," *Journal of Nutrition and Health Sciences*, 3: 1–4.
6. Li, M.-Y., Jiang, Y. & Yu, C. (2016). "Analyzation of the status quo of the approval of health food used TCM materials from 2013–2015," *Central South Pharmacy*, 14: 1139–1142.
7. Lattanzi, P. (2016). *Health Foods or Medicinal Products? The Botanicals Case in the European Union. A Food Law Perspective*, 'I diritti della terra e del mercato agroalimentare: liber amicorum Alberto Germanò,' 2 (Utet Giuridica, Turin), pp. 1321–1338.
8. Korzycka-Iwanow, M. & Zboralska, M. (2010). "Never-ending debate on food supplements: Harmonisation or disharmonisation of the law," *European Food and Feed Law Review*, 3: 124–135.
9. Lattanzi, P. (2015). "Botanicals and the regulatory framework on food supplements in the European Union: A tricky relationship," *Agricoltura, Istituzioni, Mercati*, 2: 1–20.
10. European Food Safety Authority (2012). *Compendium of botanicals reported to contain naturally occurring substances of possible concern for human health when used in food and food supplements*, available at http://www.efsa.europa.eu/it/efsajournal/pub/2663.htm. Accessed May 2017.

11. Shao, A. (2017). "Developing new functional food and nutraceutical products." In *Global Market Entry Regulations for Nutraceuticals, Functional Foods, Dietary/Food/Health Supplements*, Bagchi, D. (ed.) Chapter 15 (Elsevier, London, Waltham, San Diego), pp. 279–290.
12. Food and Veterinary Office (2015). "Overview Report on a series of fact finding missions carried out in Member States in 2013 and 2014 in order to gather information regarding the controls on food supplements," DG (Sante) 2015-7186 – MR.
13. European Commission (2015). "Evaluation of the application of the mutual recognition principle in the field of goods," Final Report, DG Int. Available at: http://ec.europa.eu/DocsRoom/documents/13381/attachments/1/translations/en/renditions/native. Accessed October 2017.
14. Gulati, O. P., Ottaway, P. B. & Coppens, P. (2014). "Botanical nutraceuticals (food supplements, fortified and functional foods) in the European Union with main focus on nutrition and health claims regulation." In *Nutraceutical and Functional Food Regulations in the United States and Around the World*, Bagchi, D. (ed.) Chapter 14 (Elsevier, London, Waltham, San Diego), pp. 221–256.
15. Biagi, M., Pecorari, R., Appendino, G., Miraldi, E., Magnano, A. R., Governa, P., Cettolin, G. & Giachetti, D. (2016). "Herbal products in Italy: The thin line between phytotherapy, nutrition and parapharmaceuticals; A normative overview of the fastest growing market in Europe," *Pharmaceuticals*, 9: 1–10.
16. de Boer, A., Urlings, M. J. & Bast, A. (2016). "Active ingredients leading in health claims on functional foods," *Journal of Functional Foods*, 20, pp. 587–593.
17. Li, J-H. & Li, D. (2011). "The status quo of Chinese legal system and standard system for health food," *Food Science*, 32: 318–343.
18. Snyder, F., Yi L. & Yazdani, G. (2014). "Traditional Chinese Medicine and European Union Law: Cultural logics, product identities, market competition, legal rechanneling, and the need for global legal and medical pluralism," *Peking University Law Journal*, 2: 129–200.

Chapter 14

The Balance Between Patients' Choice and Economic Constraints in the Use of TCM Therapies: Two European Cases*

Erik Longo and Laura Vagni

1. INTRODUCTION

The diffusion of Traditional Chinese Medicine (TCM) therapies in Europe raises the problem of their legal recognition and the regulation of their use.

The investigation of this question involves the national and sometimes the local dimension of law, as it depends on the organization of healthcare systems and the delivery of health services, which are within the competence of Member States (Article 168 TFEU). Nevertheless, the arrangements put in place by national policies on the matter are influenced by the

* Albeit its unitary conception, Erik Longo drafted Sections 1, 3, and 4 while Laura Vagni drafted the other sections.

European Union policies of orientation and coordination of Member States in the health sector (Article 168(6) TFEU).

Over the last 15 years, the European Union has developed policies for the promotion of the quality of health and the sustainability and efficiency of healthcare systems, which have inspired national healthcare policies.[1]

Moreover, the recognition at a European level of patients' rights as fundamental rights to be respected by Member States has played an important role in the gradual convergence of national health policies on a patient-centered model of care.

In this context, the process of the integration of TCM therapies into the various European systems is a matter of national law but, at the same time, is influenced by some European values, which permeate and shape national healthcare services.

The aim of this chapter is to describe this dynamic through the examples of the Italian and English legal experiences in this sector, and show how the freedom of choice and the notion of cost-containment in healthcare, developed at a European level as guiding principles in health policies, constitute the general legal framework of the national attitude toward the delivery of TCM therapies.

2. PATIENT AUTONOMY AND FREEDOM TO CHOOSE TCM THERAPIES

Since the end of the last century, patients' freedom of choice has acquired a growing relevance in most of the European legal systems. European Union policies and international sources have played an important role in this process, representing a propelling factor in the development of patients' rights, which have formed a common ground for the harmonization of national healthcare systems. In this context, the first reference is to the European Charter of Human Rights, which became legally binding for Member States with the entry into force of the Treaty of Lisbon (Article 6 TFEU).

The Charter provides for a right to benefit from medical treatments under the conditions established by national laws and practices and states that the policies and activities of the Union shall be shaped so as to ensure a high level of human health protection. The right to benefit from medical treatments has a counterpart in the right to choose the treatments on the basis of an informed consent, as stated by Article 3 of the Charter. The article provides that in the field of medicine and biology "... the free and informed consent of the person concerned, according to the procedures laid down by law..." is to be respected.

Patients' right to choose health treatments has its legal basis in other international sources. Thus, the 1994 Declaration on the Promotion of Patients' Rights in Europe, emanating from the WHO, recognizes patients' rights to self-determination. Moreover, The Convention on Human Rights and Biomedicine, also referred to as the "Oviedo Convention," states in Article 5 the right to a free and informed consent, valorizing the freedom of patients to choose their treatment. The right to freely choose which therapies to undergo and its inter-relationship with the right to be informed is specifically expressed in Article 5 of the European Charter of Patients' Rights.[2]

The right to information and the freedom of choice are the main pillars of the concept of patient autonomy. The patient's self-determination, in particular, has been founded on the requirements of providing the patient with complete and concrete information and the freedom of choice as to whether to undergo a cure or not and, in the last case, the modality, the time, and the kind of cure. These requirements are rooted in fundamental rights, which constitute the main legal framework for the empowerment of patients in the European legal systems.

The European Court of Human Rights has played a significant role in the development of the right to autonomy in healthcare. Indeed, the jurisprudence of the Court on Article 8 of the European Convention of Human Rights (ECHR) shows that the self-determination of the person constitutes an expression of the wider concept of private life and is to be preserved in all the choices of the individual, including those concerning his/her health.[a]

The application of the rhetoric of fundamental rights to the healthcare sector paved the way for the shift of the delivery of healthcare services into

---

[a]This interpretation was firmly established in the case *Pretty v. UK*, ECHR, 29 July 2002, appl. no 2346/02, para. 63; in its subsequent judgments the Court addressed the autonomy of person as a right which is protected by Art. 8 ECHR, see *Evans v. the UK*, ECHR 7 March 2006, appl. no. 6339/05; *Tysiaç v. Poland*, ECHR 20 March 2007, appl. no. 5410/03, para. 107; *Kalacheva v. Russia*, ECHR 1 May 2009, appl. no. 3451/05, para. 27; *VC v. Slovakia*, ECHR 8 November 2011, appl. no. 18968/07.

the process of EU integration, extending also to patients the freedom of movement within the common market, a right originally devised for citizens/consumers. Thus, in the famous Kohll[b] case, the European Court of Justice recognized the rights of patients to choose treatments outside their own States, stating that the public health sector, as a sector of economic activity and from the point of view of freedom to provide services, is not excluded from the application of the fundamental principle of freedom of movement. The jurisprudence of the Court of Justice was finally embedded into the directive 2011/24[c] on the application of patients' rights in cross-border healthcare. The inclusion of the health sector into the common market implied the gradual assimilation of the patient into a consumer, even if a consumer of a particular kind, with the consequent application to the healthcare sector of rules and guarantees originally developed to protect consumers' rights in the common market. In this context, the importance of patient information and freedom of choice was reinforced.

This European approach toward healthcare has a relevant impact in the delivery of TCM therapies in the European area, encouraging the enlargement of the health service offered by national systems and opening the healthcare systems to modes of self-management of care. Indeed, patient's autonomy includes the opportunity for patients to refuse conventional medicine and adhere to other forms of treatments. Therefore, the empowerment of patients' freedom of choice within and outside their own States opens the way to the acceptance of TCM therapies by the national systems and their funding.

3. COST-EFFECTIVENESS OF HEALTHCARE SERVICES: A EUROPEAN AGENDA

Over the last decade, the combined effect of the economic crisis, the continuing rise of aging population in Europe, and the increasing costs of care have put to the test the performance of healthcare systems, intensifying the

[b] *Cf.* Raymond *Kohll v. Union des caisses de maladie*, ECJ 28 April 1998, C-158/96, para. 46; see *Nicolas Decker v. Caisse de maladie des employés privés*, ECJ 28 April 1998, C-120/95.
[c] Directive 2011/24/EU of the European Parliament and of the Council of March 9, 2011, on the application of patients' rights in cross-border healthcare.

public debate on the sustainability of health expenditure.[3] Several initiatives at the EU level have put into discussion the reform of healthcare.

In 2007, the Commission started a reflection process on the sustainability of health systems,[4] which explores effective ways of investing efficiently in health.

The White Paper "Together for Health: A Strategic Approach for the EU 2008–2013" is one of the most important step of this path.[5] It paved the ways for a new "health strategy" that reinforces the importance of health in policies such as the "Lisbon Strategy for Growth and Jobs," which emphasizes the links between health and economic prosperity,[6] and the Citizens' Agenda, which recognizes people's right to be empowered in relation to their health and healthcare.[7]

Later, the 2013 Commission Staff Working Document "Investing in Health" recognized the expenditure in healthcare as growth-friendly. Cost-effective and efficient health expenditure can increase the quantity and the productivity of labor by increasing healthy life expectancy. Notwithstanding, it shows how the relatively large share of healthcare spending in total government expenditure, combined with the need for budgetary consolidation across the EU, requires "more efficiency and cost-effectiveness to ensure the sustainability of current health system models".[8]

In 2014, the European Commission communication "On Effective, Accessible and Resilient Health Systems" focuses on actions to strengthen the effectiveness of health systems, increase the accessibility of healthcare, and improve the resilience of health systems. It establishes a European agenda to support Member States to cope with the challenge of a fiscal sustainability of healthcare systems and the effectiveness of healthcare (i.e., the ability to produce positive health outcomes). In this way, the cost-effectiveness of care was pushed among the top priorities in the health sector.

4. THE DELIVERY OF TCM THERAPIES IN THE ITALIAN SYSTEM

In Italy, the duty to organize the Healthcare System (SSN) is up to Regional governments. Since the last decade, Regions have started to include CAMs (complementary and alternative medicine) therapies (and particularly TCMs) among the services offered and reimbursed by the SSN.

Quantitative and qualitative studies show the incidence of CAM usage among the population. The results of a multipurpose survey made by the Italian National Institute of Statistics (ISTAT) on "Non-conventional Therapies in Italy" revealed that 13.6% of Italians (about 8 million) used TCMs in the previous three years.[9] More women and less men use these therapies, even in combination. Most users admit to having gained amelioration or healing without side effects. Interestingly, the data shows the great awareness of possible effects of TCMs on the quality of life, environment, and personal relationships, reflecting the demand for more holistic patient-centered care. However, many users complained that the economic burden on families slows the diffusion of TCMs.

Indeed, eight years later, a survey of the same Institute on the "Protection of Health and Access to Healthcare" (2013) showed that the number of users of CAMs declined. The use of alternative cares decreased by about 40%. Only 4.9 million (8.2%) of persons declared as choosing non-conventional therapies. Homeopathy is still the most popular kind of therapy, followed by osteopathy and chiropractic (3.6%),[9] phytomedicine (1.9%), and acupuncture (1%).

One of the possible reasons of this change is the economic crisis and the lack of a clear definition of these cares into the system of healthcare reimbursement.[10]

The legal status of CAMs in the SSN is still dubious. Despite the diffusion, CAMs still lack a formal legitimacy in the Italian legal system. While invited since 1986, the Executive and the Parliament failed to pass a legislation that recognizes the practices related to CAMs. Since the 1980s, more than 100 legislative initiatives have been proposed without any tangible result by doctors who practice CAMs.[d]

---

[d]On May 18, 2002, the National Council of the Italian National Federation of Medical Doctors and Dentists Associations (FNOMCeO) issued the "Guidelines of the FNOMCeO on Non-conventional Medicines and Practices" (Resolution of Terni) that recognized nine disciplines: acupuncture, traditional Chinese medicine, ayurvedic medicine, homeopathy, anthroposophic medicine, homotoxicology, herbal medicine, chiropractic, and osteopathy.

The Constitutional reform of 2001[e] provided that the central State and the Regions have concurring legislative competence to regulate "professions". Then, Regions have taken many legislative initiatives to give professionals who practice CAMs a special status among medical professions. However, the Constitutional Court has declared these Regional statutes unconstitutional due to the impossibility of a region to create new professions, which is still a competence placed at a state level.

In other ways, Regional governments have promoted CAMs in healthcare systems.[11] The Healthcare Plans of a large number of regions now mention TCM among the levels of care and under certain conditions, offer the possibility to have reimbursement of therapies, and fund research on the efficiency and efficacy of TCMs.[12] For example, since 1996, the Strategic Regional Health Plans of Tuscany region contains references to TCMs therapies and, in particular, acupuncture. The Plans of 2004, 2008, and 2012 included a chapter on non-conventional medicine that arguably represent one of the greatest degrees of integration of such therapies in the healthcare system achieved thus far in Italy. In this chapter, TCM therapies and, in particular, acupuncture, are highly recommended for use in pain management. These Plans aim to guarantee integration in the SSN of types of non-conventional medicine which are supported by a sufficient level of scientific evidence to allow them to be defined as forms of CAM. In this context, the Tuscany region has established a Center fully dedicated to alternative cares in the town of Pitigliano (Grosseto Province, Italy).

If we set aside the example of the Tuscany region, the picture shows that Italy is considerably slower in recognizing and legitimizing TCMs: a situation that determines, in comparison with other EU countries, a strong limitation of freedom to choose alternatives therapies. Nevertheless, a bottom-up process is arising, also thanks to the vast presence of immigrants from Asia, who increasingly request such therapies.

These practices are considered to be exclusively under the professional responsibility of medical doctors and dentists.

[e] cf. art. 117 Const, as modified by Constitutional law n. 3/2001.

5. THE DELIVERY OF TCM THERAPIES IN ENGLAND

The diffusion of CAM therapies in England is quite high: surveys show that around 46% of the population is expected to access CAM therapies once or more times in a lifetime, and about 26% of the population has accessed it in the last 12 months.[13,14] Of the TCM therapies on offer, acupuncture is the most popular.[f]

Despite the citizens' increasing use of TCM therapies, these treatments are not regulated by statute in England.[g]

In 2000, the Science and Technology Select Committee of the House of Lords conducted a study on CAM practices and published a report where it investigated, among other questions, the delivery of CAMs by the National Health Service (NHS).[15] The report distinguished CAM as being divisible into three different groups. The first embraced the principal disciplines, within which were included acupuncture and herbal medicine. The second group included therapies which are most often used to complement conventional therapies and do not purport to embrace diagnostic skills, such as aromatherapy and the Alexander technique. TCM was listed in the third group, which comprised a group of alternative disciplines, based on a long established and traditional system of healthcare.

The statutory regulation of professionals working in acupuncture and herbal medicine was recommended (see para. 5.23 in Ref. 16), while

---

[f]These percentages are only indicative, as they do not take into account that most TCM therapies are offered outside the NHS and on the basis of a private interplay between the patient and the practitioner. Moreover, the delivery of TCM therapies is not uniform in the country (*cf.* Ref. 15).

[g]See The Osteopaths Act 1993 and The Chiropractors Act 1994. The Acts establish the General regulatory bodies, with the duty to develop, promote, and regulate the profession and some committees, with different functions in educational and training of professionals, in the investigation into complaints made against practitioners, in the regulations of professional standards, in health issues. The Acts are mainly devoted to the regulation of professional conduct and professional registers. *Cf.* McHale, J. V. (2015). *Legal Framework, Professional Regulation and CAM Practice in England*; Gale, N. C. & McHale, J. V. (eds.) (2015). *Routledge Handbook of Complementary and Alternative Medicine* (Routledge, Abingdon, New York).

self-regulation of professionals was considered more appropriate for the other therapies, on the basis of their stage of professional organization and evidence-base.[38–39]

The picture that emerged from the Committee's report was patchy public funding of all CAM therapies, depending on the personal attitude of the General Practitioners (GPs) toward CAM therapies. Indeed, GPs are the patients' first interface and constitute an important filter for the access to complementary therapies in primary care. The Committee considered the integration of CAM therapies with conventional therapies as still too tenuous and firmly suggested an inquiry into some key questions so as to improve the delivery of these therapies, such as their evidence base, the information provided to the public about the different therapies and the way to access them, the standardization of the process of delivery, the development of monitoring procedures, and lastly the conformity to the principle of cost-effectiveness of the services provided.

The role of GPs in the formation of an integrated system of care emerged as strategic and the GPs were considered as the gatekeepers of the CAM therapies with the role of recommending them on the basis of a precise process of referral.

Notwithstanding the Committee's recommendation, the proposal of statutory regulation for professionals of acupuncture and herbal medicine never received Parliamentary approval.[17, 41–42]

The delivery of TCMs in the NHS is today possible on the basis of their compatibility with the principles and rules introduced by the Health and Social Act 2012,[h] which reformed the NHS. The Act has been considered as the most radical innovation of the NHS since its implementation in 1948 as it introduces a completely new way to commission care within the English territory, giving strategic importance to general practitioners, who are now closer to patients and their needs.[i]

The reform keeps the centralized system introduced in 1948, but has regionalized some activities and services. In fact, together with this centralized system, the Act introduces a two-tier system, under the Secretary

---

[h] Health and Social Act 2012. The Act gained the Royal Assent in March 2012 and it came into force on April 1, 2013.[18]

[i] For a general overview, see Ref. 19.

of State for Health: the Commissioning Board and the Clinical Commissioning Groups (CCGs). The Board has the important task of the supervision and direction of CCGs, which have a great deal of power both in the choice of providers and services and in the allocation of budget for the majority of therapies, including TCM treatments.

The devolution of control to local authorities concerning the relationship between patients and healthcare providers has improved a patient-centered model of healthcare, supporting the transparency of the decision processes in healthcare and the engagement of patients in these processes. From this perspective, the CCGs constitute the attempt of the system to make the principle of patient autonomy effective. This principle has been recognized in the NHS since the end of the 1980s[20] and now permeates the NHS reform.[21–23]

Encouraging the freedom of patients favors the diffusion of TCM therapies in the legal system. Indeed, TCM therapies seem to respond better than the biomedical model to the ideas of self-management of care, which flow through the notions of patient autonomy and the personalization of care. This happens especially for the cure of chronic diseases, where the demand by patients for TCM therapies is rising, as the effects of conventional cures are largely unsatisfactory. In this context, for example, the person-centered model requires the NHS to make available a vast range of health services for patients, including also nonclinical or nonmedical services.[22] This opportunity was made effective through the implementation of the personal health budget, which was designed to allow patients to access services in addition to the comprehensive primary medical services[24] and, not by chance, starting from the end of 2014, experimenting on patients with long-term conditions.

The personal health budget consists of an individual allocation of NHS funds that can be used by the patient to meet his/her health needs, accessing also some nonmedical services. The choice of how to spend the budget for a specific service is planned by the patient together with the GP and the CCG. As the purpose of the personal health budget is to give people greater choice and control over their health, the CCG has to accept different approaches to achieving outcomes other than those used by conventional medicine. Moreover, the risks connected with health services and evidence-based considerations need to be balanced with the personal conditions and needs of the patients so as to assure the best solution in each individual case.[25]

The experience of the personal health budget in England shows a rising access to TCMs by patients who have the right to a personal budget, and in consequence the NHS is funding TCM therapies.[26,27] In fact, the evaluation made by the Department of Health on the personal health budget in the years 2009–2012 estimates a rising patient access to acupuncture and Chinese medicine.[24,28,29]

The freedom to choose TCM, however, is not unconditional. Indeed, on the one hand, this freedom is mitigated by the duty of the NHS to protect public health and avoid choices which would lead to prejudicing a patient's health[40]; on the other hand, the freedom of choice implies the idea of patient responsibility, which is the other face of the recognition of their autonomy. From this perspective, the Department of Health underlined that: "In return for greater choice and control, patients should accept responsibility for the choices they make, concordance with treatment programmes and the implications for their lifestyle" (see p. 30 in Ref. 22). Thus, patient responsibility is the link between a patient's rights and the principle of economy, efficiency, and effectiveness, which also inspired the NHS reform.[30]

Studies show the positive impact that TCM therapies can have on the containment of cost in healthcare and the capability of TCM to tackle the principle of cost-efficiency in healthcare (see Refs. 31–34).[j] However, the data collected on this matter are still controversial. The main problems seem to be the scarcity of data and the inappropriateness of the valuation of efficacy and effectiveness of TCM therapies according to methods traditionally developed for conventional medicine.

It is precisely on the basis of cost-efficiency considerations that some CCGs have recently decided to reduce the funding of some CAM

---

[j] For example, a problematic issue is that the evidence-based evaluation of CAMs by randomized controlled trials (RCTs) is inappropriate and there is the need to find alternative methods of evaluation which are more adequate to CAMs' holistic attitude toward care (*cf.* Ref. 35).

therapies in their region, with a negative effect on the egalitarian delivery of these therapies in the country.[k]

From this perspective, it is significant that the NICE[37] panel decided to withdraw acupuncture from the guidelines for low back pain and sciatica,[l] which may have an impact on GPs' acupuncture referrals. The choice was explained on the basis of the scarcity of data which indicated the cost-effectiveness of treatment. The choice was explained on the basis of scarcity of data, which indicated the cost-effectiveness of treatment; however, the British Medical Acupuncture Society criticized the choice as based on a misunderstanding of the data on the matter.[14] Therefore, it is realistic to predict that, in the years to come, a patient's freedom to access TCM therapies will depend heavily on the capability of researchers to provide evidence of the cost-effectiveness of these treatments.

6. CONCLUSIONS

The development in the European systems of a patient-centered healthcare model, focused on the protection of patients' freedom of choice and autonomy, favors the use of TCM and encourages the delivery of TCM therapies by national healthcare systems. At the same time, the emphasis on patients' freedom to access different kinds of health treatments raises a set of problems about the conditions of a patient's exercise of the freedom of choice.

Freedom of choice does not include the duty of the healthcare systems to provide a specific type of care. In fact, each Member State conserves autonomy in the management of healthcare services and in the allocation

---

[k] *Cf.* "Complementary and Alternative Therapies Evidence Based Decision Making Framework." Available at: http://www.leedswestccg.nhs.uk/content/uploads/2016/12/Complementary-and-Alternative-Therapies.pdf. A broad range of treatments and practices that are not considered standard medical treatment by NHS Leeds North CCG, NHS Leeds South and East CCG (2015–2018) are mentioned. Indeed, the funding of CAM treatments is subject to the so-called "postcode lottery" (*cf.* Ref. 36).

[l] NICE (2016). "Low back pain and sciatica in over 16s: Assessment and management," November. Rule 1.2.8 "Do not offer acupuncture for managing low back pain with or without sciatica," whereas acupuncture was recommended by the previous version of the guidelines.

of resources in healthcare (Article 168(6) TFEU). Therefore, the effectiveness of a patient's freedom to choose TCM therapies depends on the balance achieved in each State between the protection of patient freedom and other potentially conflicting principles in healthcare, such as the safety, economy, and efficiency of healthcare services. From this perspective, TCM therapies have to cope both with the challenges posed by the need to assure the high quality of health and the financial sustainability of public health. Therefore, the evidence of TCM cost-effectiveness is a contender to becoming the main gateway for TCM legal recognition and funding by national healthcare systems.

REFERENCES

1. Paoli, F. (2012). "Health systems efficiency and sustainability: A European perspective," *Eurohealth Observer,* 18(3): 14–17.
2. European Economic and Social Committee (2007). "Opinion of the European Economic and Social Committee on Patients' rights," 26 September, soc/221, Brussels.
3. Thomson, S. *et al.* (2014). *Economic Crisis, Health Systems and Health in Europe: Impact and Implications for Policy* (WHO Regional Office for Europe, Denmark).
4. Pammolli, F. *et al.* (2012). "The sustainability of European health care systems: Beyond income and aging," *The European Journal of Health Economics,* 13(5): 623–634.
5. European Commission (2007). Together for Health: A Strategic Approach for the EU 2008–2013, White Paper, COM 630. Available at: http://ec.europa.eu/health-eu/doc/whitepaper_en.pdf. Accessed June 2017.
6. Ferrera, M. (2005). *The Boundaries of Welfare: European Integration and the New Spatial Politics of Social Protection* (Oxford University Press, Oxford, UK).
7. Bonifacio, M. (2014). "Social innovation: A novel policy stream or a policy compromise? An EU perspective," *European Review*, 22(1): 145–169.
8. European Commission, Investing in Health. (2013). Accompanying the document "Towards Social Investment for Growth and Cohesion - including implementing the European Social Fund 20142020", Commission Staff Working Document, SWD(2013) 43. Available at: http://ec.europa.eu/health/strategy/docs/swd_investing_in_health.pdf. Accessed June 2017.

9. Istituto nazionale di statistica (ISTAT) (National Institute for Statistics) (2007). Le terapie non-convenzionali in Italia (Non-conventional medicine in Italy) (2005) Roma. Available at: http://www.istat.it/salastampa/comunicati/non_calendario/20070821_00/testointegrale.pdf. Accessed June 2017.
10. Istituto nazionale di statistica (ISTAT) (National Institute for Statistics): tutela della salute e accesso alle cure (2013). Available at: http://www.agenas.it/images/agenas/Agenews/newsletter4/Tutela_della_salute_accesso_alle_cure_10_lug_2014_Testo_integrale.pdf.
11. di Sarsina, R. P. & Iseppato, I. (2009). "Non-conventional medicine in Italy: The present situation," *European Journal of Integrative Medicine,* 1(2): 65–71.
12. Tognetti Bordogna, M. (2011). "Regional health system and non- conventional medicine: The situation in Italy," *EPMA Journal*, 2(4): 411–423.
13. Bishop, F. L. & Leith, G. T. (2010). "Who Uses CAM? A narrative review of demographic characteristics and health factors associated with CAM use," *Evidence-Based Complementary and Alternative Medicine*, 7(1): 11–28.
14. Hunt, J. K. *et al.* (2010). "Complementary and alternative medicine use in England," *The International Journal of Clinical Practice*, 64(11): 1496–1502.
15. Thomas, K. J. *et al.* (2001). "Use and expenditure on complementary medicine in England: A population based survey," *Complementary Therapies in Medicine*, 9(1): 2–11.
16. Select Committee on Science and Technology, House of Lords (2000). Sixth Report — Complementary and Alternative Medicine (London).
17. Barber, S. (2014). Regulation of Herbal Medicines, House of Commons Standard Note SN/SC/6002.
18. Davies, A. C. L. (2013). "This time, It is for real: The Health and Social Care Act 2012," *Modern Law Review*, 76(3), pp. 564–558.
19. Department of Health (2013). Guide to the Healthcare System in England, (London), 76(3): 564–558. Available at: https://www.gov.uk/government/publications/guide-to-the-healthcare-system-in-england.
20. Department of Health (1989). Working for Patients' (London: HMSO, Cm 555).
21. Department of Health (2010). Equity and Excellence: Liberating the NHS (London: HMSO, CM7881).
22. Department of Health (2012). Liberating the NHS: Greater Choice and Control — A Summary of Responses (London).
23. Department of Health (2012). NHS Constitution for England, updated on 14 October 2015.

24. Department of Health (2011). Personal Health Budget: Early Experiences of Budget Holders, Fourth Interim Report (London).
25. NHS England (2014). Guidance on the "Right to Have" a Personal Health Budget in Adult NHS continuing Healthcare and Children and Youth's People Continuing Care.
26. Rogers, J. (2011). "Personal health budgets: A new way of accessing complementary therapies?" *Complementary Therapies in Clinical Practice*, 17(2): 76–80
27. Sheppard, M. K. (2015). "The paradox of non-evidence based, publicly funded complementary alternative medicine in the English National Health Service: An explanation," *Health Policy*, 119(10): 1375–1381.
28. Department of Health (2012). Personal Health Budget: Experiences and Outcomes for Budget Holders at Nine Months, Fifth Interim Report.
29. Department of Health (2015). Personal Health Budget: National Progress Update May 2016.
30. Veitch, K. (2010). "The government of health care and the politics of patient empowerment: New labour and the NHS reform agenda in England," *Law & Policy*, 32(3): 313–331.
31. Maxion-Bergemann, S. *et al.* (2006). "Complementary and alternative medicine costs - a systematic literature review," *Forsch Komplementärmed*, 13(suppl. 2): 42–45.
32. Kim, S. *et al.* (2012). "A systematic review of cost-effectiveness analyses alongside randomised controlled trials of acupuncture," *Acupuncture in Medicine*, 30(4): 273–285.
33. Kooreman, P. & Baars, E. W. (2012). "Patients whose GP knows complementary medicine tend to have lower costs and live longer," *European Journal of Health Economics*, 13: 769–776.
34. Herman, P. M. *et al.* (2012). "Are complementary therapies and integrative care cost-effective? A systematic review of economic evaluations," *BMJ Open*, 2: e001046. doi: 10.1136/bmjopen-2012–001046.
35. Hansen, C. & Kappel, K. (2010). The proper role of evidence in complementary/alternative medicine," *Journal of Medicine and Philosophy*, 35: 7–18.
36. Jackson, E. (2013). *Medical Law*, Third Edn. (Oxford University Press, Oxford, UK).
37. Lay, L. (2016). "NICE should reconsider its recommendation to withdraw acupuncture from its 2016 guidelines on low back pain and sciatica," *European Journal of Integrative medicine*, 8: 329–331.
38. Department of Health (2009). A Joint Consultation on the Report to Ministers from the DH Steering Group on the Statutory Regulation of Practitioners of

Acupuncture, Herbal Medicine, Traditional Chinese Medicine and Other Traditional Medicine Systems Practised in the UK (London).

39. Department of Health (2011). Statutory Regulation of Practitioners of Acupuncture, Herbal Medicine, Traditional Chinese Medicine and other Traditional Medicine Systems practised in the UK, Analysis Report on 2009 Consultation.
40. Ernst, E. (2004). "Patient choice and complementary medicine," *Journal of the Royal Society of Medicine*, 97(1): 41.
41. McHale, J. V. (2015). "Legal framework, professional regulation and cam practice in England." In *Routledge Handbook of Complementary and Alternative Medicine*, Gale, N. C. and McHale, J. V. (eds.) (Routledge, Abingdon, New York), ch. 4, pp. 41–60.
42. Walker, D. R. (2015). Report on the regulation of herbal medicines and practitioners. Available at: http://www.dcscience.net/Report_on_Regulation_of_Herbal_Medicines_and_Practitioners.pdf. Accessed June 2017.

Chapter 15

Understanding Traditional Chinese Medicine from a Legal and Semantic Perspective

Saisai Wang and Kim Van der Borght

1. INTRODUCTION

The mainstream opinion in Western convention medicine generally regards Traditional Chinese Medicine (TCM) as a non-science-based medicine. The criticism is that TCM is based on anecdotal information due to the difficulties in figuring out the complexities of biology, physiology, anatomy, biochemistry, genetics, infection and disease pathophysiology, and epidemiology.

However, much research has been conducted to establish scientific evidence on the safety and efficacy of traditional Chinese medicinal products (TCMPs). An example is the drug Artemisinin. It is a non-quinine-based drug that was used by the Chinese army during China's brief war with Vietnam in 1979. From this initial version of the antimalarial pill, the later drug was developed.[1]

Scientists at the Shanghai Institute of Materia Medica, where Artemisinin was first isolated, have further refined the compound into the most effective antimalarial drug to date.[2] TU Youyou was awarded the Nobel Prize in Medicine in 2015 for this discovery.[a] Similar positive cases are recorded in the professional literature, where a combination of scientific research methods and Chinese traditional medicines has led to effective treatments for various kinds of diseases.[3]

The merit of TCM in this respect has been acknowledged but there is a lack of scientific data to prove the safety and efficacy of most compounds.

2. TCM VERSUS WESTERN CONVENTIONAL MEDICINE

MacIntosh[4] explained about the different medicines in the West. The following section references the sequence of thought in her paper to make a comparison between the medicines understood by the West and TCM.

2.1. *Conventional, orthodox, allopathic, or biomedical medicine*

MacIntosh explains that the term "conventional medicine" as understood in the US is used synonymously with various terms, including allopathic medicine, orthodox medicine, traditional medicine, and biomedical medicine.

The first appearance of the word "allopathic" was in the late 18th century in reference to the use of therapeutic modalities which were based on the assumption that symptoms need to be treated. The word "allopathic" is more appropriate when describing the characteristic of the conventional medicine in the current western world, since "[t]he focus on treating symptoms appeared to have developed as one of the guiding treatment principles in orthodox medicine."

However, the terms "conventional" and "orthodox" was thought to have a "high degree of credibility" — even though they do not appropriately describe the practice of that form — so they are still widely used in practice. As MacIntosh[4] noted, "[t]he power of those terms are so great

[a] Official website of the Nobel Prize. "Youyou Tu — Biography." Available at: www.nobelprize.org/nobel_prizes/medicine/laureates/2015/tu-bio.html. Accessed 3 April 2017.

that to some extent they lead to negating the existence of any other system of medicine".

MacIntosh mentioned that traditional medicine was often used synonymously for orthodox medicine in the West, but "[i]n the sense that allopathic medicine would claim its basis to be scientific, rather than cultural or spiritual, traditional medicine should not be used synonymously with orthodox medicine." Therefore, recalling the wording of TCM, it is not difficult to understand why TCM is linked to Chinese culture rather than to medical science in the West. If "traditional" stands for "the handing down of opinions, doctrines, practices, rites, and customs, especially by oral communication," as MacIntosh writes, then TCM is not "traditional" medicine. Not only does TCM include knowledge of diagnosis but it also is a therapeutic method, in contrast to allopathic medicine. Many ancient Chinese books and the current scientific research studies record the rational and scientific essence of TCM. The rational essence encompassed by TCM is continuously explored and researched by scientists. Regarding the entirety of "traditional medicine" as a counter-scientific phenomenon could be just a linguistic ploy reflecting of a bias of superiority by Western conventional medicine. If TCM is regarded as non-scientific in the Western world, it is important to force a change of assessment by highlighting the scientific factors encompassed by TCM.

The term "biomedical" was also compared with "conventional" by MacIntosh: "It was also often used to refer to conventional medicine" due to its accurate, scientific, and proven feeling adhered to the word by Western medical doctors.[5]

2.2. *Alternative, complementary, natural, and integrated medicine*

MacIntosh also analyzed the second group of medical terms which include alternative, complementary, natural, and integrated medicine. TCM is categorized into this group in the West. She distinguishes the system of medicine and the practice of medicine. The former was ruled by American Medical Association (AMA) to be truly credible with a theoretical basis,[6] while the latter was defined in the dictionary as the "scientific study of diagnosing, treating, or preventing disease without including a system of medicine".[4] TCM belongs to the latter category in the West.

She discussed whether the therapeutic aspect of alternative medicine should be given more attention than its diagnostic aspect in the reality. She suggested that if the term "alternative medicine" is simply used to mean therapies, which can be used to treat illness, but are not the "standard of care," then the paradigm for practice of alternative medicine is the same as orthodox medicine".[4] As a kind of alternative medicine, TCM is not only about therapies but also includes a series of diagnostic procedures. The curative effect of TCM therapies have been verified in many cases, but TCM's merit is more than that. Ancient books on TCM, such as *Huang Di Nei Jing*, did record abundant knowledge on diagnosing symptoms, and they are profound on health check and have raised wide attention of the West.[7] In addition, the issue of TCM prescription must consider the TCM diagnostic mechanism.

Complementary medicine has been defined to be similar to alternative medicine, but it is conceptualized as medicinal systems used in conjunction with allopathic therapy. The term "alternative medicine" stands for medicinal systems that are more controversial in practice. In contrast, complementary medicine is more tolerated even though it too consists of nonstandard treatments.[4]

Natural medicine is considered "the science and art of preventing, curing or alleviating ill health using treatment modalities in harmony with the laws of nature".[4] Naturopathic medicine is a synonymous with natural medicine. Recognized by the West, the concept was introduced in the US in the early 1900s by a German-born healer, Benedict Lust.[8] Based on the information, TCM is not the natural medicine recognized by the West, even though it also pays attention to the relation between nature and human health.

Homeopathy is treated as another type of natural medicine. MacIntosh observed that homeopathic medicine has both a systematized theoretical and a therapeutic basis. This medicinal system was developed by the German physician Samuel Hahnemann in the late 1800s.[4] Hahnemann believed that the substance which causes the disease was the substance which can cure the disease by administering very small doses of the substance in a highly diluted form.[9] But this healing method is also controversial and its efficacy is rejected by its critics.[10,22]

MacIntosh rejects the term "holistic medicine" as an archaic and confusing term. She argues that "natural medicine" was probably a more appropriate term instead of holistic medicine, since there was no system of medicine known as holistic medicine.[4] In contrast, holistic thinking is one of the main theories in TCM, guiding the physician to treat and adjust the body's health as a whole instead of only focusing on the target. The holistic approach of TCM has raised the attention for its conceptual and philosophical underpinnings. TCM concerns the relationship between nature and the human body as well as seeing the human body as a whole, where different relationships of the parts of the body are central in understanding its functioning and health.

Finally, integrative medicine is a medicine used by a single medical practitioner who is familiar with both allopathic armamentaria and therapies and alternative medicine modalities. Nowadays, more and more TCM doctors combine TCM and the western conventional medicine. They read the check-up report produced via their armamentaria as well as use the traditional diagnostic methods, including observation, auscultation and olfaction, interrogation, and palpation, to decide the symptoms. They give prescriptions combining both western medicinal products and TCMP. In addition, lots of herbal officinalis are developed containing chemical components.

TCM is perceived differently in the West and in China. According to the terms used in the West, TCM can be categorized as traditional and holistic medicine. Following Western definitions, TCM is not orthodox medicine due to the lack of a scientific basis. It is categorized as part of CAM. In contrast, in China, TCM is orthodox medicine based on experimentalism. Changing the way TCM is viewed in the West is not an easy task but the current classification leads to confusion. It is therefore important to clarify what exactly TCM entails.

3. TERMS RELEVANT TO TCM IN CHINA

The World Health Organization defined traditional medicine as "the sum total of knowledge, skills and practices based on the theories, beliefs and experiences indigenous to different cultures that are used to maintain health, as well as to prevent, diagnose, improve or treat physical and mental illnesses". The description covers the characteristics of

TCM and it concerns traditional medicine as a combination of a diagnostic mechanism and a therapeutic method. However, the explanation is too general and broader than necessary to comprehensively capture the various elements of TCM.

3.1. *Classifications of TCM and its products*

TCM can stand for either a diagnostic mechanism or a therapeutic method. Referring to the therapeutic method, TCM can be classified into physiotherapy and drug therapy. The former is, for instance, acupuncture and massage, while the later includes different TCMPs. TCMPs can be classified from different angles. For instance, according to the function of the medicine, TCMPs can be classified into products for detoxification, products for clearing heat, products for regulating the flow of vital energy and removing obstruction, and products for promoting blood circulation and removing blood stasis, and so on. According to the part(s) of the plant that is/are used by producing the TCM, the herbal medicinal product can be classified into a product made from the root of the plant; the leaf, the flower, and stem of the plant; and so on. According to the nature of the raw materials, TCMPs can be classified into herbal medicine, animal medicine, and mineral medicine.[11]

The above classifications mainly contribute to the medical research area. They are important for physicians and practitioners who apply TCM to cure diseases and also important for pharmacists who distribute the TCMPs in the market. Although, when doing legal research, until now, TCM as a whole is not an object of EU law, TCM practitioners and various TCMPs are under subject to various regulations.

In law, TCMPs can be classified as registered and nonregistered products. The products can be dispensed either by pharmacists or by practitioners. Both registered TCMPs and nonregistered TCMPs but dispensed by registered medical practitioners are legally considered medicine.[12]

Registered medicine can be divided into proprietary medicinal products and generic medicinal products. A proprietary medicinal product is "[a]ny ready-prepared medicinal product placed on the market under a special name and in a special pack".[13] It is normally still in the protection period based on patent law. Therefore, it is also called a patent medicinal product. However, many traditional Chinese officinal products cannot apply for patent protection. Instead, the producers hold the formula secret. Then under such circumstances, the trademark law or other intellectual property rights (IPR) protection provisions can be applied to the product.

A generic drug is "a pharmaceutical product, usually intended to be interchangeable with an innovator product that is manufactured without a license from the innovator company and marketed after the expiry date of the patent or other exclusive rights".[14] Both proprietary medicinal product and generic drug include ethical drug and over-the-counter (OTC) drug. An ethical drug is that which can only be dispensed with a doctor's prescription, while OTC is prepared and packaged for the public's immediate use and has been found "to be safe and appropriate for use without the supervision of a health care professional such as a physician".[15]

Nonregistered TCMPs may be legally used as well. Many herbal medicines might be sold or imported in a form of raw materials or preparations, since Chinese doctors can combine several herbal materials or preparations to cure the disease based on the principles of formulating a prescription. In such cases, either the doctor or the practitioners should have a license.

3.2. *Terms used in Chinese legislation*

Medicine Registration and Administration Measure of China (Short for the Measure)[13] is promulgated according to the Drug Administration Law of China and the Implementing Regulation of the Drug Administration Law of China (State Council Regulation 360, 2002) to ensure the safety, efficacy, and quality control of drugs and standardize drug registration in mainland China. It applies to all drug research and clinical studies. The Measure uses the term "Chinese Medicine" to represent the TCM discussed in this chapter in order to distinguish TCM and Western medicine.

In a Notification made by China Food and Drug Administration (CFDA[16–18]), three concepts relating to TCM products were noted and these represent the forms of TCM seen in the market.[19] They are Chinese Crude Drugs, Traditional Chinese Medicine Decoction Pieces, and *Zhong Cheng*

Yao. Chinese Crude Drugs consist of the raw material of Traditional Chinese Medicine Decoction Pieces and *Zhong Cheng Yao*. China has enacted Good Agricultural Practice for Chinese Crude Drugs for regulating this part.[19] The reason why Chinese Crude Drugs are considered a medicine instead of plant or part of the body of the animals or mineral materials is that all crude drugs need to be sorted, washed, cut, and finished, so that the part of plant, animal body, or mineral material with the medicinal function can be separated efficiently (see Ref. 19, Article 30). However, crude drugs usually cannot be used by patients directly.

Traditional Chinese Medicine Decoction Pieces (hereinafter Decoction Pieces) are drugs that can be used by doctors to formulate the TCM for patients and are processing drugs. They can be given to the patients directly for decocting or to be used for producing *Zhong Cheng Yao*. It is notable that the Decoction Pieces only could be used under the supervision of Chinese doctors based on the principle of the formula rule of the TCM. The way of processing crude drugs is regulated in Chinese Pharmacopoeia,[20] and for guaranteeing the safe use of TCM, the crude drugs need to be cleaned, cut, and qualified and prepared into small pieces ready for the decoction, and formula granule is a typical decoction piece which is popularly used in current practice due to its convenient way of use by the patients.

Zhong Cheng Yao is affiliated to proprietary medicine in the Hong Kong Chinese Medicine Ordinance (HKCMO). HKCMO states that

> "[P]roprietary Chinese medicine (Zhong Cheng Yao) means any proprietary product formulated in a finished dose and known or claimed to be used for the diagnosis, treatment, prevention or alleviation of any disease or any symptom of a disease in human beings, or for the regulation of the functional states of the human body. It is composed either solely of the following as active ingredients or any Chinese herbal medicines, or any materials of herbal, animal or mineral origin customarily used by the Chinese".[21]

It is notable that HKCMO treats *Zhong Cheng Yao* as proprietary medicine: in other words, from the legal aspect, it can be protected via patent law and trademark law. But actually, *Zhong Cheng Yao* can be either a proprietary medicinal product or a generic drug. In the market, it is important to put OTC on the package of the *Zhong Cheng Yao* if a certain kind of *Zhong Cheng Yao* can be sold without the doctor's prescription. Third, *Zhong Cheng Yao* can be either a proprietary medicinal product or generic drug.

TCM practitioners may provide different services, such as acupuncture, massage, or General Practitioners (GP). For each type of service, a license to practice is needed. In China, the professionals need to be trained and educated in TCM subjects if they use TCM to treat patients.

4. INSPIRATIONS FROM THE ABOVE DISCUSSIONS

First, there might be some notions and theories in TCM which are difficult to be understood and accepted by the West at present, which is understandable since there is a big difference in the historical development of medicine between China and the West. However, a lack of understanding should not lead to a rejection of TCM by the West as it would lose out on its merits. A part of the responsibility rests on scholars, practitioners, and doctors to assist in a better understanding of TCM in the West as well as to promote reciprocal collaboration, especially in the field of scientific methodologies to ensure further scientific evidences on the safety and efficacy of individual TCMP is produced.

Second, from the aspect of law and regulation of TCM, legislations in the EU and its Member States can be divided into two groups: legal rules for practitioners and legal rules for products. The separation of rules on practitioners and products is not well-suited in the use of TCM. The products that are being regulated are mainly crude Chinese drugs and decoction pieces but Chinese medicinal practice requires the use of these products to be result of a consultation process with practitioners as described in this chapter. Regulating these products only and releasing them into the marketplace will give direct access to patients. This is not the method for a safe and effective use of these products. Patients need to be diagnosed and products need to be tailored to their individual needs and situation by a practitioner. Therefore, these products and the use by practitioners should be controlled by hand-in-glove regulation.

The other kind of legislation regulates the import and use of *Zhong Cheng Yao*, which is currently covered by EU pharmaceutical laws.

Accurate instructions on the symptoms of using *Zhong Cheng Yao* and the instructions on using the medicinal products *per se*, such as side effects, need to be shown clearly.

Third, this chapter does not pay much attention to the Chinese practitioner, since as for the term practitioner *per se*, there is not much confusion in practice. However, different types of services should be regulated by different market access rules. Acupuncture has been comparatively better accepted and regulated in the West, but Chinese GP as the executor for realizing the combination between diagnostic and therapeutic functions of TCM is hardly regulated due to a severe lack of understanding of TCM. An additional hurdle for Chinese practitioners is the difficulty in importing and regulating TCMPs. Without the products, the practitioners cannot perform their role. Without practitioners, the products cannot be safely and effectively used in the West.

REFERENCES

1. Elegant, S. (2010). "Herbal healing," *Time*, 18 November. Available at: http://lenguasmodernas.ucr.ac.cr/sites/default/files/2017–02/4.Reading%20practica%20paraphrasing.pdf. Accessed 25 April 2017.
2. Gu, J. *et al.* (1999). "The radical transformation in artemisinin: A DFT study," *Journal of Physical Chemistry A*, 103(46): 9364–9369.
3. Jiang, W. (2005). "Therapeutic wisdom in traditional Chinese medicine: A perspective from modern science," *Trends in Pharmacological Sciences*, 28(11): 558–563.
4. MacIntosh, A. (1999). "Understanding the differences between conventional, alternative, complementary," *Townsend Letter for Doctors and Patients*. Available at: http://tldp.com/medicine.htm. Accessed 25 April 2017.
5. Benjamin, S. *et al.* (1997). "Exploring the other health care systems," *Patient Care*, pp. 133–169.
6. Lynoe, N. (1989). "Theoretical and empirical problems in the assessment of alternative medical technologies," *Scandinavian Journal of Social Medicine*, 17(4): 257–263.
7. Paul, U. (2011). Unschuld and Hermann Tessenow in collaboration with Zheng Jinsheng. *Huang Di Nei Jing Su Wen — An Annotated Translation of Huang Di's Inner Classis*, (University of California Press, USA), Volume I.

8. James, C. Whorton (2003). "Benedict lust, naturopathy, the theory of therapeutic universalism," *Iron Game History*, 8(2): 22–29.
9. Schwabe, W. "History of Homeopathy and biography of Dr. Samuel Hahnemann." Available at: http://www.schwabehealth.com/wcm/mb/schwabe/en-in/home/index.html. Accessed 6 April 2017.
10. NIH (2009). "Homeopathy: An introduction." Available at: http://nccam.nih.gov/health/homeopathy. Accessed 10 November 2014 (last updated May 2013).
11. MCDMS PRC (Ministry of Commerce of the People's Republic of China Department of Market Supervision) (2012). "Analysis report on important varieties of raw materials of Chinese medicinal product 2012." Available at: http://sczxs.mofcom.gov.cn/article/dyplwz/bh/201305/20130500136736.shtml. Accessed 21 April 2017.
12. PRC (2007). Directive 2001/83/EC, Art. 5(1): Measures for Administration of Prescription.
13. Directive 65/65/EEC (1965), O.J 022, pp. 0369–0373.
14. Alfonso-Cristancho, R. *et al.* (2015). "Definition and classification of generic drugs across the world," *Applied Health Economics & Health Policy*, 13(Suppl 1): 5–11.
15. U.S. FDA (2015). "What are over-the-counter (OTC) drugs and how are they approved?" Available at: http://www.fda.gov/AboutFDA/Transparency/Basics/ucm194951.htm. Accessed 7 April 2017.
16. CFDA, Decree 28, (2007). Medicine Registration and Administration Measure of China.
17. NPC Standing Committee, (revision 2001). The Drug Administration Law of the PRC.
18. Guo Shi Yao Jian An (2003). No. 251.
19. CFDA (2002). "Good agricultural practice for chinese crude drugs." Available at: http://eng.sfda.gov.cn/WS03/CL0768/61642.html. Accessed 5 July 2017.
20. Chinese Pharmacopoeia Commission (2015). *Pharmacopoeia of the PRC*, Vol. 1 (China Medical Science and Technology Press, Beijing).
21. HKCMO, (2007). Chinese Medicine Ordinance. c 549 s 2.
22. James, G. (1993). "Homeopathy: An energy level therapy," *Journal of Professional Nurse (London, England)*, 9(1): 54–57.

Chapter 16

Female Doctors in Ancient China: Comparative Studies Through Literature and Science

Elena Santilli

When the heart opens, the eyes open too. If the heart closes, the eyes close too.

Tai Shang Huang Ting Nei Jing Yu Jing, by Wei Hua Chun.

Mutual integration between Eastern and Western healthcare visions can be pursued according to a humanistic approach. By following the hermeneutic and methodological principles outlined in the philological sources inspired by (neo) Lachmann's procedures,[1–7] an in-depth review of the relevant sources of Traditional Chinese Medicine is feasible in order to highlight the semantic, social, and integrated visions of the medical field. The use of literary techniques has the advantage to redeem the historical role of books on Chinese Medicine, positioning them in a multifaceted perspective. Indeed, avant-garde *comparativism*,[8–10] up until now only used in humanistic subjects, can be employed to enhance the value of one part of literary production often neglected by scientific manuals. This is the strategy that has been adopted for this research.

Gender investigation through classics of Traditional Chinese Medical Literature produced until the Ming Dynasty has led to a more comprehensive understanding of the opportunities of integration between different cultural systems according to the goals established by the guidelines of the Chetch Project. In cooperation with the Department of Literature of the Nanjing University of Chinese Medicine, headed by Mr. Chen Renschou, and with the active support of Mrs. Schen Jie,[a] systematic research work was carried out. The research was based on a shared method of analysis of ancient texts written by female doctors and used as training guides in Traditional Chinese Medicine. The research also entailed an in-depth review of the original materials kept at the Beijing National Library and the China Academy of Chinese Medical Science Library in Beijing. Codicological, pragmatic, and textual evidence came to light, thus leading to new joint strategies for the definition of Chinese medical and social knowledge.

More specifically, using Traditional Chinese Medical books as historical sources was possible by applying critical parameters, deemed useful for philological editing of texts. Therefore, they became the background for a social survey on links between women, medicine, culture, and political power during the centuries.

The hermeneutic value of literary analysis of the stylistic, lexical, and prosodic approach became clear, thanks to a pioneering approach on content and stylistic strategies used in passing on traditional medical knowledge, taking into account the full spectrum of supremacy of female medical culture. Expectations related to this case study were more than

---

[a] Mrs. Schen Jie is the Deputy Director of the Institute of Literature in Chinese Medicine of NJUCM, Executive Council Member & Secretary General of Specialty Committee of TCM Literature and School Research of WFCMS, Deputy Secretary General of Medical History and Literature Branch of China Association of Chinese Medicine, Council Member of Specialty Committee of Famous Schools Research of Jiangsu Association of Chinese Medicine (JSACM), Council Member of Specialty Committee of Basic Theory and Literature Research of JSACM. Mrs. Schen Jie is the author of the paper titled "Female Doctors in History," as yet unpublished. It will be printed in the III issue of *QuìiNang* series. The current chapter has been inspired by her work.

exceeded. It was therefore deemed essential to work on an integrated method and common topics by creating a multidisciplinary working group involving the University of Macerata and the Nanjing University of Chinese Medicine. This group will start its work in Summer 2017. Its goal will be to extend gender studies to technical literature, and this chapter is a preliminary endeavor of dealing with this topic.

1. INTRODUCTION: GENDER MEDICINE

In all traditions, the relationship between medicine and culture is evident since time immemorial. Most of all, medicine represented a collective *vasus* into which practical needs and philosophical theories flowed. It is no coincidence that the Greek philosopher Teofrasto[b] (fourth century B.C.), contrasted natural philosophy and medical remedies, summarizing the convergence of pragmatic and metaphysical approaches. Moreover, Galeno (second century A.D.), a physician who lived in Rome but was born in Greece, sanctioned the intimate teleology inside medicine, the requirement for Western medieval medical approach. This dual nature of medicine was cultivated in different areas and various manners. Scholars have recently underlined the fact that practical medicine was a prerogative of women. By contrast, philosophical speculation was typical of men. This "gender understanding" of the medical field is a key to interpreting our ancient sources. It also offers the opportunity to access the social structure and historical development of habits and customs.

Thanks to its innovative vision on ancient medicine, the recent essay titled "*Medichesse, La vocazione femminile alla cura*," by Erika Maderna,[11] sheds new light on our Western classical past. The essay shows the deep connection between women and medicine: after all, it is a well-known fact that therapeutic skills are delegated to the *oikos* and, because of it, women were employed to provide medical assistance in their communities. Even though the limitations of archetypical planning would entail a review of this topic, the historical accuracy of characters and events cannot be discussed. However, the full list of literary references provides a strong

---

[b] Teofr., *De sensibus*, I.

case for a multifaceted perspective on medicine. In fact, by collecting medical information, this chapter could overcome the conventional view of medicine and describe the bond between women and care, women and poetry, and women and divination. Western attitudes highlighting extra-linguistic and thematic polysemy on female gender and medicine actually strengthened in contemporary academic and non-academic debates and can also be applied to Chinese Medicine. Gender typological analysis in Chinese Medicine is justified by the marginalization of the origin of diseases: for women, in fact, it is focused on blood cycles despite the level of qi (relevant for men). It involves instability of energy, considered necessary for pregnancy, and defining a critical body–space relationship to regulate energy that is different from men's symptomatic conditions. Additionally, the dearth of systemic dissertations on female practitioners in ancient Chinese Medicine created the conditions to carry out an in-depth analysis of these mysterious figures on whom traditional medical literature is based. Consequently, the task of the authors was to draw up a preliminary list of female doctors and their writings once they had been philologically reviewed. A new anthology based on scientific criteria can identify innovative sources that are not yet available and have not yet been translated in Western countries. Some translated extracts from original texts were included in this chapter in order to show the authors' original words. All of this will hopefully lead to more systematic investigations and greater social awareness of this subject matter.

2. FEMALE DOCTORS IN CHINA

There were many female doctors in China before the Ming Dynasty, and they managed to occupy important positions in society and politics. The first female doctors were already practicing during the Han Dynasty, i.e., from second century B.C. to second century A.D. Historical sources mention *Yì Xù*,[12] a young physician who came from the Shan Xì province. Very talented in acupuncture and the preparation of decoctions generally applied from the navel to the chest, *Yì Xù*'s fame is due to her role at the Imperial Court where she was asked to tend to Empress-Mother. Given the reluctance by female members of the royal lineage to be examined by male doctors, female doctors were considered a necessity. Furthermore, this was a standard practice among common people. There is no significant information on her: what is known is that she distinguished herself because of her skills and honesty. As is typical in Chinese literary records, moral skills reflected practical abilities. There is an interesting anecdote about *Yì Xù*: one day she was asked by the empress whether her brother was worth recruiting as an army officer. *Yì Xù* prayed her mentor not to intervene in his favor because of his questionable morality.

By contrast, *Chùn Yù Yàn*,[13] compromised by politics and morally corrupted, worked as a midwife and oncologist. A contemporary of *Yì Xù*, she practiced her medical art at the Royal Palace but she was quickly dropped from court because, in order to advance her husband's career, she assassinated the Empress by administering a poisonous herb. She was found out and prosecuted.

Wèi Huà Cùn[14,15] was the most representative female doctor during the Ying Dynasty. Her name is associated with Daoist Medicine because of her interest in the work of Laozi and Zhuangzi. She is alleged to have lived between 252 and 334 A.D. and her fame grew thanks to the recognition given by Emperors of subsequent Dynasties who described her as a superhuman character. She came from the upper class (her father, *Wei Shu*/ 魏舒, was a court official) and was well educated. She married *Liu Wen* (刘文), with whom she had two sons. She later separated from her husband (318 A.D.) and lived on her own, practicing medicine for the rest of her life. *Huàng Tìng Jìng*, the title of *Wèi Huà Cùn*'s text, is divided into *Huàng Tìng Nèi Jìng Jìng*, focusing on internal organs, and *Huàng Tìng Wài Jìng Jìng*, relating to general medicine and the Daoist vision of *salus medica*. Even though scholars believe that she is not the author of the whole text, it is likely that she used it and changed its structure and content. Therefore it is fair to assume that she was somehow involved in passing this book on to posterity. After all, the link between medical texts and women is clear in the Shanqing School's hagiography that highlights the role of female doctors in developing a bodily perspective, whereby the body is perceived as an energy microcosm united with deity. In fact, her disciple, *Yang Xi* (杨羲), elevated her to the role of his soul guide, thus fostering her cult in the Maoshan Mountain, in south Nanjing.

For the purposes of this chapter, inclusion of an extract from a section on the "heart" in *Wèi Huà Cùn*'s work taken from a manuscript that was philologically restored was deemed relevant. In spite of the arduous interpretation of the text, due to its ancient poetic style that sometimes compromises its reading and hermeneutic value, the fundamental role played by the heart stands out. According to Traditional Chinese Medicine, this organ is the nucleus and the key to balanced health. It is "the monarch, the king of the whole body and other organs. If the heart starts to think, it originates all activities and, if the heart doesn't reflect, men can't have anything in mind but chaos." Human feelings are judged in the same way as the heart and as *ying* and *yang*. Therefore, the heart determines daily human activities. The medical relevance of the cardiac organ is clearly epitomized by the following poetic comparison: "The eyes are the heart's mind and if the heart is destroyed inside, eyes cannot see. The heart's mind benefits the essence of the eyes. When the heart opens, the eyes open too. If the heart closes, the eyes close too." The simple stylistic structure of these verses is linked to the content's naturalness and the logical organization of the medical description. Even though the heart is presented with a long series of metaphors, the aim of the text is achieved. The author associates the organ to a "lotus that has yet to blossom" with seeds, nourishment, and protection inside itself. Blood and qi are considered servants of the heart that is depicted as a golden bell with red ribbons (*alias* vessels). The connection of the organ with the whole body is further strengthened by references to peacefulness. "If the body's mind is peaceful, the body is quiet and diseases don't threaten. The heart dominates the tongue and the mouth. It is able to regulate human fluids and distinguish different flavours."

Bào Gu[16,17] was the most famous female doctor in China during the Jing Dynasty. She was also well known for her marriage to the inventor of a remedy against malaria, Doctor *Gè Hong*. According to records, she was the first physician to use moxibustion. However, her actual work is only recorded in literary sources. She is also remembered as a fairy-doctor, thus becoming part of popular myths not only in medical culture but also in social traditions. This meant that literary documents had to be read even more critically in order to identify the historical limitations of this woman and evaluate the role of *tales* in passing on medical and traditional knowledge. For instance, fairy tales narrate how *Bào Gu* was the inspiration behind the etymology of sagebrush or how she invented the moxibustion technique: one day, on her way back home, she met a sad girl who was crying because of her appearance. Indeed, her face was covered with tumorous masses and as a result, she was derided by her peers. *Bào Gu* was moved to pity and decided to practice moxibustion on her, releasing the girl from her pain. *Bào Gu* is alleged to have had magic powers, which she used through sagebrush's twigs. It is clear that all anecdotes are based on her fame as a female doctor but we can never consider them as historical sources. After all, there is no literary evidence of *Bào Gu*'s work although it is conceivable that some of her medical notes (about 99 on medical herbs) ended up in her husband's writings. There again, the professional relationship between *Bào* and *Gè Hong* is cemented by their interest in medicine and alchemy: despite coming from the southern Chinese district (*Bao* was born in Changzhi, in Shanxie Province, and her father *Bao Liang* was the Director of the Nanhai Prefecture), they usually spent time traveling in the Guangdong territory, expanding their skills and knowledge on the natural power of trees and water. Medicine was a life choice for both of them: *Gè Hong* left his official position to become a hermit in Mount Luofu.

The natural approach practiced by *Bào Gù* and her husband was taken up by *Hù Yin*. She is an important person from a historical point of view because she was the first female doctor to attend the Royal School of Medicine, where there were only four places a year just for men. She was the most innovative female doctor because she applied scientific criteria to the analysis of medical diseases, releasing medicine from its traditional religious and philosophical legacy. As a Daoist follower, *Hù Yin* wrote *Hùang Tìng Vèi Jing Wuzang Lin Fu Bu Xiè Tù*, a treatise on internal organs and their operating principles, liberating medical literature from contemporary mystic and religious lore. Indeed, she believed in the biological origin of diseases and, therefore, there was no connection with divine confluences and energies. It is no coincidence that the text became one of the most important medical references of the time. Divided into five chapters, each section is introduced by an iconic reference whose purpose is to symbolize the *origo mali*. This dissertation contains an extract from this treatise that is considered her most famous writing. A section on the gallbladder was added. From the version of the original manuscript kept at the *National Library* of Beijing, the section on "heart," introduced by a red bird, symbol of the instability of ascending and descending heat movements, associated to the natural element of fire, was selected.

The poetic structure is further enhanced by the first few lines focusing on the pronunciation of the heart's ideogram requiring an intense guttural outbreath. This type of airflow has numerous medicinal consequences. This is how the author describes, almost abruptly, the rigorously biological and scientific angle of her treatise. However, she still uses literary similes but mainly for educational and practical purposes: the heart's color is "silky red" and its shape is similar to that of a "flower that has yet to blossom"; its place in the body is clearly outlined as are its conditions and possible remedies. There is a reference to the link between the cardiac muscle and (i) the tongue ("If a patient is sick because of airflows acting on the heart, he is unable to speak. If the blood in the veins and arteries is obstructed, the patient's tongue looks ill.... The patient repeats his words..., has difficulty in breathing, is mournful"); (ii) the memory ("he whose beats are low will give long speeches and show fallacious memory"); and (iii) the spirit. Hence a holocentric structure of the cardiac activity can be inferred. *Hù Yin* uses the following terms: "This organ is connected to the rest of the body through veins. It manages to reach even the fingertips. It is the engine of life and action. It is the governor of all other organs; it is the home of the spirit. It is the monarch of the body." The stability of body fluids depends on the heart's functionality: "A patient with heart problems can suffer from losses of body fluids. The small intestine is an active aide of the heart and plays the role of receptor. The tongue too is connected to the heart and therefore is able to savour flavours. If the heart is sick, the tongue does not recognise flavours and shrinks, thus restricting its own functionality. The heart is also connected to the veins. If the blood is sick, it pollutes all other organs and the heart is the first to die." The paratactic style and the simple lexicon show a type of functionality that, although breaking away from the patterns of the most ancient poetry, is a source of medical pragmatic rationality offering a thematic sequence revolving around physiological, pathological, diagnostic, and corrective aspects. This does not imply a contrastive attitude toward interdisciplinary medical culture, as is also shown by the loyalty to the *Yin* and *Yang* philosophy, constantly referred to in the text. Furthermore, the heart is perceived as a living being because it interprets the ability to exist both in biological and metaphysical terms. To this end, the descriptions of the vital cycles of the heart, its habits, and peculiar features are significant: "The heart is connected to the summer and *tian gan*.... In musical scales, the heart is connected to the G note (*zhi*) that, by nature, is connected with the expansion of the fire element. Its colour is red, its flavour is bitter; its smell is that of fried food. The nature of the heart is polite and the emotions generated by the heart are associated with joy. It can be depicted as Mount Hengshan in southern China. At cosmic level, it is associated with the planet Mars." This description of the heart is followed by an in-depth explanation of its diseases and possible remedies. The author states that April and May are the best months to treat the heart or, more specifically, the fourth and fifth months of the lunar calendar. "On 7th, 8th, 22nd and 23rd days of these two months, there is a quarter moon: in the morning of these four days and with the face looking south, you must sit down and chatter teeth nine times and swallow your saliva three times. Then, you must meditate. Afterwards, breathe in red air from lit incense sticks. Move your mouth, swallow your saliva (three times) and hold your breath for thirty standard breathing acts. This practice can reinvigorate the heart and its functions."

Specific prescriptions are given for heart attack: "In this circumstance the patient's colour is red and the veins dilate. A heart attack often entails damage to the mouth. The chest, the shoulder, the upper abdominal part and the back and the arms all feel strong pain. The patient dreams of people dressed in red, with red knives or touching fire. People thus seen (in dreams) cause (in the patient) a state of profound fright. If the patient's heart is sick, the chest, the abdomen and the leg are associated with one single pain." The following is the advice given to prevent this disease: "For these heart problems, light food that is not too spicy must be eaten. To reinvigorate the heart, bitter flavours are preferable. To reduce the painful effect, however, sweet flavours are useful too. Hot food and being warmly dressed are advisable. The body, in fact, will reject water and cold."

The versatility and knowledge of *Hù Yin* is shown not only by the number of different heart diseases that are illustrated and their thorough descriptions but also by the references to the herbs used in prescriptions that were available at the time. The following is the best example of this aspect: for heart diseases shown by patients through "rigidity of the tongue, strong pain to the muscle and the need to ingest food," administering *Wu shen wan* is suggested. Patients who also show poor memory and frequently dream of the sky, must therefore take *qin jiao*, *ren shen*, *dan shen*, *xuan shen*, *gan jiang*, *sha shen*, *suan zao ren*, and *ku shen*. These herbs must be put in packets, mixed with honey to make tablets out of them, and administered on an empty stomach with a ginseng decoction (about 20 pills, twice a day)".

The preventative attitude suggested by the author is interesting. At the end of each section of her treatise, she includes a series of precautions that each man can decide to follow in his daily life. In the case of the heart, the author says: "In April (lunar calendar), eating garlic is prohibited because, if ingested, hair becomes white and falls more frequently. In May (fifth months of the lunar calendar), eating leeks is prohibited because it could be toxic for the heart. Eating animals' hearts is also prohibited. For heart problems, eating barley and apricots and *agastache rugosa* is preferable. Eating other types of fruit is also prohibited." Physical activity remains crucial: "The following exercises must be performed only in April and May of the lunar calendar: first, sit down with your palms up and then move the hands up and then down 5/6 times. For the second exercise, sit down and bring one hand up thinking that you are holding the stones of the sky and then change hand, adopting the same position. Finally, the third exercise. Cross your hands as if to form a net and then put them under your feet at the same time 5/6 times. This position manages to create wind in the heart and provides relief. This exercise must be carried out while breathing. At the end of it, shut your eyes for a while and swallow your saliva 3 times and chatter your teeth three times. And then stop."

During the Song Dynasty (960–1279 A.D.), there were only three women who distinguished themselves in the medical field. The first one to be found in literary sources is *Zhàng Xiao Niang Zi*, known for her services to the imperial household. More specifically, she distinguished herself for her fruitful studies on cosmetics that, according to contemporary accounts, were able to give "renewed and undying youthfulness" to the emperor's wife. In spite of the qualitative and quantitative limitations of written statements, it looks as if this female doctor received the secrets of aesthetics and dermatology from an old doctor in payment for the kindness and courtesy she showed him. Once again, this is a demonstration of an anthropological crystallization of the Greek *kalokagatia* acting as an etiological source for training a female doctor.

Other interesting characters were *Feng Shi* and *Li Xue*. Although the former is known to have been employed by the imperial court and was responsible for treating the Empress-Mother, distinguishing herself for her skills in preparing decoctions and handling herbs, every trace of the latter has gone lost. The very few and fragmented sources available for this period of time are mainly drawn from the cultural attitude that characterized the Song Dynasty. Even today, the conservative and harsh policy of the time, in fact, makes it hard to fully understand Chinese Middle Ages.

By contrast, the Ming Dynasty is like a ray of light for the history of Chinese female medicine. The most famous female doctor of medieval China, *Tàn Yun Xian*,[18,19] lived during this period. She lived in the Nanjing province between 1461 and 1556. She came from a family of army officers. Information on her biography can be obtained from the preface of her personal medical text that was written in prose.[c] Her grandfather had become a doctor after quitting his military position. In order to strengthen his practices and knowledge in the medical field, he had married a woman who came from a family of physicians for many generations. They had two sons but none of them were interested in pursuing the medical profession and chose military careers instead. *Tàn Yun Xian* was therefore introduced to medicine to compensate for the need to pass on family knowledge in spite of the gender restrictions this discipline was suffering from. According to the words of this author, she had shown, since she was very young, a promising talent that, unlike her sisters, made it easier for her to follow the difficult path of practicing medicine. It must be pointed out that, in the case of female doctors, learning the medical art was made arduous mainly because of the difficulty in finding patients who were willing to be treated by an apprentice doctor. This reluctant attitude toward women in social professions also meant that it was impossible to practice medicine outside one's home. At any rate, *Tàn Yun Xian* did not hesitate to cultivate medicine and used herself and her children as guinea pigs, showing great determination in having her career and fulfilling the

---

[c]A translated version of the miscellaneous book has been available since 2015. See Ref. 20.

dreams she had as a child who, accustomed to practicing the poetic art and reading classical literature, was always fascinated by books on traditional medicine.

The real mentor of this female doctor when she was young was her grandmother who ensured that the young *Tàn Yun Xian* learned the typical methods of Traditional Chinese Medicine. Just before her death, she made sure that *Tàn Yun Xian* received her instruments and formulary. She asked her to study her own medicine extensively and to treasure it. *Tàn Yun Xian* found it very difficult to deal with the loss of her grandmother, who according to her accounts, died at 73. For seven months she suffered both internally and externally while vegetating in a state of total apathy. The author herself states that it was her grandmother who rescued her from this unproductive state: she visited her in a dream and told her not to be saddened by her loss because she was not really dead but continued to live. She told her what remedies to take to recover from this state of affliction. She also told her that all the treatments to alleviate her suffering were to be found in the collection of remedies she had put together when she was alive. She therefore ordered her to recover and, subsequently, to make herself useful to society through her medicine. This story soon spread in the community (especially among its women) who found the sex of this doctor and her gender medicine an extra opportunity to receive medical care.

The outcome of *Tàn Yun Xian*'s medical experience is contained in a treatise whose *codex unicus*, kept at the Library of the Chinese Academy of Traditional Medicine in Beijing, was autoptically studied during this research. It was written all in one go in 1510 when *Tàn Yun Xian*, according to what she stated in the preface, was already 50 years old. After reviewing her grandmother's medical manual, to which she had added her own contributions, she decided to publish a first version of the text. This version was first copied by the only son she had (she also had three girls) and was then sent to her nephew for publishing. The text saw the light in 1511 as a *unicum* in the history of medical literature: in fact, not only was it drafted by a woman as a development of a medical text written by another woman, but it also contained exclusive references to diseases and medical cases related to women.

The treatise has 31 chapters, with each one of them dedicated to a medical case. The inquiring approach of this scrupulous author is evident from the various introductions with details about female patients. As well as scientific information, attention is paid to patients' social and family dynamics. Age, job, social status, and emotional conditions are detailed in the various pages of this treatise thus reconstructing, from a social and historical point of view, the lives of patients who were given traditional treatments.

A stylistic comment of the treatise would lead to a description of the author's medical prose as fundamentally sterile, devoid of literary interest and free from redundant poetic embellishments that characterized other documents written at the time. Although the presence of a rigid structure cannot be denied, the intimate connection between the textual organization and the literary purposes of the text must be reiterated. This text was conceived as a true account of medical cases and was mainly meant to be a practical consultation guide. By contrast, the methodical and rigorous presentation of medical cases and the scrupulously detailed content are worth highlighting. In the introductions to patients, which clearly show the profound closeness between this female doctor and her patients, the type of medicine that *Tàn Yun Xian* was practicing comes to the fore. In fact, she believed that lowering the emotional filter and communicating with patients were essential to practicing medicine. The opportunity her patients had to confide in this professional interlocutor enabled them to describe the main features of their symptoms exhaustively. On the other hand, it was the small details of their daily lives and their emotional discomfort that could lead the doctor to come up with more rounded diagnoses and administer treatments that were more in line with the specific responsiveness of her patients to treatments. It is not surprising to find that the *causa mali* of many women was their husbands' adulterous behavior!

From a structural point of view, each case is illustrated and explained according to some rationale that had nothing to do with contemporary medical literature. The author presents her patients and then outlines symptoms, treatments, and outcomes, without omitting notes on timings and bibliographic references. Alongside this innovative approach, there is a more conservative attitude involving constant reference to medical texts consulted in order to prescribe. All this implicitly bears witness to the validity of the chosen treatments.

Some examples of the prose and medical attitude of *Tàn Yun Xian* have been included below. The first of the 31 cases described by the doctor is that of a patient who coughs up blood and suffers from frequent retching.

"The patient is 32 years old and her husband is a merchant. Consequently, the spouse makes good money and she is financially comfortable. This woman has reported unstable temperature after following her husband in some trips and, therefore, is sick. She has vomited two bubbles of blood and coughs. The cough has been going on for three years and has never gone in spite of treatments and remedies. The patient has therefore decided to come here." The doctor decides to use "some herbs whose function is that of containing and stopping the discharge of blood, decoctions to regulate qi and subsequently some tablets to reinvigorate the body. The formulations include *sishengwan*, *bawutang* and *dabuyin wan*." The formulation in question can be attributed to a very well-known medical text titled *Fu ren da quan liang fang*. However, the doctor changes the formulation by leaving out *sheng heye* and adding *huang*, *bian bai ye*, *huang lian*, *shan zhi ren*, *xing ren*, and *bei mu* (2 *liangs* for each herb). This decision clearly shows the creativity and professional independence of the author who carries on describing how to take these remedies. It is necessary to "put the herbs in a container and mix them with honey to make some tablets. They have to be taken orally with mint as decoctions." The treatment is successful and, as the author maintains, "once the treatment is over, the patient is cured and in good health."

If this chapter shows the herbal skills of *Tàn Yun Xian*, there is no denying that the doctor was also highly skilled in other techniques. In one of the cases linked to the conditions that can follow childbirth, she states: "The patient is 27 years old and laments alternating between being cold and being feverish following childbirth.... The patient has already tried a number of remedies but to no avail.... The moxibustion technique is used and then acupuncture (type gv 14 and bl13(2) and bl 43 (2) and st36(2)). The patient is then prescribed 10 decoctions (*Tiao zhong yi qi tang* type) based on the remedy from the book titled *Dong yuan shi xiao fang*."

Listing all significant occurrences in the treatise written by *Tàn Yun Xian* in historical, philological, and medical terms would be impossible.

However, even the small number of cases that were described clearly demonstrates the quality and level of popularity of medieval medicine among female practitioners. Although it was often characterized by a "gender vision," this medicine seems to feed on traditional medical notions but not in a hierarchically binding fashion.

At times, female medicine enriches and outdoes contemporary traditions becoming a model and a reference for the entire medical literature.

3. CONCLUSIONS

The potential of gender interpretation of Chinese medical literature does not certainly end with the 15th century. Subsequently, *Zeng Yi*, who had lost her father and lived during the Qing Dynasty, managed to contain at least four epidemics thanks to her medical self-training, which she managed in spite of the fact that she lived in the countryside with her mother. *Wang Hèng Qi* and *Gu De Hua*, who lived in the Nanjing province, as well as *Lian Van* and *Yue Lin*, were described as female doctors with unrivalled medical skills. The latter two doctors were nuns: *Lian Van* had a fiancé but decided to become a nun devoting herself to the medical art and distinguishing herself in kung-fu as well as orthopedics and obstetrics. *Yue Lin* pursued the aspirations of a family that for generations had had physicians in their midst. *Ma Jun Shu* too played a fundamental role in contemporary pediatric literature, thanks to her skills in massage techniques and the publication of *Tui na Jie Jing* (1930), a text on anatomy, the functions of the organs, acupuncture, and massage techniques. It is a document that clearly shows faith in a type of medicine that safeguarded patients (children in particular) from invasive techniques typical of traditional and experimental medicine. The fame of this book has extended to this century, thanks to its heavy promotion in the 1950s (see Refs. 21–27).

Although there are other female doctors, no systematic and systemic review of sources and archives has been carried out in their cases. This review would definitely be worth attempting and useful in order to understand the weight and applicability of this type of documents in describing history and the history of women in a country like China where comparativist and thematological interpretations are still rare.

And not just that: creating a thematic account of Traditional Chinese Medicine would be a starting point to study interrelated dynamics between male and female schools of medicine and healthcare professionals. It would also be possible to study, in a synchronic and diachronic context, the clear constraints between the popularity of medicine and philosophical, religious, and political contexts. What, in this chapter, is outlined as a suggestion could be the hard core of a transthematic interpretation of Chinese medicine. Traditional medicine, i.e., the union between philosophy and science, finds its themes *right* in the fulfillment of women aspirations. However, it still suffers from neglect and misunderstanding but can be interpreted in a different manner.

By stressing once again the potential of scientific and literary methods, an invitation is made to open up to senses and tools, to relax parameters used in cataloguing and researching, to look for integration of analyses that can ensure that the profound purpose of theoretical and practical culture acquires meaning and truth.

REFERENCES

1. West, M. L. (1973). *Textual Criticism and Editorial Technique Applicable to Greek and Latin Texts* (Teubner, Stuttgard).
2. Maas, P. (1982). *Critica del testo* (Le Monnier, Florence) [in Italian].
3. Pasquali, G. (1988). *Storia della tradizione e critica del testo* (Le Lettere, Florence) [in Italian].
4. Montanari, E. (2003). *La critica del testo secondo Paul Maas: testo e commento* (SISMEL Edizioni del Galluzzo, Florence) [in Italian].
5. Timpanaro, S. (2004). *La genesi del metodo del Lachmann* (UTET, Turin) [in Italian].
6. Malato, E. (2008). *Lessico filologico, un approccio alla filologia* (Salerno Editrice, Rome) [in Italian].
7. Reynolds, L. D. & Wilson, N. G. (2016). *Copisti e Filologi. La tradizione dei classici dall'antichità ai tempi moderni,* (edizione 4) (Medioevo e Umanesimo, Edizioni Antenore, Roma-Padova) [in Italian].
8. Gnisci, A. (2002). *Letteratura comparata* (Bruno Mondadori, Milan) [in Italian].
9. Trousson, R. (1965). *Un problème de littérature comparée: les études de thèmes, essai de méthodologie* (M.J. Minard, Lettres Modernes, Paris) [in French].

10. Detienne, M. (2005). *I Greci e noi* (Raffello Cortina Editore, Milano).
11. Maderna, E. (2012). *Medichesse, La vocazione femminile alla cura* (Aboca, Arezzo, Italy).
12. 汉·司马迁.史记·卷一二二·酷吏列传第六十二.北京:中华书局, 1959.
13. 汉·班固.汉书·卷九十七上·外戚传第六十七上.北京:中华书局, 1962.
14. 明·张宇初.道藏.影印本.天津：天津古籍出版社, 1987.
15. 张继禹.中华道藏.北京:华夏出版社, 2004.
16. 宋·李昉,等.太平广记.北京:中华书局, 1961.
17. 杨顺益.晋代女针灸家鲍姑及鲍姑艾.中国针灸, 1989 (2), pp. 42–43.
18. 郑金生.明代女医谈允贤及其医案《女医杂言》.中华医史杂志，1999, 29(3), pp. 153–156.
19. 汪剑.谈允贤《女医杂言》评按译释.北京:中国中医药出版社, 2016.
20. Wilxon, L. & Lu, Y. (2015). *Miscellaneous Records of a Female Doctor* (Chinese Medicine Database, USA).
21. 李经纬.中医人物词典.上海:上海辞书出版社, 1988.
22. 李云.中医人名辞典.北京:国际文化出版公司, 1988.
23. 严世芸.中国医籍通考.上海:上海中医学院出版社, 1991.
24. 陈道瑾,薛渭涛.江苏历代医人志.南京:江苏科学技术出版社, 1985.
25. 清·裘庆元.珍本医书集成·医案杂著类.北京:中国中医药出版社, 1999.
26. 胡翘武,胡国俊.曾懿女医晚年医学轶事.四川中医, 1985, (10), pp. 6–7.
27. 邓玉海,赵毅.女推拿学家马君淑.按摩与导引, 2000, 16(6), pp. 69–70.

Part 3

Traditional Chinese Medicine: Evidences from the Medical Field

Chapter 17

Using International Perspective to Develop Traditional Chinese Medicine

Xiaolin Yuan and Xu Zhang

1. INTERNATIONALIZATION IS THE INEVITABLE TREND OF THE DEVELOPMENT OF CHINESE MEDICINE

With the development of globalization, the concept of human health and the medical model is undergoing an epoch-making change. The dialogue of crosstalk and fusion from different regions, societies, and cultural traditions becomes increasingly obvious. In an era of modern medicine, with the complementary and common development of Chinese medicine learning from each other, globalization has arrived, and internationalization is the inevitable trend in the development of Chinese medicine.

The development of modern science and technology has led to a change in the modern medical model from biomedicine to the medical, biological, psychological, social, and environmental factors model. The purpose of medicine has shifted from the infinite pursuit of disease and its treatment to prevention. Such an adjustment in direction is gradually coincident with the Traditional Chinese Medicine (TCM) as a whole, system theory, treatment based on pattern differentiation, and health care ideas. In other words, the direction of the development of Chinese medicine is consistent with the future development of medical trends. At the same time, with social and economic development and improvement in people's living standards, people's concept of health is also quietly changing. They not only want to get medical treatment but also hope that they can prevent themselves from getting sick, or get sick less frequently. The change in this concept of health and health needs adheres to the basic tenets of Traditional Chinese Medicine, which emphasizes the ideas of "preventive treatment of disease, disease prevention, and prevention of recurrence after healing".

More importantly, the process of the internationalization of Chinese medicine has also coincided with the World Health Organization (WHO) adjusting its global strategy, thereby providing an historic opportunity. The WHO's new global strategy (2014–2023) aims to "build knowledge base for active management of traditional and complementary medicine (T&CM) through appropriate national policies to strengthen the quality assurance of traditional and complementary medicine by regulating products, practices and practitioners to promote universal health coverage by integrating T&CM SERVICES appropriately into health service and self-health care." This is a new, open, and friendly approach to traditional medicine, involving knowledge-based traditional medicine systems and policies, emphasizing the potential of traditional medicine, informed choice, and self-care and urging member countries to integrate traditional medicine into the their respective national health service systems. The WHO has initiated a program to integrate traditional medicine into the International Classification of Diseases (ICD) system and to become a member of the WHO International Fraction Family (WHO-FIC) at the same time. The successful advancement of the program means that the first authoritative international disease classification standard will emerge from ancient Traditional Chinese Medicine.

Traditional Chinese Medicine based on the theoretical basis of the Chinese medicine classification system will witness global promotion and meet international standards, while the WHO platform will help promote Chinese medicine as a health and wellness service for mankind more accurately, positively, and widely, resulting in far-reaching impact. According to this idea, China has insisted on the use of Traditional Chinese Medicine resources for research, exploitation, and application for a long time, which is not only a pragmatic measure but also a forward-looking view. At the same time, WHO's new strategy has also opened the door to not only promote the spread of Chinese medicine and the acceptance of Member States but also propose new requirements on the standardization of Traditional Chinese Medicine research and intellectual property protection, further promoting sustainability of the resource development and use and the effectiveness of products, training, and services.

In addition, the internationalization of Chinese medicine is also an economic and cultural strategy in line with China's national interest. In recent decades, the achievements of China's economic development have attracted increasing worldwide attention. At the same time, there is an increasing attention to Chinese culture and the Chinese medicine industry, which embodies the essence of Chinese culture. Chinese medicine has become a "business card" of Chinese culture, and the process of internationalization of Chinese medicine has become an important part of China's national strategy.

President Xi Jinping pointed out: "Chinese medicine embodies the profound philosophy and the health concepts and experience of the Chinese nation for thousands of years. It is not only the treasure of ancient Chinese science but also the key to the treasure trove of Chinese civilization." Wang Goqiang, the Director of the State Administration of Traditional Chinese Medicine, also stressed that "China will actively implement the strategy to promote Chinese medicine development outside China, which will help us achieve the goals of 'the Belt and Road Initiatives'."

Wang Shen, Vice President of the Chinese Academy of Traditional Chinese Medicine also believes that: "The internationalization of Chinese medicine is the only way to develop Chinese medicine and the window to the world."

The next decade will be a critical period for the internationalization and prosperous development of Chinese medicine in the world. The *Strategic Plan for the Development of Traditional Chinese Medicine (2016–2030)* issued by the State Council also identified the "government support, civil operation, local services, mutual benefit and win-win" as the principles behind the building of overseas Chinese medicine centers. The success of the internationalization of TCM depends on the smooth progress of the national strategy.

Finally, the rapid development of Chinese medicine in the world also shows that the trend of internationalization is irresistible. According to incomplete statistics, at present, Chinese medicine has spread to 183 countries and regions in the world, and Confucius Institute of Chinese Medicine has been established in four countries. China has signed 83 agreements with foreign governments and relevant international organizations on medicine cooperation. Worldwide, there are nearly 100,000 medical institutions, with the number of practitioners of Chinese medicine reaching 300,000. Ma Jianzhong, Deputy Director of the State Administration of Traditional Chinese Medicine, pointed out that: "The background of the times provides a good opportunity for the exchange and cooperation of Chinese medicine; the scientific and orderly development of Chinese medicine has laid a solid foundation for the exchange and cooperation of Chinese medicine and the characteristics of Chinese medicine itself, exploring more room for the exchange and cooperation." *The Strategic Plan for Development of Traditional Chinese Medicine (2016–2030)* will also take on the tasks of the development of Chinese medicine as one of the priorities in the next few years, which include participation in international cooperation and competition, promotion of the localization of social services, and Chinese medicine international education, including Chinese medicine development overseas. This shows that, "going out of the country, to the world" internationalization strategy is not only the inevitable trend in the development of Chinese medicine but also provides a strong external impetus for the development of Chinese medicine.

2. THREE ASPECTS OF THE INTERNATIONALIZATION PROCESS OF CHINESE MEDICINE

The internationalization process of Chinese medicine has taken place since the 1970s, and a significant aspect of the process is that it has gone through gradual change, from nongovernmental exchanges to governmental cooperation. It was pointed out that "The Government play a very important role to promote the trade services development of Chinese medicine under current situation. The internationalization of Chinese medicine industry is not high, hence the government must have strong hands to promote international development." TCM researchers and professionals have put forward in more detail the strategic model of internationalization strategy of Chinese medicine, namely the five-dimensional development framework: "the technology clearing the way, the culture paving the way, the medical converging, industry advancing, talent output". Further development agenda as include "international standardization of TCM, international academic exchanges, information sharing and personnel exchanges, international trade in services and international training" and other means. All these indicate that the trend of internationalization of Chinese medicine has not only been the general consensus in the industry but also many practitioners have provided feasible suggestions and direction for its implementation.

At present, the internationalization of Chinese medicine must be supported and the government must provide opportunities to carry out joint research projects, as only in this way could we fully reflect the strategic intent of internationalization. Chinese medicine practices clinical efficacy and its scientific research potential can be fully exploited and the resulting development of Chinese medicine could also be guaranteed. In this process, the internationalization of the Chinese medicine industry is the main body, the internationalization of scientific research is a vanguard, and internationalization of education provides a strong backing. These three aspects, by supporting each other, constitute the complete chain of the internationalization of Chinese medicine.

First, the internationalization of industry is the main body and core of the internationalization of Chinese medicine. The primary aim behind the internationalization of Chinese medicine is to provide effective Chinese medicine products and services to people around the world; strive to solve the various diseases, pain, and discomfort of patients; and eventually deliver quality products to consumers, which is the key to the survival of the Chinese medicine industry. Therefore, the core of the internationalization of Chinese medicine and the main body is the international industry in line with the law of the market economy. After decades of development, the role of the current Chinese medicine industry in the economic status of the system is more important, and its development is more mature. With the international Chinese medicine market originally spreading due to the demand of the Chinese people residing in Southeast Asia and then to Europe and the United States, there has been a gradual convergence to the main gathering of the developed countries. The overseas Chinese medicine industry generates business from the commission of foreign sales agencies to set up joint venture sales. Market competition also arises from the extensive price competition to the technology, quality, and service competition. The development of the enterprise also pay more attention to attract foreign capital shares and set up production, sales, and overseas research and development (R&D) base, focusing on technology R&D and personnel training. Therefore, the internationalization of the Chinese medicine industry has become an inevitable trend and already has a considerable foundation for the development of Chinese medicine industry. Thus the internationalization of the effect will be directly related to the success of the process of internationalization of Chinese medicine.

Second, the internationalization of scientific research is the forerunner and pioneer of Chinese medicine internationalization. As early as 2006, an acupuncturist who has worked in the United States for many years appealed that scientific research must be the first to develop for the internationalization of the Chinese medicine. In 2015, the Chinese scientist Tu You-you won the Nobel Prize in Physiology or Medicine for his research on artemisinin, which proves that the scientific research on Chinese medicine can not only stand at the forefront of international academic research but also be a powerful leader in promoting the internationalization of Chinese medicine. Compared to a few decades ago, we have made great progress on the scientific research of Chinese medicine in terms of government funding, staff strength, the expansion of research, and the results output of the project, but there are still some problems that require attention, such as narrow research areas, uneven research resources distribution, backward evaluation system, and other issues. In particular, the process of linking the research work of Chinese medicine in China with that of the international academic community is not in place, which renders the research work of Chinese medicine science still at a low level of repetition, inadequate clinical and interdisciplinary integration. To break away from this situation, we must follow closely the pace of the international academic community, be familiar with the current international medical community's hot, difficulty and the key point and master the multidisciplinary theory, technology, and methods, tapping the academic value and research potential of Chinese medicine in an in-depth manner and encouraging innovation, crosstalk, and an effective scientific research and evaluation system. It will not only push the internationalization of Chinese medicine industry but also play a leading role in further promoting the internationalization of Chinese medicine education.

Third, the internationalization of education is the internationalization of Chinese medicine backing and protection. The essence of the internationalization of TCM education lies in the dissemination of TCM culture and the cultivation of Chinese medicine talent. On one hand, the premise of internationalization of Chinese medicine is the recognition of Chinese culture and its fundamental identification with the Chinese culture, since without this cultural identity, the Chinese medicine industry cannot really be accepted on a global platform. And once the people of other countries in the world are aware of the identity of the Chinese medicine culture with the help of the various sources, such as TCM classics, Chinese medicine clinics, Chinese medicine schools, pharmacies and other entities, TCM expositions, Chinese medicine culture festivals, or Chinese medicine websites, the Chinese culture will in turn become a powerful guarantee to promote the internationalization of Chinese medicine. On the other hand, both the management and decision-making of the Chinese medicine industry, or the exploration and application of Chinese medicine research, are inseparable from the international perspective of talent. Therefore, the cultivation of Chinese medicine is the fundamental guarantee of the internationalization process. The operation of modern pharmaceutical enterprises requires not only international strategy and courage of the decision-makers but also an understanding of both the government and professional community. Furthermore, it requires communication and leadership skills of senior personnel and its international operations need to have the requisite resources for technology, marketing, leadership, implementation and other professional skills of the echelon. According to incomplete statistics, by the end of 2012, the number of Chinese engaged in the international exchange of Chinese medicine personnel reached 30, and the number of expatriates reached 3,800. The number of TCM training institutions operating overseas was 30 and their affiliated institutions were present in more than 30 countries and regions. The talent team selection and training must be performed keeping in mind that they are being done for both domestic and overseas roles. Therefore, an international talent team must be chosen, such that its presence and growth will also continue to promote the process of internationalization of Chinese medicine.

In the specific implementation, the presumption of the combination of industry, scientific research, and education is an effective "international integration of Chinese medicine production and research alliance." The internationalization of Chinese medicine production and research alliance was suggested in 2010. "Now the Chinese medicine industry has a reasonable structure and large scale. Particularly, the group of advanced manufacturing enterprises is guided by the science and technology. It is the right time to go out" said the proposal. Through the establishment of an industry–university–research alliance, once can integrate domestic and foreign advantages of resources to form a joint force, which forms the basis of a tailored roadmap for the worldwide spread of a traditional national industry. One researcher also believes that: "The combination of production, education and science is a fundamental solution to the problem of school education and social dislocation." In this process, the creation of business-oriented international entities provides a viable exploratory direction. For example, "Traditional Chinese Medicine Global Alliance (TCMGA)," is a "market-oriented operation that the enterprises and research institutes union voluntarily to project as a link, to provide professional services to the interests of the fair and reasonable distribution of the cooperative organization under the government guidance." The first consortium includes 12 companies and six research institutes. The establishment of the Union, direct communication of the clinical application of Chinese medicine, and basic scientific research, further connected to the efficacy analysis and quality control, provides a substantive beneficial exploration for the internationalization of Chinese medicine.

3. SEVERAL PROBLEMS IN THE INTERNATIONALIZATION OF CHINESE MEDICINE

Although the TCM industry, scientific research, and overseas education have made some progress, they are still in the early stages of internationalization. We have to respond positively to some of the problems encountered before ensuring the smooth progress of the next stage of internationalization in order to achieve further development and expansion. The current problems are elucidated below.

The first is the standard of the Chinese medicine industry, including the access standards of the Chinese medicine industry and the quality standards of Chinese medicine products. As mentioned earlier, the targets markets of Chinese medicine industry have been the Middle East, Southeast Asia, other Asian countries, and gradually, Europe, United States, South America, Africa, and further expansion to other countries. Hence, the Chinese medicine industry will inevitably encounter product access qualification issues. Take the United States for example: the US Food and Drug Administration (FDA) stresses on the strict implementation of the drug classification system, especially for the state to implement strict application of drug testing and technical testing. In the FDA approval standards, the Chinese medicine is only identified as a "complementary and alternative medicine," which means it cannot be compared with mainstream medicines and can only be taken in the form of health food, health products, and food additives in the US market. Although later this rule has been relaxed, the problem of access of Chinese medicine has not been completely solved. The other is the quality standards of Chinese medicine products: the production of TCM products involves cultivation, active ingredient extraction, toxicology efficacy testing, drug manufacturing, packaging, and other aspects that must conform to the relevant international standards. Therefore, the lack of uniformity in quality norms will greatly limit the pace of internationalization of Chinese medicine. To solve these problems, an in-depth study of the international quality standards of common pharmaceutical products and countries on the basis of specific provisions to develop realistic Chinese medicine industry norms and product quality standards is an important step to promote the process of internationalization.

The second is the problem of the localization of Chinese medicine. The development of medicine in China for thousands of years shows that this is in line with China's special national conditions and social needs of the disease diagnosis and treatment. Its greatest feature is consideration of individual's constitution, environment, and climatic and seasonal conditions in the treatment of diseases. Chinese medicine can play its unique role in resolving specific diseases in specific areas, and it can obtain the recognition of the local people and the government in order to take root in the local area. Internationalization can also be effectively promoted. At present, a remarkable achievement of the process of localization of Chinese medicine is the flourishing of overseas Chinese medicine education and research. For example, the author participated in the fourth "Ministration of Education's training for Chinese Medicine Teachers Teaching International Students in English" in May 2016 and had the honor to listen to a number of well-known scholars from the United States, Britain, Canada, Australia, and other countries on national education and Chinese medicine multicultural classroom introduction, thereby proving that the vision of internationalization is wide open. Prof. Sun Zhongren, Vice President of Heilongjiang University of Traditional Chinese Medicine, also proposed to use "the platform of the Confucius Institute to train local Chinese medicine talents to contribute to the development of Chinese medicine and international competitiveness." Therefore, the effective measures of Chinese medicine internationalization is using local animal and plant resources, exploring new sources of drugs, and continuing to strengthen the potential of indigenous medicine resources research to cultivate local social and cultural knowledge of Chinese medicine talent. Thus a solid advancement in localization is the source of vitality of Chinese medicine internationalization.

The third is the clinical efficacy of Chinese medicine. As early as 2006, someone pointed out: "The efficacy of Traditional Chinese medicine has brought vitality to Chinese medicine for thousands of years and made a great contribution to China's prosperity." It was further added that the value of TCM depends on its clinical efficacy. TCM is used not only for the treatment of general diseases and difficult illnesses, but more importantly, it can solve clinical difficulties that the Western medicine still cannot solve, reflecting the advantages of TCM, which is the clinical research and basic research of basic point and starting point. Further scientific research on the clinical applications of TCM put forward a higher claim. In the context of the discourse on Western medicine, the study of Chinese medicine has encountered great difficulties, but clinical research can be more easily achieved with the experience accumulated over thousands of years in China's historical practice. The Science Citation Index data of relevant TCM literatures also show that the international academic circles are more interested in the research of acupuncture and moxibustion, decoction, and medicinal properties than medical history research and theoretical research. In this regard, for the rapid integration of TCM with the mainstream medical community through the scientific research and clinical applications, we must start with clinical efficacy. These two aspects of the internationalization of Chinese medicine are important parts of the process.

Fourth is the popularization of Chinese medicine. Some researchers pointed out that "the premise of internationalization of Chinese medicine industry is the cultural identity of Chinese medicine, without cultural identity, the Chinese medicine industry cannot really go out." Cultural acceptance is the main problem that hinders the popularization of TCM. Professor Sun Zhongren said, "People are deeply affected by the culture and receive the direct benefits. Publicity targeted at the public is the key to success. We can truly influence a country's culture only by influencing its people." TCM is accompanied by the history of Chinese culture and its formation. It is not only a science and technology to deal with but also a distinctive feature and rich connotation of human culture. Chinese medicine is rooted in Chinese culture and its model is based on the integration of the ancient natural and human sciences, under the influence of Chinese cultural traditions, while also involving the formation of the basic characteristics of TCM and prevention concepts, as well as clinical practice in accordance with the development model. Therefore, spreading the essence of Chinese medicine requires the popularization of Chinese culture. In this respect, both national and nongovernmental forces can play their respective roles in specific fields.

To sum up, the internationalization of Chinese medicine is not only a national strategy for China so as to participate in the development of economic globalization, enhancing its international competitiveness and international image, but also a historic opportunity to promote the upgrading of the TCM industry and promote the scientific research of TCM and the transformation of TCM education. The process of internationalization of Chinese medicine must adhere to the industrial, scientific research, and education troika to keep pace with each other, and promote common development model and state, in order to achieve economic, cultural, and social benefits of balanced development. At present, we are still in the early stage of internationalization of Chinese medicine, during which the problems of standardization, localization, clinicalization, and popularization are not only a reflection of the achievements and deficiencies of the previous stage but also provide the opportunity and direction for the further advancement of the later stage.

BIBLIOGRAPHY

1. Zhang, B. L. & Zhang, J. H. (2015). "Twenty years' review and prospect of modernization research on traditional Chinese medicine," *Zhongguo Zhong Yao Za Zhi*, 40(17): 3331–3334.
2. Shang, H. C., Zhang, B. L. & Li, Y. P. (2008). "Thinking and methods in practical assessment of TCM clinical therapeutic effect," *Zhongguo Zhong Xi Yi Jie He Za Zhi*, 28(3): 266–268.
3. Wang, G. & Song, J. (2010). "Technical standards of traditional Chinese medicine industry," *Zhongguo Zhong Yao Za Zhi*, 35(12): 1644–1647.
4. Yang, X., Xiao, S., Guo, Z., Wang, Z. & You, Y. (2012). "Analyses on positive influence of harmonious development of traditional Chinese medicine compounds' researches and patent protection," *Zhongguo Zhong Yao Za Zhi*, 37(1): 9–12.

5. Yuwen, Y., Han, X. J., Wang, L. Y., Shi, N. N., Wang, Y. Y. & Lü, A. P. (2011). "Thinking on methods for formulating development strategy of traditional Chinese medicine standardization," *Zhong Xi Yi Jie He Xue Bao*, 9(5): 483–48.
6. Yi, X. F. & Chang, B. Y. (2014). "Improving the TCM international power of communication by the localization of TCM," *China News of Traditional Chinese Medicine*, January 16, p. 3.

Chapter 18

Cancer-Related Digestive Symptoms

Qijun Fang, Yujuan Wang and Tianshu Xu

1. INTRODUCTION

Digestive symptoms such as nausea, vomiting, abdominal pain, and diarrhea are most common adverse reactions of cancer patients undergoing radiotherapy and chemotherapy using medication such as Cisplatin and Pacilitaxel. Clinical evidence has shown that 70–80% of cancer patients who underwent chemotherapy treatment experienced nausea and vomiting.[1] When simultaneously treated by orally prescribed antagonistic drugs, patients can always present obvious side effects and have a remarkably decreased quality of life.

As proved by previous animal and clinical experiments, acupuncture could improve digestive symptoms through a variety of mechanisms, such as regulating gastric electrical-rhythm disorders by increasing the storage of serotonin and gastrin in the gastric antrum and reducing their release into the serum. This chapter is primarily concentrated on specific manual techniques and related mechanisms of acupuncture for the improvement of cancer-related digestive symptoms, especially nausea and vomiting.

2. ACUPUNCTURE

2.1. *Body acupuncture*

Prescription:

Main points: Neiguan (PC6), Zusanli (ST 36), Zhongwan (CV12).

Manipulation:

First, the acupunturist should wash hands. Second, keep the patient in a supine position, sterilize the skin comprising the acupoints, and insert the needle (0.25 mm × 40 mm) into the acupoints using the mild reinforcing and reducing method by lifting-thrusting and twirling-rotating. When the patient feels ache, numbness, heaviness, or distension around the acupoint, then hold the needle in the acupoints for 20–30 mins. The treatment is given once per day and lasting for 14 days.

Modifications:

For asthenia-cold in the spleen and stomach, Pishu (BL20) and Weishu (BL21) are added; for insufficiency of stomach yin, Taixi (KI3) and Sanyinjiao (SP6) are added; for liver qi invading the stomach, Tai-chong (LR3) and Qimen (LR14) are added; for fullness and distension in the epigastrium and abdomen, Zhangmen (LR 13), Burong (ST19), and Pishu (BL20) are added.

Cautions:

(a) The selection of needling methods should be made according to the patient tolerance. For patients who are nervous or weak, mild manipulation can be used after the procedure for their recovery.
(b) Acupoints close to vital organs or large blood vessels should be carefully needled.
(c) Acupoints on the areas with infection, ulcer, scar, or tumor should not be needled.
(d) Patients experiencing blood coagulation and having hemorrhagic tendency should not be punctured.

(e) It is inadvisable to provide acupuncture treatment to women during their menstruation period.
(f) For patients fitted with a cardiac pacemaker, electroacupuncture should be forbidden.

Progression:

A total of 26 patients were admitted to Zhang's clinical research group, except the routine treatment for vomiting (metoclopramide 20mg, im, bid, and Ondansetron 8mg, iv, qd 30 min before chemotherapy), they were punctured at bilateral Neiguan (PC 6) and Zusanli (ST 36) twice a day before the chemotherapy lasting until three days after the chemotherapy, with each treatment lasting for 30 min. All the patients were adapted to the self-comparison approach, i.e., the needling therapy was used either in the first or the second treatment course. Finally, the patients undergoing the acupuncture treatment were found to have a lower rate and degree of vomiting than the control group (57.7% vs. 73.1%, $p < 0.01$) and an improved life quality.[2] Animal experiments showed that electroacupuncture on Zhongwan (CV12) and Neiguan (PC6) could inhibit 5-HT secretion in the central nervous system (CNS) of rats exhibiting nausea or vomiting induced by chemotherapy.[3] Zhang *et al.* found that acupuncture could improve gastrointestinal symptoms through a variety of mechanisms, such as regulating gastric electrical-rhythm disorders by increasing the storage of serotonin and gastrin in the gastric antrum and reducing their release into serum.[4]

2.1.1. *Abdominal acupuncture*

Prescription:

Main points: Zhongwan (CV12), Xiawan (CV10), Qihai (CV6), Guanyuan (CV4).[5]

Manipulations:

First, the acupunturist should wash hands. Then tell the patients to maintain a supine position, and then sterilize the skin comprising the acupoints.

Insert the needle (0.22 mm × 40 mm), with the depth of needle depending on the position of the disease. These acupoints should be inserted by slight twirling and rotating or just twirling without rotating. The depth of CV12, CV6, and CV4 should be deep, while CV10 is Middle, then hold the needle in the acupoints for 20–30 min. The treatment is given once per day, lasting for six days. The order should be as followed: CV12, CV10, CV6, CV4.

Modification:

For constipation, Tianshu (ST 25) is added; for diarrhea, Shuifen (CV9) is added. For abdominal pain, Daheng (SP 15) is added, and for deficiency of stomach yang, moxibustion on Shenque (CV8) is added.

Caution:

Besides the cautions to be taken while performing body acupuncture, some others also should be noted as followed:

(a) The order of removing the needles should be the same as that in which they were inserted.
(b) Patients with acute peritonitis pain or abdominal tumor should be forbidden from undergoing this procedure.

Progression:

In Xing's clinical research, 30 in-patients preparing to receive Cisplatin-based chemotherapy for at least two cycles were divided into an observation group and a control group (by the envelope-concealing method) to conduct a self-controlled crossover study. The observation group was treated by abdominal acupuncture together (CV12, CV10, CV6, CV4) with Tropisetron hydrochloride, and the control group were treated only by Tropisetron hydrochloride. From the chemotherapy days one to six, the gastrointestinal reactions (nausea and vomiting), other adverse reactions to chemotherapy, as well as blood routine, liver, and kidney function examinations before and after treatment were recorded. At last, compared to group that only used Tropisetron hydrochloride, abdominal acupuncture plus Tropisetron hydrochloride was found to reduce nausea and delayed vomiting more effectively. (96.7% vs. 73.3%; 96.7% vs. 93.3%).[6]

3. MOXIBUSTION

Manipulations:

Mild-Warming Moxibustion

Guanyuan (CV4), Qihai (CV6), Zusanli (ST36), Zhongwan (CV12), and Shenque (CV8) are selected as the main acupoints. Take a lighted moxa and point it to the former acupoint with 3 cm distance, without moving. The exact distance is set such that the patients just feel warmth but not scorching heat. Each acupoint can be moxibusted for 15 min until erythema of the skin appears. This treatment is given once per day, lasting for seven days.

Ginger Moxibustion

A slice of fresh ginger about 2–3 mm thick is cut, punched with several holes in its center, and then placed on the selected acupoint. Place a lighted moxa on ginger: when the moxa burns out completely, remove it and replace with a new one until the local skin turns reddish but without the formation of blisters. Generally, three cones are used for each point per treatment session. Repeat this treatment one another day, three to four times per week, with the whole treatment lasting four weeks. Guanyuan (CV4),

Zusanli (ST36), Shenque (CV8), Zhongwan (CV12), and Neiguan (PC6) are mostly often selected as the main acupoints for treating vomiting and nausea.[7]

Thunder-Fire Moxibustion

Neiguan (PC6), Zusanli (ST36), and Zhongwan (CV12) are mostly chosen as main acupoints. Take a cylinder-shaped moxibustion at a suitable distance from the skin such that patients can bear the heat. ST36 and CV12 usually use rotational moxibustion, with eight rounds comprising one group. The interval time between every group is 5 s. The treatment should be stopped when the patients feel the temperature of local skin too high to bear. CV12 is treated by sparrow-pecking moxibustion, and the moxa stick is ignited and kept about 2–3 cm above the skin. When the patients feel a burning sensation in their skin, the moxa stick is moved away quickly, and after 5 s, the above movement is repeated. Moving the moxa stick away seven times is considered as one cone, and five cones are applied on each point. The treatment was given once a day, with seven times comprising one course.[8]

Direct Moxibustion

In order to increase the adhesion of moxa cone to the skin, some garlic juice, Vaseline, or some another medicine should be placed on both Geshu (BL17) and Zusanli (ST36). With a moxa stick measuring about 0.5 cm × 0.8 cm made up of mugwort wool is ignited. And when the stick is burned until one-third of its size, replace with a new one, and repeat this procedure for three times. The treatment was given once a day, with seven times comprising one course.[9]

Cautions:

(a) For patients with numbness of limbs or bradyesthesia, moxibustion should be moderate to avoid scalding.
(b) For patients whose skin is broken or infected or have allergy to some traditional Chinese medicines, moxibustion is not advisable.
(c) For patients who are famished or suffer from overheating or extreme exhaustion, fear, or thirst, moxibustion is not advisable.
(d) It is inadvisable to provide acupuncture treatment to women undergoing menstruation.

Progression:

Ruan *et al.*[10] divided the gastric-cancer patients who received S-1 plus oxaliplatin chemotherapy into two groups, the treatment group were given herb-partitioned moxibustion at the same time they began chemotherapy, and the treatment lasted 14 days following a latency of 7 days. So one treatment course was 21 days. The vomiting degree, vomiting times, associated symptoms, Karnofsky score, the European Organization for Research and Treatment of Cancer, and Quality of Life Questionnaires were observed after two treatment courses. Zhongwan (CV12), Guanyuan (CV4), Neiguan (PC6), Zusanli (ST 36), Tianshu (ST25), and Daheng

(SP15) were selected as main the acupoints, and the herb-partitioned moxibustion was made up of Banxia, Jupi, Huanglian, Wuzhuyu, and Dingxiang, with the juice of fresh ginger. Compared to the control group, the vomiting degree decreased significantly in the treatment group on the 1st, 7th, and 14th day of chemotherapy ($p < 0.05$), and compared with the 1st day, the vomiting degree decreased significantly on 14th day in the treatment group. Compared to the control group, stomach pain, fatigue, and poor appetite were significantly relieved in the treatment group on the 14th day of chemotherapy ($p < 0.05$). The scores of karnofsky Performance Status (KPS) and European Organization for Research and Treatment Quality of Life Questionnaires (EORTC QLQ) in the treatment group were superior to those in the control group ($p < 0.05$)

4. ACUPOINTS-MOUNTING

Acupoint selection:

Neiguan (PC6), Zusanli (ST36), Zhongwan (CV12), Pishu (BL20), Weisu (BL21), Shenque (CV8), and Yongquan (K11) are selected as the main acupoints.

Manipulations:

Chinese herb medicine is broken into powder, which performs the function of warming the spleen and stomach to descend adverse-rising qi. Then the powder is made into a box shape using the juice of fresh ginger, with the size being 1 cm × 1 cm × 1 cm. Then they are pasted using medical tape and placed on the selected acupoints. Four hours later, the powder and tape are removed. The whole treatment lasts 14 days.

Cautions:

(a) For patients whose skin is broken, infected, or allergic to some Traditional Chinese Medicine or tape, this treatment is not advisable.
(b) It is not advisable to take a bath and do strenuous exercise during the treatment.
(c) Patients with acute peritonitis pain should be forbidden from undergoing this treatment.

Progression:

Zhou and Li[11] collected 80 cases of breast cancer with chemotherapy and divided them into a control group (using only tropisetron) and a treatment group (using tropisetron plus acupoints-mounting), with every group having 40 cases. PC6, ST36, CV12, and K11 were selected, and the pill was made up of powder of the Chinese herbs Shufuzi, Rougui, Ganjiang, and Wuzhuyu. The treatment of acupoints-mounting was given once per day for one hour, with six days comprising a course. After one course of treatment, the rate of relief from vomiting and nausea in the treatment group was 92.5% whereas in the control group it was just 52.5%.

5. ACUPOINT CATGUT-EMBEDDING THERAPY

Acupoint selection:

Major acupoints: Tianshu (ST25), Weisu (BL21), and Zusanli (ST36). Adjunct points: Shenmen (HT7) and Sanyinjiao (SP6) are used for insomnia and dreaminess. Zhongwan (CV12), Guanyuan (CV4), Qihai (CV6), and Gesu (BL17) are used for dizziness and fatigue. Shangjuxu (ST37) and Gongsun (SP4) were used for diarrhea. Dachangxu (BL25) was used for abdominal distension and constipation.

Manipulation:

In major points, 1 cm of catgut (size 0) is used, while 0.2–0.5 cm of catgut is used in adjunct points and 0.2 cm catgut is used in Shenmen (HT7). Disinfect points with complex iodine, and put the proper catgut into No. 6.5 pinhead, which is used as casing. Hold the needle with the right hand, prick the needle to a proper depth, push the needle core with the left hand, and pull the pinhead with the right hand, which leaves the catgut in the subcutaneous tissue or muscle under points. Finally, press the pinhole for a moment with a cotton ball. The local aching pain appearing two to three days after the treatment is normal response, so special treatment will be unnecessary. The treatment frequency is once a week, a course is four times, and the whole treatment included six courses.[12]

Cautions:

(a) The procedure should obey the principle of aseptic technique.
(b) For the patients with allergies or when the patient's skin around the catgut-embedding is infected, acupoint catgut-embedding therapy should be forbidden.
(c) Patients experiencing a tuberculosis activity period or those who have an out-of-control blood glucose level should be forbidden from undergoing acupoint catgut-embedding therapy.
(d) To avoid the needle from breaking under the skin, acupoint catgut-embedding therapy should be done lightly, with a average force.

Progression:

Rong *et al.*[13] used catgut-embedding therapy on the acupoints of both Zhongwan (CV12), Zusanli (ST36), Tianshu (ST25), Shangjuxu (ST37) 24 hours before the patients underwent chemotherapy. The control group was treated only with Granisetron hydrochloride. In the end, 50.65% of patients who underwent acupoint catgut-embedding therapy group did not experience vomiting and nausea, while in the control group, the percentage was just 19.48%.

6. OTOPOINT–PELLET PRESSING THERAPY

Main acupoints:

Shenmen (TF4), Jiaogan (AH6a), Liver (CO12), Spleen (CO13), Stomach (CO4), Endocrine (CO18), and Adrenal gland (TG2p).

Manipulation:

After the skin is sterilized routinely, Wang Bu Liu Xing Zi is fixed on the acupoints with medical tape and then pressed to stimulate the points, and the patients are advised to press the acupoints several times every day. Each acupoint is pressed for 1–2 min every time. Two days later, it is changed to the other ear using the same acupoints with equal pressure. The treatment lasts 10 days.

Cautions:

(a) It is not advisable to use the therapy to treat the aged and patients with weak constitution and overt strain.
(b) Do not press the points with excessive force to avoid damage to the skin.
(c) Pill pressing should not be used if inflammation or chilblain is present on the auricle.
(d) For slight inflammation, timely application of 2.5% alcohol is advisable.
(e) It is not advisable to perform this method on those who are allergic to tape.
(f) The tape on ears should be changed more often in summer due to accumulation of sweat.

Progression:

In clinical treatment, acupoint catgut-embedding therapy is always combined with Western medicine or other external therapy. Related research found that the vagus nerve had a rich distribution in the acupoint of TF4, and otopoint–pellet pressing can regulate the tension of the vagus nerve and reduce the vagus nerve's impulse-afferent so that the occurrence of reflex vomiting is reduced. Another study states that stimulating the acupoints of the ear can inhibit the vomiting nerve center and reduce the rate of morphine-induced central vomiting.[14]

REFERENCES

1. "Effective interventions for CINV: NCCN Antiemesis Clinical Practice Guidelines in Oncology," *ONS News*, 2004, 19(9 Suppl), pp. 17–18.
2. Zhang, H. Wu, W. & Chai, X. (2006). "Effect of puncturing Neiguan (PC 6) and Zusanli (ST 36) on chemotherapy-related vomiting from platinum-involved therapeutic project: A report of 26 cases," *Journal of Acupuncture and Tuina Science*, 4(4): 233–235.
3. Cui, Y., Shi, G., Fei, P. *et al.* (2016). "Effect of electro-acupuncture on 5-HT level in brain stem of cisplatin-induced nausea and vomiting in rats," *Liaoning Journal of Traditional Chinese Medicine*, 43(2): 415–417.

4. Zhang, A., Chen, R., Kang, M. *et al.* (1997). "Explore the effect of rotational acupuncture on expression of 5-HT and gastrin in experimental rabbits," *Chinese Acupuncture and Moxibustion*, 17(5): 299–302.
5. Guo, D. & Yang, L. (2011). "Research of using abdominal acupuncture to treat the adverse effect of malignant bone tumor after chemotherapy," *Journal of New Chinese Medicine*, 43(10): 84–86.
6. Xing, J., Li, X. & Ren, X. (2013). "Therapeutic observation of abdominal acupuncture in preventing nausea and vomiting caused by cisplatin-based chemotherapy," *Shanghai Journal of Acupuncture and Moxibustion*, 32(12): 1046–1048.
7. Xu, S., Yang, J. & Zhao, B. (2014). "Possible therapeutic effect of ginger-partitioned moxibustion on chemotherapy induced toxic side effects and quality of life scale: A clinical observation," *Global Traditional Chinese Medicine*, 12(7): 901–905.
8. Chen, Z. & Li, L. (2011). "Clinical observation of effect of Thunder-fire moxibustion on vomiting and nausea caused by chemotherapy of cisplatin," *Journal of New Chinese Medicine*, 42(12): 88–89.
9. Liu, S. (2010). "Clinical observation of direct moxibustion in treating adverse effects caused by chemotherapy." Doctoral Thesis, Traditional Chinese Medicine of Guangzhou University, Guangzhou, China.
10. Ruan, Y., Zhang, W., Wang, X. *et al.* (2014). Effect of herb-partitioned moxibustion on chemotherapy-induced nausea and vomiting of gastric cancer," *Chinese Archives of Traditional Chinese Medicine*, 32(11): 2664–2666.
11. Zhou, S., Li, Y. & Shi, J. (2015). "Clinical effectiveness and safety of acupoint application in the treatment of chemotherapy-induced nausea and vomiting," *World Journal of Integrated Traditional and Western Medicine*, 10(9): 1259–1261.
12. Meng, S. & Lu, J. (2012). "Twenty-seven cases of adverse reaction in postoperative chemotherapy of breast cancer treated with acupoint catgut-embedding therapy," *World Journal of Acupuncture-Moxibustion*, 22(2): 64–67.
13. Rong, H., Yu, W. & Wu, C. (2016). "Clinical observation of acupoint catgut-embedding therapy on avoiding and treating vomiting and nausea caused by chemotherapy," *China Practical Medical*, 11(11): 178–179.
14. Chen, X. & Er, Z. (2014). "Combined ear acupuncture with azasetron to avoid and treat nausea and vomiting caused by intravenous anesthesia," *Chinese Journal of Surgery of Integrated Traditional and Western Medicine*, 12(6): 646–648.

Chapter 19

Cancer-Related Fatigue

Qijun Fang, Yujuan Wang and Tianshu Xu

1. INTRODUCTION

Cancer-related fatigue can be observed in all the stages of cancer, which is distressing and persistent, with a subjective sense of physical, emotional, and/or cognitive tiredness related to cancer or cancer-related treatment, and is not relieved by rest and interferes with usual daily activities.

It is difficult to find the concept of cancer-related fatigue in ancient Chinese classic medical books. According to the symptoms and clinical experience, people have found that cancer-related fatigue belongs to asthenic overstrain in Traditional Chinese Medicine (TCM). It is the deficient symptoms of five Zang organs and six Fu organs. The main pathogenesis is that deficient Yin, Yang, *qi*, and Blood causes the deficiency of Zang and Fu organs, and the extreme deficiency is called asthenic overstrain. The basic principle of treatment is reinforcing according to the patients. The methods include nourishing Yin, reinforcing Yang, tonifying qi, enriching blood, and so on.

Previous animals and clinical experiments proved that acupuncture treatment which is safe and economic can effectively relieve the syndrome of cancer-related fatigue, such as non-specific weakness and systemic decline, without any side-effects. Acupuncture works through a variety of mechanisms, such as regulating cytokines and the hypothalamus–pituitary–adrenal axis, which can release hormones and serotonin; correcting Th1/Th2 imbalance; and regulating the immune system. The main acupuncture methods include moxibustion, general acupuncture, otopoint-mounting, and acupoints-mounting. This chapter is primarily concentrated on specific manual techniques and related mechanisms of acupuncture on the improvement of cancer-related fatigue.

2. METHODS

2.1. *Moxibustion*

Indications: Patients who have a deficiency of Yang or Qi or Blood, except patients who have a deficiency of Yin.

Manipulations:

Grain Moxibustion

It is one kind of direct moxibustion. First, lay a thin scutellarin ointment between the moxa cone and the selected acupoint. Then, place a moxa cone on the acupoint (ST36 both sides, GV7) and ignite it for moxibustion. The moxa cone is like a grain, about 3 mm in diameter and 5 mm high. When the patient complains of burning pain, slightly remove the moxa with a tweezer. Repeat this for seven times to complete one treatment. Repeat one treatment every alternate day three to four times a week. The whole treatment will last four weeks.

Du Moxibustion with Chinese Herb

It is one kind of indirect moxibustion. It is especially used in patients who have deficiency in Yang. Keep the patient in a prone position, clean the skin on the back, and then place the gauze on the DU meridian. Place the medicinal cake which has been heated to a temperature of 37°C on the gauze. Press out a groove in the middle of the cake, then put moxa in the channel and ignite it. When the patient complains of burning pain, properly lift the gauze and cake. After two cones, remove the cake and use gauze to clean the skin. Warn patients to keep warm. Perform one treatment a week. The whole treatment lasts four, weeks.

The medicinal cake is made of Shen Jincao, Hai Tongpi, Tou Gucao, Ji Xueteng, Baizhi, Ru Xiang, Mo Yao, and so on.

Ginger Moxibustion

If the patient has obvious symptoms of digestive tract disorder, ginger moxibustion provides better efficacy. Cut a slice of raw ginger about 2–3 mm thick, with the size as large as that of the moxa cone used, punch several holes at its center, and place it on the selected acupoints. Then, place a moxa cone on the ginger and ignite it for moxibustion. When the patient complains of burning pain, slightly lift the ginger and the moxa cone for a short time and place them down again, or replace the moxa cone and reignite it. Repeat this procedure until there is a local erythema of the skin. Generally, three cones are used for each point selected during one treatment session. Repeat the treatment every alternate day, three to four times a week, with the whole treatment lasting four weeks.

Mild-Warming Moxibustion

Ignite one of the ends of the moxa stick, hold the stick, and keep the ignited end above the selected acupoints from a distance without moving. The acupoints include CV8, CV12, CV4, CV5, ST25, ST36, and KI1. When the patient complains of burning pain, properly lift the ignited end of the moxa stick. Apply moxibustion until there is erythema of the skin. It will take 30 min for one treatment. Repeat the treatment on alternate days, three to four times a week, with the whole treatment lasting four weeks.

Efficacy characteristics:

Moxibustion can help improve blood circulation, reinforce Yang, lift the deficiency of Qi, Blood and Yang, adjust Yin and Yang, and move the meridian. It can reduce uncomfortable symptoms for patients with cancer. In addition to the Yin-deficient patients, every patient can be treated using this method. It is easy to perform and the effect is significant.

Cautions:

All types of moxibustion must be performed in strict accordance with the direct operation of moxibustion procedures. Do not treat the patients who are allergic to the smoke of moxibustion by this procedure. It is inadvisable to apply moxibustion to patients who are famished, overheated, tipsy, over fearing, over angry, over thirsty, or in terror. Do not deal with the reddish color and burning heat of the local skin area that appear after moxibustion, but wait for them to disappear as they may occur due to excessive or prolonged moxibustion. In case of small blisters on the skin, do not break it but leave it to disappear of its own accord, whereas in case of the large ones, break it with a sterilized needle to drain the fluid out, cover it with sterilized dressing and fix the dressing on the skin.

Development:

A total of 46 patients were randomly divided into two groups: one group was treated using grain-moxibustion and drugs, and the other one was treated only by drugs, which were the same as used by the grain-moxibustion group. Then the differences between KPS score scale, EORTC QLQ-C30 score scale, Piper fatigue scale of the two groups were observed before and after the treatments. Zhang[1] and her partners have concluded that grain-moxibustion can solve the cancer-related fatigue problem by improving the amount of blood cells and releasing clinical symptoms caused by malignant tumors, such as vomit, nausea, constipation, and pain.[1] Huang *et al.*[2] proved that moxa grain-moxibustion can effectively upregulate T lymphocyte proliferation activity and balance Th1/Th2 in tumor-bearing mice, suggesting an enhancement of the body's anti-tumor ability after moxibustion by performing animal experiments.

2.2. *General acupuncture*

Indications: All patients.

Manipulations:

Keep the patient in a supine position, sterilize the selected area with a 75% alcohol cotton ball, wash hands, and insert the needle (0.25 mm × 40 mm) into the acupoints (the main acupoints are CV4, CV6, CV17, ST36, SP6, KI10, SP10). Using the mild reinforcing and reducing method, hold the needle in the acupoints after the use of needling manipulation for 30 min, lift and thrust as well as twirl and rotate the needle evenly and gently at a moderate speed every 15 min. Perform general acupuncture once a day. The whole treatment lasts 14 days.

Efficacy characteristics:

The main acupoints which belong to Kidney meridian (foot shaoyin), *Ren* meridian, and Stomach meridian (foot yangming) can regulate the balance of qi, Xue, Yin, and Yang, tonifying the kidney Jing and reinforcing the Spleen qi. When treating the patient with moxibustion (CV4, CV6, CV12, KI1), it will work better.

Cautions:

It is advisable to delay giving acupuncture treatment to the patients who are very nervous. It is inadvisable to give acupuncture treatment to women during pregnancy or women undergoing menstruation. Acupoints on the areas with infection, ulcer, scar, or tumor should not be needled. Patients with irregularity in blood coagulation and with hemorrhagic tendency should not be punctured. Acupoints close to the vital organs or large blood vessels should be carefully needled. For patients who are very nervous or weak, mild manipulation can be used.

Development:

Suya *et al.*[3] divided 60 cases of cancer patients with spleen and kidney deficiencies exhibiting fatigue into two groups: treatment group and control group, each group consisting of 30 subjects. The control group was treated with nutritional support and symptomatic treatment. The treatment group was treated with acupuncture in addition to nutritional support and symptomatic treatment. KPS score, Piper fatigue scale score, and peripheral blood and other indicators were observed before and after treatment. The results showed that the treatment group showed better improvement in their lymphocyte count and fatigue state compared to the control group.

Dean-Clower *et al.*[4] conducted a study to investigate the efficacy of acupuncture in improving symptoms and quality of life (QOL) in patients with advanced ovarian cancer or breast cancer as a palliative treatment. Experimental studies have shown that a periodical eight weeks of acupuncture treatment is effective and feasible, which shows that acupuncture can improve the fatigue of cancer patients.

2.3. *Acupoints-mounting*

Indications: All patients.

Manipulations:

The main acupoints are GV14, BL23, SP10, ST36, CV8, and BL24. Break the Chinese herb medicine (He Huanpi, Huang Qi, Dang Gui, Zhi Mu, Dan Shen, Gan Song, Wu Weizi, Gui Zhi, Ren Shen, Fu Zi, Bing Pian, etc.) into power. Then make the powder into a box shape (1 cm × 1 cm × 1 cm) and place it on the acupoints which are selected, paste with medical tape, and remove the powder and tape after four hours. The whole treatment lasts 14 days. (Adjust the acupoints and the composition of drugs according to the patient yin and yang blood deficiency and perform further adjustment based on symptoms.)

Efficacy characteristics:

It is easy to operate, the patient has no obvious discomfort, and the drug is safe. This method is used especially for patients with poor appetite, as it is difficult for them to ingest the Chinese herb medicine soup. In this method, drugs can be directly absorbed through the skin and is safe and effective.

Cautions:

It is inadvisable to perform acupoints-mounting on those who are allergic to tape. If patient feels hot and experiences pain in the area where the tape and powder is pasted, remove it earlier. Avoid bathing and participating in a lot of sports during the treatment.

Development:

A total of 61 patients were randomly divided into the control group and treatment group by Hong *et al.*[5] The control group comprised 30 subjects and was treated with routine chemotherapy. The treatment group had 31 subjects and was treated with routine chemotherapy, Shenqi Fuzheng injection, and acupoints-mounting on PC6, ST36 from the first day of chemotherapy. The treatment lasted 10 days. Cao and his partners observed the patient's symptoms from the 1st day to the 21st day. The results showed the leukocyte and platelet count of control group decreased significantly ($p < 0.05$), and the incidence rate of fatigue, vomiting, and nausea of the treatment group was lower than that of the control group ($p < 0.05$).[5]

2.4. *Otopoint-mounting*

Indications: All patients.

Manipulations:

This method is also termed "pill pressing." Prescription: CO2-4, TF4, AH6a, CO12. Modification: CO10, CO11, CO14. If the above-mentioned points are ineffective, add sensitive points. Search for the tenderness point using the probe's pressure; it is a sensitive point if the patient feels pain. Choose the most obvious selection of tenderness or two or three points as the treatment points. Paste Wang Buliuxing Zi on the points with medical tape, then press it to stimulate the points. The patient will have a hot and painful feeling on the local area of the skin. Apply the treatment to one ear, then change to the other ear after two days, using the same pressure. During the period, the patient should be urged to press the auricular pressure point several times a day, each for a period of 1–2 min per point. The treatment lasts 10 days.

Efficacy characteristics:

It is easy to perform.

Cautions:

Keep the tape dry. Do not press the points with excessive force to avoid damage to the skin. Pill pressing should not be used if inflammation or chilblain is present on the auricle. It is inadvisable to perform this method on those who are allergic to tape. For slight inflammation, 2.5% alcohol should be applied in timely manner. It is inadvisable to treat the aged and patients with weak constitution and those who are overstrained using this method.

Development:

A total of 36 cases of ovarian cancer patients with chemotherapy who suffered from cancer-related fatigue were treated by Liu *et al.*[6] with otopoint-mounting. After the treatment, the patients' fatigue symptoms and QOL were found to improve significantly.[6]

Yu *et al.*[7] conducted a study to investigate the efficacy of auricular acupoints on the symptoms, QOL, and Piper fatigue scale score in breast cancer patients undergoing chemotherapy treatment. The experimental studies have shown that a periodical eight days of therapy using of otopoint-mounting is effective and feasible, which shows that otopoint-mounting can improve the QOL and provide relief from fatigue in cancer patients.[7]

REFERENCES

1. Zhang, X., Huang, W. & Xu, T. (2016). "Effect of grain-sized moxibustion on cancer-related fatigue and quality of life in patients with malignant tumor," *Shanghai Journal of Acupuncture and Moxibustion*, 35(6): 659–662.
2. Huang, W., Wan, Q. & Xu, T. (2014). "Effect of moxa-grain-moxibustion on serum Th 1/Th 2 type cytokines in Lewis tumor-bearing mice," *Acupuncture Research*, 39(6): 477–481.
3. Su, Y., Zhu, Y. & Xia, L. (2016). "Clinical study on acupuncture for cancer-related fatigue due to spleen-kidney deficiency," *Shanghai Journal of Acupuncture and Moxibustion*, 35(7): 830–832.
4. Dean-Clower, E., Doherty-Gilman, A. M., Keshaviah, A. *et al.* (2010). "Acupuncture as palliative therapy for physical symptoms and quality of life for advanced cancer patients," *Integrative Cancer Therapies*, 9(2): 158–167.
5. Cao, H., Li, Z. & Wang, L. (2015). "Observation on the efficacy of Shenqi Fuzheng injection combined with acupoint application to reduce the toxicity after chemotherapy," *Modern Traditional Chinese Medicine*, 35(1): 14–42.
6. Liu, Q., Liu, X-y. & Tu, M. (2013). "Effect of aerobic exercises and auricular acupoint pressing on cancer-related fatigue among oophoroma patients during intermittent chemotherapy," *Journal of Nursing Science*, 28(15): 44–45.
7. Yu, L., Zheng, S. & Tao, L. (2012). "Auricular acupoint pressure relieving cancerous fatigue in patients with postoperative chemotherapy for breast cancer," *ACT General Nursing*, 10(10): 2689–2691.

Chapter 20

An Introduction to Zhou Zhongying's Experience in Diagnosing and Treating Osteoarthritis with GuBi Decoction Based on the Pattern Differentiation of Kidney Deficiency and Collateral Obstruction

Xueping Zhou and Jing Wang

1. INTRODUCTION

Zhou Zhongying (b. 1928), is a tenured professor, supervisor of doctoral degree candidates, master of Chinese medicine, and one of National Representative Inheritors of "TCM Diagnostic Method" in the Intangible Cultural Heritage Project. Professor Zhou Zhongying has been engaged in the medical practice, education, and research of Traditional Chinese Medicine (TCM) Science of Internal Medicine for nearly 70 years and excels in the diagnosis and treatment of acute symptoms and intractable diseases. He maintains that emphasis should be placed upon the pathogenesis during the determination of treatment based on the differentiation of symptoms and signs. He advocates that "Pathogenesis Syndrome Element is the core of determination of treatment based in pathogenesis obtained through differentiation of symptoms and signs." As the Editor of *TCM Pathogenesis Dialectics*, he aims to melt multiple dialectics into one and activates the dialectics to enhance the diagnosis and treatment capacity of complex refractory disease.

Osteoarthritis (OA) is a multifactorial disease that often develops in middle-aged and elderly individuals around the world. The incidence of OA is positively correlated with older age. The incidence of OA among the population aged 55 years is 44–70%. Among the population older than 65 years, the incidence of OA is approximately 60% in men and as high as 70% in women.[1] With an increase in the aging and longevity of the population, the incidence of OA is increasing annually (OA was the fourth most common cause of hospitalization in the United States in 2009[2]). OA is mainly characterized by articular cartilage degeneration, osteosclerosis, and osteoproliferation; its primary clinical manifestations include gradually progressive arthralgia, joint swelling, joint stiffness, and joint dysfunction. This disease leads to joint deformation and loss of joint function and has become a public health issue that severely affects social labor forces and is associated with significant economic burden.[3] To date, however, there are no curative treatments or ideal medicinals for OA.[4] Treatment of OA using TCM has the advantages of outstanding therapeutic effects, low costs, and fewer toxic side effects. Therefore, it is of great importance to refine, disseminate, and employ the clinical thoughts and experiences of well-known veteran TCM practitioners.

2. TREATMENT STRATEGY AND PRESCRIPTION ANALYSIS

The clinical manifestations of OA indicate that this disease belongs to the category of "GuBi" (bone impediment) in TCM. Professor Zhou Zhongying believes that the etiology of OA is kidney deficiency due to aging, invasion by external pathogens, excessive strain, and joint trauma. Its pathogenesis is characterized by kidney and blood deficiencies and impediments in the meridian vessels. The mechanism of OA development is believed to be rooted in deficiencies in the essence of blood in the liver and kidney, while wind-dampness and the impediment of meridian vessels due to static blood also contribute to OA development. The pathological nature of OA is characterized by deficiencies in the root causes and deficiency in origin and excess in superficiality, intermingled with deficiency and excess. Although the disease is distributed in the sinews and bones, the pathology originates from the viscera and bowel, primarily the liver and kidney, with the kidney being the dominant organ. Taking the kidney, blood deficiencies, and impediments in the meridian vessels into consideration, Professor Zhou established a primary treatment method that can be used to tonify the kidney, nourish the blood, eliminate impediments, and free the collateral vessels. According to this method, Professor Zhou combined various medicines and independently developed a medical formula for treating bone impediments that consisted of Sangjisheng (*Taxillus chinensis*), Jixueteng (*Caulis spatholobi*), Huainiuxi (*Achyranthes bidentata Blume*), Chuanduan (*Radix dipsaci*), Gusuibu (*Rhizoma drynariae*), Qiannianjian (*Rhizoma homalomenae*), Tubiechong (*ground beetle*), and Yousongjie (*pine nodular branch*).

In the formula, Sangjisheng (*Taxillus chinensis*) can help replenish the liver and kidney to dispel wind-dampness and strengthen the sinews and bones. Jixueteng (*Caulis spatholobi*) can help nourish the blood in the liver to emolliate the sinew vessels, and harmonize the blood and collateral vessels. Both Sangjisheng (*Taxillus chinensis*) and Jixueteng (*Caulis spatholobi*) are sovereign medicinals. Huainiuxi (*Achyranthes bidentata Blume*) can help to tonify the liver and kidney, strengthen the sinews and bones, dissipate blood stasis, and disperse abscesses and swelling. Chuanduan (*Radix dipsaci*) can help to tonify the liver and kidney and strengthen the sinews and bones. Gusuibu (*Rhizoma Drynariae*) can help to replenish the kidney to cure trauma, strengthen the sinews and bones, and to activate the blood to relieve pain. Huainiuxi (*Achyranthes bidentata Blume*), Chuanduan (*Radix dipsaci*), and Gusuibu (*Rhizoma drynariae*) are minister medicinals. Qiannianjian (*Rhizoma homalomenae*) can help to dispel wind-dampness, strengthen the sinews and bones, relieve pain, and disperse swelling. Tubiechong (*ground beetle*) can help to dissipate blood stasis and strengthen the sinews and bones. Both Qiannianjian (*Rhizoma homalomenae*) and Tubiechong (*ground beetle*) are assistant medicinals. Yousongjie (*Pine Nodular Branch*) can help dispel wind-dampness and free the collateral vessels to relieve pain and is a courier medicinal in this formula owing to its direct therapeutic effects on the joints. All of the aforementioned medicinals in combination have therapeutic effects in tonifying the liver and kidney and eliminating impediments and freeing collateral vessels. This formula tonifies the liver and kidney, replenishes the essence and blood, and strengthens the sinews and bones; most importantly, it is completely based on the therapeutic principle of treating the root cause of disease.

OA primarily occurs in middle-aged and elderly individuals. Due to deficiencies in healthy qi, pathogens, including external wind, cold, and dampness, can easily enter the meridians, collaterals, and joints; this impedes the qi and blood, obstructs the circulation, and leads to stasis in the long term. OA is primarily associated with internal damage and deficiency, and the deficiency in kidney essence is the root cause of this disease. Therefore, practitioners should devote special attention to including tonification procedures in treatments when using medicinals to free the collateral vessels. It is important to tonify the kidney and strengthen the bones and, more importantly, to emolliate the liver, nourish the blood, and moisten the sinews. Even at the onset of severe pain, tonification of the liver and kidney should still be emphasized to cure the root cause of this disease. Attacking the pathogens should not be overemphasized; otherwise, the pathogenesis would be affected adversely. Given these reasons, a treatment based on syndrome differentiation is of vital importance.

The GuBi concoction is focused on tonifying the kidney and nourishing the blood. However, given that kidney deficiency and collateral obstructions are the pathogenic basis of this disease, the formula not only contains medicinals that tonify and replenish the liver and kidney but also those that dispel wind and eliminate dampness to activate the blood to dissipate blood stasis, to disperse swelling to relieve pain, as well as to relax sinews and free the collateral vessels. The medicinals in combination are mainly aimed at curing the root cause of disease; therefore, strongly toxic medicinals are not included in the formula.

The compound formula neither contains medicinals that are pungent and hot by nature, or those that have a warm-dryness character such as Chuanwu (*Aconitum carmichaeli Debx*) or Caowu (*Radix aconiti kusnezoffii*), nor does it contain medicinals made of poisonous bugs such as Qaunxie (*scorpion*) and Wusong (*centipede*). Therefore, the formula not only avoids essential qi damage caused by the aforementioned pungent, hot, or warm-dryness medicinals but also toxicity-induced damage to healthy qi.

3. COMPATIBILI1TY APPLICATION

The clinical syndromes will vary with changes in pathogen levels, patient physique, and the pathophysiology of disease; therefore, the formula should vary accordingly. If the wind pathogen is in excess, it will attract other pathogens that migrate to the muscles and joints, and the pain will disperse and move throughout the body. Therefore, Qinjiao (*Radix gentianae Macrophyllae*), Fangfeng (*Radix saposhnikoviae*), Haifengteng (*Piper kadsura*), and Xungufeng (*Herba aristolochiae Mollissimae*) should be used to dispel wind and free the collateral vessels. If the cold pathogen is in excess, the syndromes will manifest as cold pain in the joints as well as cold hands and feet. Therefore, Zhichuanwu (*Radix aconiti Praeparata*), Zhicaowu (*Radix aconiti Kusnezoffii Praeparata*), Guizhi (*Ramulus cinnamomi*), Xixin (*Herba asari*), Shenjincao (*Herba lycopodii*), and Tougucao (*Garden Balsam Stem*) should be used to warm the meridians and disperse cold as well as free the collateral vessels to relieve pain. If the dampness pathogen is in excess, the syndrome will include swelling, soreness and pain in the joints as well as widespread swelling and numbness. In this case, Chaocangshu (*fried Rhizoma atractylodis*), Tianxianteng (*Dutchmanspipe vine*), Lulutong (*Fructus liquidambaris*), Mugua (*Carica papaya*), and Sigualuo (*Retinervus luffae fructus*) can be used to resolve dampness and free the collateral vessels. If chronic impediment pain and phlegm stasis impediment are present, the syndrome will involve stiffness in the joints and restricted movement. If there is an obvious sharp pain, Zhichuanshanjia (*roasted pangolin*), Sanqi (*Panax notoginseng*), and Sumu (*Caesalpinia sappan*) can be used to dissipate blood stasis and free the collateral vessels. For syndromes such as intractable joint deformation and swelling, Baijiezi (*White mustard seed*),

Zaojiao (*Chinese honeylocust spine*), Zhinanxing (*processed Pinellia pedatisecta*), and Zhijiangcan (*roasted Bombyx batryticatus*) can be used to disperse the swelling and nodules. If the qi and blood are deficient due to exterior deficiency, weak defense, or nutrient–defense disharmony, the syndrome will manifest as aversion to cold in the entire body, occasional sweating, and dull pain in the joints. The treatment strategy should be to replenish the qi and nourish the blood, as well as harmonize the nutrients and free the collateral vessels. Therefore, Guizhi (*Ramulus cinnamomi*), Baishao (*Radix paeoniae Alba*), Chuanqiong (*Ligusticum wallichii*), Huangqi (*Radix astragali*), Fangfeng (*Radix saposhnikoviae*), and Baishu (*Rhizoma atractylodis Macrocephalae*) can be used to replenish the qi and nourish the blood, as well as activate the blood and free the collateral vessels. In patients with kidney yang deficiency, the syndrome will manifest as cold pain in the waist and knees, with an aversion to cold, and coldness in the limbs. Yinyanghuo (*Herba epimedii*), Bajitian (*Radix morindae Officinalis*), and Lujiaopian (*sliced deer antlers*) can be used to warm the kidney and assist the yang. In patients with insufficient kidney essence who experience syndromes such as tinnitus or deafness, Zhihuangjing (*processed Rhizoma polygonati*), Shanyurou (*Fructus corni*), and Zhishouwu (*Polygonum multiflorum Thunb*) can be used to tonify the kidney and replenish the marrow.

REFERENCES

1. Pereira, D., Peleteiro, B., Araujo, J. *et al.* (2011). "The effect of osteoarthritis definition on prevalence and incidence estimates: A systematic review," *Journal of Osteoarthritis Cartilage*, 19(11): 1270–1285.
2. Murphy, L. & Helmick, C. G. (2012). "The impact of osteoarthritis in the United States: A population-health perspective," *American Journal of Nursing*, 112(3 suppl 1): 13–19.
3. McCarberg, B. & Tenzer, P. (2013). "Complexity in the pharmacologic management of osteoarthritis pain," *Current Medical Research and Opinion*, 29: 539–548.
4. Snijders, G. F., Cornelia, H. E., Piet, L. C., van Riel, M. *et al.* (2011). "The effects of doxycycline on reducing symptoms in knee osteoarthritis: Results from a triple-blinded randomized controlled trial," *Annals of Rheumatic Diseases*, 70: 1191–1196.

APPENDIX: A CASE PRESENTATION TO VERIFY THE FORMULA

A 69-year-old woman made her first visit on July 10, 2003. The patient's disease had developed for more than 10 years and her bilateral knee arthralgia was gradually becoming more severe. Recently, she experienced a sore swelling and painful bilateral symptoms in her lower limbs and found it difficult to walk and squat. The symptoms were significantly more severe in her left foot than her right. The patient also experienced other symptoms, including bilateral knee-joint stiffness, which led to flexion and extension restriction and knee joint deformation. The patient disliked cold and wind, and her symptoms were alleviated at warmer temperatures. The patient consumed a normal diet, with normal gustation, urination, and defecation. She had a dark purple tongue with a thin, yellow, greasy coating and a fine pulse. The pattern differentiation of this patient was wind-dampness impediment, binding of phlegm and stasis, and deficiencies of the kidney and blood.

Formula: Sangjisheng (*Taxillus chinensis*) 15 g, Jixueteng (*Caulis spatholobi*) 15 g, Chuanduan (*Radix dipsaci*) 15 g, Gusuibu (*Rhizoma drynariae*) 10 g, Yousongjie (*Pine nodular branch*) 15 g, Huainiuxi (*Achyranthes bidentata Blume*) 12 g, Qiannianjian (*Rhizoma homalomenae*) 15 g, Tubiechong (*ground beetle*) 5 g, Zhijiangcan (*toasted Bombyx batryticatus*) 10 g, Zhinanxing (*processed Pinellia pedatisecta*) 10 g, Zhiquanxie (*toasted scorpion*) 5 g, Bajirou (*Lonicera japonica Thunb*) 10 g, Xianlingpi (*Herba epimedii*) 10 g, Mufangji (*Cocculus orbiculatus*) 12 g, Weilingxian (*Radix clematidis*) 15 g, Shenjincao (*Herba lycopodii*) 15 g, Mugua (*Carica papaya*) 12 g, Xixiancao (*Herba siegesbeckiae*) 15 g, Chouwutong (*Clerodendron trichotomum*) 15 g.

After a one-month treatment course using the above formula, which was subject to modification according to symptom variation, the patient experienced significant relief in her bilateral lower-limb soreness and pain, as well as bilateral knee-joint stiffness, and the flexion and extension of her limbs became significantly easier. The patient continued using this formula to stabilize the disease, which continued to be alleviated.

Note: The disease in this case was diagnosed to be bone impediment, which often develops in fatigued and elderly patients, and is caused by the invasion of the external wind-cold dampness pathogen. The long-term course of bone impediment may include invasion of the collateral vessels, phlegm stasis, and impediment. Therefore, the course of bone impediment may be a combination of deficiencies of the kidney and blood, wind-cold-dampness, and phlegm stasis. There is a tendency for yang deficiency and cold congealing, as well as a tendency toward transformation into heat from the long-term stagnation of the aforementioned pathogen. The bone impediment patterns manifest as arthralgia, joint stiffness, and deformation; aversion to cold; and a dark purple tongue with a thin yellow greasy coating. Therefore, the treatment strategy for bone impediment should be to dispel wind and eliminate dampness, tonify the kidney and nourish the blood, warm the yang and dissipate cold, activate the blood and dissipate blood stasis, resolve phlegm, as well as to clear heat and free the collateral vessels. The formula to treat bone impediment consists of Jiangcan (*Bombyx batryticatus*), Nanxing (*Rhizoma arisaematis*), Bajirou (*Lonicera japonica Thunb*), and Xianlingpi (*Herba epimedii*), all of which are combined as components of the Xitong pill.

Chapter 21

The Crisis of European Healthcare Systems in the 21st Century: The Patient with Chronic Disease and the Potential Role of Acupuncture in the National Healthcare Systems

Carlo Maria Giovanardi, Mauro Devecchi, Giuseppina M. Farella, Alessandra Poini and Giuseppe Tallarida

1. INTRODUCTION

Chronic diseases represent the new challenge for the healthcare providers in the third millennium: to combat this challenge, the WHO created the Chronic Diseases and Health Promotion department in order to prevent and control this type of diseases and promote health. On the other hand, the WHO, in its 2014–2023 strategy for traditional medicine (TM), recommends the member states to "recognize TM as a resource that could contribute to the improvement of health care services, particularly Primary Healthcare (PHC), and that TM is relevant to improved health outcomes." In this chapter, we will explore the critical issues of healthcare related to the changing health needs and the potential benefits of adding acupuncture to the routine care in public settings

2. DEFINITION OF CHRONIC PATIENTS: PARTICULAR REFERENCE TO CHRONIC PAIN AND RESULTING COSTS

Pain is "[A]n unpleasant sensory and emotional experience associated with actual or potential tissue damage, or described in terms of such damage… pain is always subjective. Each individual learns the application of the word through experiences related to injury in early life".[1]

Dueñas *et al.*[2] have not only put in evidence the problem of the reported pain to the single patient but, above all, the impact of pain on the global daily life (job, family, etc.), observing the concept of pain that we could define "global."

Chronic pain also substantially influences the healthcare system. According to Azevedo *et al.*,[3] "[A]n important set of benchmarks are presented regarding health services utilization in chronic pain subjects, comprising useful tools for public health policy and decision-making."

Several papers have faced the problem of chronic pain costs, in Europe and noticing an increasing number of accesses from the General Practitioners and from experts in the treatment of pain (also nine accesses in six months).[4–6]

The cost of chronic pain in the US has been estimated at $560–$635 billion.[7] Particularly, chronic pain can be associated with psychological consequences, such as depression, anxiety, and insomnia.[8] Nowadays chronic pain is a great problem under different points of view: many patients suffering from chronic pain are elderly patients with high rate of comorbidities and poly-pharmacotherapy.

A routine monitoring of pain treatment is needed because it has opioid use as the cornerstone treatment. There have been several studies regarding the specific indication and management of opioid use.

There are both pros and cons to the use of opioids in pain treatment. During the opioid Consumption, respiratory depression and, besides, an increase in the mortality in patient affected by Chronic Obstructive Pulmonary Disease (COPD) has been correlated. Not least, opioids are an absolute contraindication during pregnancy.[9,10] Another important side effect of opioids consumption is addiction: in the United States, around 2.1 million suffer from substance use disorder related to abuse of prescription opioids for pain relief.[11] The problem is growing also in Europe: in 2012, there were 1.3 million problem opioid users reported.[12] Even if abuse of prescription opioids has not been regarded as a major problem in Europe, there is a growing interest in among the public and in the field of science.

A recent study[13] reported the distribution of prescription opioid abuse in five European countries (France, UK, Germany, Italy, and Spain) and its associated costs. The results showed that the major prevalence of prescription opioid abuse (for chronic pain) was in France (13.7% per 10,000 individuals aged 15–64 years) and UK and Germany (11.0% and 10.7% per 10,000 individuals aged 15–64 years, respectively). The study also show the overall healthcare burden of abuse by country: across the five European countries, the annual healthcare costs ranged from EUR 2.0 million to EUR 152.9 million (France, EUR 97.9 million; Germany, EUR 152.9 million; Italy, EUR 4.3 million; Spain, EUR 2.0 million; UK, EUR 65.7 million). The aggregate costs for the healthcare systems of abuse of prescription opioids per 1,00,000 individuals aged 15–64 years ranged from EUR 6,264 to EUR 279,927 (France, EUR 238,691; Germany, EUR 279,927; Italy, EUR 10,901; Spain, EUR 6,264; UK, EUR 160,835).

Florence *et al.*[14] have recently analyzed the costs of opioid abuse, over-prescription, and dependence in the United States. Costs were analyzed from a societal perspective (i.e., direct costs of healthcare system, loss of productivity and related costs, and costs to the criminal justice system). Data of two million Americans, responding to inclusion criteria for prescription opioid abuse and dependence in 2013, were analyzed. Cumulative costs for prescription opioid overdose, abuse, and dependence were estimated at over USD 78.5 billion (in 2013 dollars). From the total spending for healthcare and substance abuse (USD 28 billion), the great part was covered by insurance, amounting to USD 26 billion. The costs for loss of productivity (including reduced productive hours and lost production for incarcerated individuals) and non-fatal cases was USD 20 billion. It is interesting to note, as the authors[14] report, that "two-thirds of the total economic burden was due to health care, substance abuse treatment, and lost productivity for non-fatal cases. Fatal overdoses accounted for $21.5 billion."

3. CONVENTIONAL AND COMPLEMENTARY APPROACHES TOGETHER IN A COORDINATED WAY: THE INTEGRATIVE MEDICINE

In the 21st century, the concepts of "personalized" and "integrated" have assumed a notable importance.

In medicine, these concepts are already used on a large scale. In surgery, it speaks of hybrid technique, i.e., mininvasive methods associated with percutaneous techniques (fast growing field).[15] In oncology, recently, it speaks of target therapy, or a personalized therapy addressed to oppose the carcinogenic mechanisms.[16] Modern medicine has resorted to the association of different methods or an "integrative" approach to oppose two great variables that predominate in the management of a patient with chronic disease: the adverse effects and the standardization of the therapy.

Besides the creation of these methods which are the ones at the forefront, appropriate guidelines need to been formulated to guarantee the correct use. In the field of chronic pain, how we can manage these variables with integrative medicine? As mentioned earlier, chronic pain is more difficult to manage, in addition to having a notable impact on the population. In Europe the diseases that more represent chronic pain are migraine[17] and lower back pain.[18] There are many scientific evidences on the effectiveness of acupuncture in the treatment of these two chronic diseases. In the West, in fact, the population resorts to complementary and alternative medicine (CAM), particularly to acupuncture, for the treatment of the chronic pain, gynecological diseases, and stress management.[19]

In our opinion, acupuncture can be a valid aid in the treatment of these pathologies. One of the many examples is the study performed by Li *et al.*,[20] who have compared acupuncture and moxibustion in the treatment of the fibromyalgia syndrome versus tramadol and amitriptyline, obtaining some good results for the first ones. Very significant victories are obtained by combining conventional medicines with CAM. The question, therefore, is: when to use an integrative medicine?

It is necessary that the practitioners of both the fields (conventional and complementary medicine) produce some detailed guidelines to be able to get an optimization in terms of time taken, results attained, and effectiveness of the integrative medicine for the best management of the patient with chronic pain, not least in terms cost-effectiveness.[21] Surely, on the base of Evidence Based Medicine (EBM), chronic pain is one of the fields where conventional and complementary therapy can collaborate for determining the best approach to treat the patient.

As mentioned earlier, chronic pain has a strong impact on the quality of life[2] and there is always an increasing interest, both from the patients and from the practitioners, on integrative medicine for the added value that it can give.[22] According to Robinson *et al.*,[23] "[C]omplementary Medicine in primary care may be a cost effective addition to standard General Practitioner care but sufficient follow up and rigorous mixed methods approaches are needed to assess whether it can help achieve wider public health goals in health improvement and preventing ill health."

In conclusion, treatment using integrative medicine should have, in the first place, a non-pharmacological approach; if it controls well, it reduces the costs of management of the patient, eliminates adverse effects, and improves the quality of life. Besides, there is an increasing interest in the population on the CAM method and to an approach that is more people centered. Therefore, as in isolated Italian realities, it is necessary to introduce CAM in a real way into the National Healthcare Systems to make integrative medicine accessible to more people.

REFERENCES

1. International Association for the Study of Pain (IASP) (2012). Taxonomy. Available at: http://www.iasp-pain.org/Taxonomy. Accessed April 2017.
2. Dueñas, M. *et al.* (2016). "A review of chronic pain impact on patients, their social environment and the health care system." *Journal of Pain Research*, 9: 457.

3. Azevedo, L. F. *et al.* (2013). "Chronic pain and health services utilization: Is there overuse of diagnostic tests and inequalities in non-pharmacologic treatment methods utilization?" *Medical Care*, 51(10): 859–869.
4. Woolf, A. D. *et al.* (2004). "Musculoskeletal pain in Europe: Its impact and a comparison of population and medical perceptions of treatment in eight European countries," *Annals of Rheumatic Diseases*, 63(4): 342–347.
5. Pérez, C. *et al.* (2015). "Modeling the predictive value of pain intensity on costs and resources utilization in patients with peripheral neuropathic pain," *Clinical Journal of Pain*, 31(3): 273–279.
6. Von Korff, M. *et al.* (2007). "Frequency and priority of pain patients' health care use," *Clinical Journal of Pain*, 23(5), pp. 400–408.
7. Gaskin, D. J. & Richard, P. (2012). "The economic costs of pain in the United States," *Journal of Pain*, 13(8): 715–724.
8. Castro, M. *et al.* (2011). "Comorbid depression and anxiety symptoms in chronic pain patients and their impact on health-related quality of life," *Archives of Clinical Psychiatry (São Paulo)*, 38(4): 126–129.
9. Dureja, G. P. *et al.* (2017). "Evidence and consensus recommendations for the pharmacological management of pain in India," *Journal of Pain Research*, 29(10): 709–736.
10. Vozoris, N. T. *et al.* (2016). "Incident opioid drug use and adverse respiratory outcomes among older adults with COPD," *European Respiratory Journal*, 48(3): 683–693.
11. Substance Abuse and Mental Health Services Administration (2013). *Results from the 2012 National Survey on Drug Use and Health: Summary of National Findings*, NSDUH Series H–46, HHS Publication No. (SMA) 13–4795. (Substance Abuse and Mental Health Services Administration, Rockville, MD, USA).
12. European Monitoring Centre for Drugs and Drug Addiction (2014). *European Drug Report 2014: Trends and Developments* (Publications Office of the European Union, Luxembourg).
13. Shei, A. *et al.* (2014). "Estimating the health care burden of prescription opioid abuse in five European countries," *Clinico Economics and Outcomes Research*: *CEOR*, 7: 477–488.
14. Florence, C. S. *et al.* (2016). "The economic burden of prescription opioid overdose, abuse, and dependence in the United States, 2013," *Medical Care*, 54(10): 901–906
15. Bergquist, P. J. *et al.* (2017). "Cardiac applications of PET-MR," *Current Cardiology Reports*, 19(5): 42.

16. Forster, J. C. *et al.* (2017). "A review of the development of tumor vasculature and its effects on the tumor microenvironment," *Hypoxia (Auckland)*, 5: 21–32.
17. Woldeamanuel, Y. W. & Cowan, R. P. (2017). "Migraine affects 1 in 10 people worldwide featuring recent rise: A systematic review and meta-analysis of community-based studies involving 6 million participants," Journal of Neurological Science, 372: 307–315.
18. Dubois, J. *et al.* (2017). "Chronic low back pain patients' use of, level of knowledge of and perceived benefits of complementary medicine: A cross-sectional study at an academic pain center," *BMC Complementary and Alternative Medicine*, 17(1): 193.
19. Robinson, N. *et al.* (2012). "Exploring practice characteristics and research priorities of practitioners of traditional acupuncture in China and the EU–A survey," *Journal of Ethnopharmacology*, 140(3): 604–613.
20. Li, D. *et al.* (2016). "Fibromyalgia syndrome treated with acupuncture at the acupoints of the affected meridians and heavy moxibustion at painful points: A randomized controlled trial," *Zhongguo Zhen Jiu*, 36(2): 147–151.
21. Institute of Medicine (US) Committee on the Use of Complementary and Alternative Medicine by the American Public (2005). *Complementary and Alternative Medicine in the United States* (National Academies Press, Washington (DC), USA).
22. Ruggie, M. (2004). "Marginal to mainstream: Alternative medicine in America," *Journal of Royal Society of Medicine*, 97(12): 605–606.
23. Robinson, N. *et al.* (2006). "Auditing outcomes and costs of integrated complementary medicine provision — the importance of length of follow up," *Complementary Therapies in Clinical Practice*, 12(4): 249–257.

Chapter 22

Focus on Headache, Migraine, Low Back Pain, and Infertility: Effectiveness and Cost-Effectiveness of Acupuncture in Chronic Diseases

Mauro Devecchi and Giuseppina M. Farella

1. INTRODUCTION

The recent developments in the medical field have enabled a longer life expectancy, especially in developed countries. At the same time, however, there has been an increase in chronic conditions, such as diabetes, cancer, and cardiovascular diseases, against which governments are running for cover with information policies, prevention, and health promotion. Other chronic conditions, although perceived as less important and not as life-threatening, however, are also very frequent. They affect especially the young adult population and are highly disabling, with a high social cost.

They are some of the most recurrent pain conditions: headache, migraine, and low back pain.

Moreover, in Western countries, fertility problems are spreading, and an increasing number of couples require the contribution of Assisted Reproductive Technology (ART).

Acupuncture has been used in the West for treating painful conditions since its first diffusion; recently, it has also become increasingly popular in the fertility field, not only to assist natural fertility but also as a support for ART procedures.

In this chapter we briefly analyze the most recent evidence on the effectiveness and cost-effectiveness of acupuncture as a treatment for headache, migraine, low back pain, and infertility.

2. HEADACHE AND MIGRAINE

In 2000, the World Health Organization (WHO) published a report, in which migraine is ranked 19th among disorders causing year lived with a disability for both sexes (ranked 9th in women), with the disability during a severe migraine attack that can be considered on level with active psychosis, tetraplegia, and dementia.[1]

According to Stovner *et al.*,[2] in the European countries, the one-year prevalence rates for headache, including men and women, range between 29% and 77%, while for migraine, the overall values vary between 9.6% and 24.6%. Different studies also report the proportion of people suffering from headache, in which headache causes absence from work or school: from the 7% of the general population recorded in San Marino and Finland,[3,4] to the 14% of the Danish population.[5]

The effectiveness of acupuncture in relieving headache and migraine has been investigated in many clinical trials, and recently, two updated reviews have been published by the Cochrane group, both lead by Linde.

In the first paper,[6] the potential role of acupuncture for the *prevention of tension-type headache* was evaluated: they included randomized trials with a post-randomization observation period of at least eight weeks, which compared the clinical effects of an acupuncture intervention with a control (treatment of acute headaches only or routine care), a sham acupuncture intervention, or another prophylactic intervention in adults with episodic or chronic tension-type headache. The reviewers included 12 trials with 2,349 participants (median 56; range 10–1,265) and concluded, with a "moderate" level of evidence, that "available results suggest that acupuncture is effective for treating frequent episodic or chronic tension-type headaches, but further trials — particularly comparing acupuncture with other treatment options — are needed".[6] This because only two of the 12 trials compared acupuncture with routine care, as actually suggested by the "Pragmatic Trial" design. The authors also underlined as they "do not consider sham-controlled trials a priority for the future."

The second review[7] focused on acupuncture for *prevention of episodic migraine*: it included 22 randomized trials of at least eight weeks duration that compared an acupuncture intervention with a no-acupuncture control (no prophylactic treatment or routine care only), a sham-acupuncture intervention, or prophylactic drug in participants with episodic migraine. The subjects in this review numbered 4,985 participants in total (median: 71; range 30–1,715), and there was a moderate quality of evidence.

The authors concluded, on the basis of the available evidence, that adding acupuncture to the symptomatic treatment of migraine attacks seems to reduce their frequency and may be at least as effective as treatment with prophylactic drugs.

As we can see from these two reviews, acupuncture can be an interesting treatment option for these very disabling conditions, and it has been shown to be not only effective but also cost-effective.

Witt *et al.*[8] assessed the costs and cost-effectiveness of additional acupuncture treatment in patients with headache compared with patients receiving routine care alone. They included 3,182 patients in total and performed a multicenter randomized controlled trial (RCT): in acupuncture patients, the overall cost difference between baseline and the end of the three-month treatment period was EUR 362.05 (95% CI; 293.78, 430.32) compared with EUR 7.05 in control patients. On the other hand, they evaluated the Quality of Life using the SF-36 questionnaire, and if at baseline, they found no significant difference, at the end of the observation, highly significant differences were assessed in favor of acupuncture-treated patients. Calculating the cost-effectiveness of the intervention on the base of these data, they observed again of 0.0301 ± 0.004 Quality Adjusted Life Years (QALY) in the acupuncture group compared with the control group, with an incremental cost-effectiveness ratio (ICER) of EUR 11.657 (overall) and EUR 12.140 (diagnosis-specific) per QALY gained. Therefore, for the assumed threshold value of EUR 50.000, the additional acupuncture intervention would appear to be cost-effective.

A similar trial was conducted in the UK by Wonderling *et al.*[9] with a threshold per QALY of £30.000, consistent with decisions that have been taken by the National Institute for Clinical Excellence(NICE): 401 patients aged 18–65 years who reported an average of at least two headaches per month were recruited from general practices to receive up to 12 session of acupuncture or standard treatment alone. They found an improvement in QALYs over the 12 months in the acupuncture group but not in control, with the difference between groups reaching significance ($p = 0.02$). They estimated the mean health gain to be 0.021 QALYs, equivalent to eight quality-adjusted days, with a mean incremental cost of the acupuncture intervention to the NHS of £205 per patient but with a small reduction in direct patient costs (in medications and visits to practitioners of complementary and alternative medicine (CAM)).

Overall this equates to an additional cost of £9.180 per QALY gained, including patient costs, and considering the threshold of £30.000 per QALY, then acupuncture in the treatment of chronic headache is highly likely to be cost-effective.

The results of the two European studies are consistent with those of the Chinese papers published by Deng *et al.*[10] and Wu *et al.*,[11] where acupuncture is widely integrated in the public healthcare system, suggesting the feasibility of a possible evolution in this direction also in the Western countries.

3. LOW BACK PAIN

Low back pain (LBP) is one of the most common causes of pain that drives patients to the use of acupuncture. In a recent cross-sectional survey[12] in Switzerland, 238 patients with chronic LBP were asked about their use of complementary medicine (CM): 77.3% reported the use of some CM, with the most common therapies used being osteopathy (48.8%), massage (45.2%), and acupuncture (31.6%).

With regard to these non-pharmacological treatments, Kizhakkeveettil *et al.*[13] recently compared the effectiveness of acupuncture with that of spinal manipulative therapy with a group receiving both treatments: they found all the treatments ensuring clinically meaningful improvements in the primary outcome measures, but without differences among groups.

The wide use of the non-pharmacological techniques has prompted the medical societies to review the existing literature and to produce guidelines for physicians: the 2007 *American College of Physicians* guideline already addressed non-pharmacologic treatment options for LBP, and in its 2017 update, acupuncture was confirmed to have a better effect on pain intensity and function in chronic LBP compared to pharmacological treatments and to sham acupuncture. With regard to acute LBP, authors found limited evidence of the effect of acupuncture.[14]

Based on this evidence, they produced the following new recommendations for physicians[15]:

> Recommendation 1:
>
> Given that most patients with acute or subacute low back pain improve over time regardless of treatment, *clinicians and patients should select non-pharmacologic treatment* with superficial heat (moderate-quality evidence), massage, ***acupuncture***, or spinal manipulation (low-quality evidence). If pharmacologic treatment is desired, clinicians and patients should select nonsteroidal anti-inflammatory drugs or skeletal muscle relaxants (moderate-quality evidence). (Grade: strong recommendation).
>
> Recommendation 2:
>
> For patients with chronic low back pain, clinicians and patients should *initially select non-pharmacologic treatment* with exercise, multidisciplinary rehabilitation, ***acupuncture***, mindfulness-based stress reduction (moderate-quality evidence), tai chi, yoga, motor control exercise, progressive relaxation, electromyography biofeedback, low-level

laser therapy, operant therapy, cognitive behavioral therapy, or spinal manipulation (low-quality evidence) (Grade: strong recommendation).

The findings of the American group are consistent with those of MacPherson *et al.*[16] on chronic pain and acupuncture: they found not only that it is effective in all the various pain conditions, including LBP, but also that it is cost-effective.

One of the most interesting aspects of this treatment is its safety: it makes it a very important option for LBP treatment for sensitive patients, such as elderly or pregnant women. In a recent review[17] investigating the effectiveness of different CAMs for the management of low back and/or pelvic pain (LBPP) in pregnancy, reviewers found for acupuncture both clinically important and statistically significant results, while for other CAMs, the evidence was unclear.

A critical topic that Yuan *et al.*[18] underline is the one of co-intervention: moxibustion and cupping were not commonly used in clinical studies for LBP, although reported by textbooks and clinical practice. According to their opinion, this could be due to the effort to control for confounders in RCTs by examining one component of the practice. However, as most Traditional Chinese Medicine practitioners use co-interventions to improve the effectiveness of acupuncture, they suggest the design of pragmatic trials to test acupuncture plus common co-interventions, as it usually happens in clinical practice. The importance and the effectiveness of such techniques, as cupping, has been investigated and confirmed also by Huang *et al.* in their review.[19]

4. FERTILITY AND ACUPUNCTURE

About 10–15% of couples face problems of conceiving during their reproductive life and seek the guidance of fertility care specialists.[20] One of the most widely used treatment options are the techniques of ART, but despite modern technologies having improved the treatment, the *in vitro* fertility (IVF) success rates remain low, with only 30% of courses resulting in live births in the US.[21] Many patients choose CAM to increase the success rate of their IVF treatment,[22] and among them, acupuncture is the most common technique chosen by couples seeking a baby and referring to US fertility clinics.[22,23] Also, in the UK, fertility problems are the second most common medical condition, after pain, leading people to undergo acupuncture treatments.[24]

There has been an increasing attention in recent years on the role that acupuncture could play in the fertility process: the results of adjuvant acupuncture are still under debate, and this could be due to a lack of homogeneity in the methodology of clinical trials' design.

Qualitative research suggests that acupuncture may help patients in reducing stress and psychological consequences resulting from IVF treatment.[25,26] In a recent survey conducted by Nedeljković *et al.*[27] among fertility centers listed on the websites of the Swiss, German, and Austrian National Fertility Associations, they found that acupuncture was offered by 33 (38.4%) of the clinics, and the providers of treatments were mainly physician-acupuncturists (84.8%). The authors also concluded that treatment provision by non-acupuncturists should be omitted in future trials to increase the external validity and clinical effectiveness of acupuncture research in ART.

Several systematic reviews were conducted in the last 12 years, and the results were uncertain and dependent on the criteria of inclusion of the trials and comparison of acupuncture, if sham acupuncture or usual care. Zheng *et al.*[28] concluded that adjuvant acupuncture improves the Clinical Pregnancy Rate (CPR) and Live Birth Rate (LBR). They chose to exclude the Streitberger Sham Needle-controlled Trial, based on the evidence that this device is not an inert control and may confuse more rather than clarify the interpretation of the effects of IVF adjuvant acupuncture.[29]

In a recent systematic review and meta-analysis by Qian *et al.*,[30] excluding sham studies and comparing only to usual care, the authors conclude that acupuncture improves CPR among women undergoing IVF, and optimal positive effects could be expected using acupuncture in IVF during controlled ovarian hyper-stimulation (COH).

Humaidan and Stener-Victorin[31] investigated the possibility of applying electroacupuncture (EA) due to its analgesic effects in patients who undergo ovarian pick-up, comparing it to conventional medical analgesia (CMA) and demonstrating the feasibility of this technique and the improvement in time and costs of EA compared to the CMA.

Male infertility factors contribute to 25% of all causes of subfertility,[32] with poor semen quality being the most common contributor to male infertility.[33] A recent systematic review and meta-analysis of four RCTs (n = 500)[34] examined the effect of acupuncture on semen quality and found that acupuncture increased sperm count with rapid progression and sperm concentration; however, this did not translate into increased clinical pregnancy rates.

Two smaller studies were not included in this meta-analysis. First is a small, prospective, randomized study of men with semen abnormalities who received acupuncture and moxa or sham acupuncture.[35] Patients in the treatment group had a significant increase in the percentage of normal-form sperm compared with those in the control group.

In the second trial involving a prospective controlled study, 40 men with idiopathic oligospermia, asthenospermia, or teratozoospermia received acupuncture or no treatment.[36] At the end of treatment, significantly more sperms without ultrastructural defects were found in the acupuncture group compared with the no-treatment group. However, cost-effectiveness in this field has not been investigated yet.

5. CONCLUSIONS

There are many fields in which acupuncture has been scientifically investigated in the last years, and the overall quality of papers is steadily increasing. Both efficacy/effectiveness and cost-effectiveness have been assessed for conditions of primary interest for the healthcare providers, in order to assess the feasibility of providing acupuncture in public hospitals and settings as it happens in the East.

LBP, headache, and migraine are some of the most recognized indications for acupuncture and it is also very commonly used to treat diseases in the Western countries. There is also an emerging interest and evidence in the adjuvant effects of acupuncture in female and male infertility and its support to ART procedures.

According to the papers reviewed in this chapter, many guidelines recommend acupuncture as a first-step intervention to propose in these common conditions, due to its safety, low evidence of side effects, and affordable costs.

For other applications acupuncture has a growing attention but evidence is still not definitive in many fields, due to some unresolved methodological problems, such as the placebo problem.

As a step forward, it would be desirable for clinicians, researchers, and reviewers to work together to achieve consensus on some points that actually represent potential bias in acupunture trials, such as:

- Application of the STRICTA criteria;
- Avoiding the use of sham controls;
- The use of pragmatic trials, in order to investigate the technique in a more realistic environment.

REFERENCES

1. Mathers C. D., Stein, C., Fat, D. M. *et al.* (2002). Global Burden of Disease 2000: Version 2, methods and results. World Health Organization. Available at: http://www.fic.nih.gov/dcpp/ppts/gbdpaper.pdf.
2. Stovner, L. J., Zwart, J. A. *et al.* (2006). "Epidemiology of headache in Europe," *European Journal of Neurology*, 13: 333–345.
3. Nikiforow, R. & Hokkanen, E. (1979). "Effects of headache on working ability: A survey of an urban and a rural population in Northern Finland," *Headache*, 19: 214–218.
4. Benassi, G., D'Alessandro, R., Lenzi, P. L., Manzaroli, D., Baldrati, A. & Lugaresi, E. (1986). "The economic burden of headache: An epidemiological study in the Republic of San Marino," *Headache*, 26: 457–459.
5. Rasmussen, B. K., Jensen, R. & Olesen, J. (1992). "Impact of headache on sickness absence and utilisation of medical services: A Danish population study," *Journal of Epidemiology and Community Health*, 46: 443–446.
6. Linde, K., Allais, G., Brinkhaus, B., Fei, Y., Mehring, M., Shin, B. C., Vickers, A. & White, A. R. (2016). "Acupuncture for the prevention of tension-type headache," *Cochrane Database of Systematic Reviews*, 4, Art. No.: CD007587. doi: 10.1002/14651858.CD007587.pub2.
7. Linde, K., Allais, G., Brinkhaus, B., Fei, Y., Mehring, M., Vertosick, E. A., Vickers, A. & White, A. R. (2016). "Acupuncture for the prevention of

episodic migraine," *Cochrane Database of Systematic Reviews*, 6, Art. No.: CD001218. doi: 10.1002/14651858.CD001218.pub3.

8. Witt, C. M., Reinhold, T., Jena, S., Brinkhaus, B. & Willich, S. (2008). "Cost-effectiveness of acupuncture treatment in patients with headache," *Cephalalgia*, 28: 334–345.
9. Wonderling, D., Vickers, A. J., Grieve, R. & McCarney, R. (2004). "Cost effectiveness analysis of a randomised trial of acupuncture for chronic headache in primary care," *BMJ*, 328(7442): 747.
10. Deng, Z. Q., Zheng, H., Zhao, L., Zhou, S. Y., Li, Y. & Liang, F. R. (2012). "Health economic evaluation of acupuncture along meridians for treating migraine in China: Results from a randomized controlled trial," *BMC Complementary and Alternative Medicine*, 12: 75.
11. Wu, H., Hu, Z. & Lu, J. (2010). "Health economics evaluation in comprehensive therapy in the treatment of chronic tension-type headache of feng-tan type," *China Medical Herald*, 7: 19–20.
12. Dubois, J., Scala, E., Faouzi, M., Decosterd, I., Burnand, B., & Rodondi, P. Y. (2017). "Chronic low back pain patients' use of, level of knowledge of and perceived benefits of complementary medicine: A cross-sectional study at an academic pain center," *BMC Complementary and Alternative Medicine*, 17: 193.
13. Kizhakkeveettil, A., Rose, K. A., Kadar, G. E. & Hurwitz, E. L. (2017). "Integrative acupuncture and spinal manipulative therapy versus either alone for low back pain: A randomized controlled trial feasibility study," *Journal of Manipulative and Physiological Therapeutics*, 40(3): 201–213.
14. Chou, R., Deyo, R., Friedly, J., *et al.* "Non-pharmacologic therapies for low back pain: A systematic review for an American College of Physicians Clinical Practice Guideline," *Annals of Internal Medicine*, 166(7): 493–505.
15. Wilt, T., McLean, R. M. & Forciea, M. A. (2017). "Noninvasive treatments for acute, subacute, and chronic low back pain: A Clinical Practice Guideline From the American College of Physicians," *Annals of Internal Medicine*, 166(7): 514–530.
16. MacPherson, H., Vickers, A., Bland, M., *et al.* (2017). "Acupuncture for chronic pain and depression in primary care: A programme of research," *Programme Grants for Applied Research*, 5(3). PMID: 28121095.
17. Close, C., Sinclair, M., Liddle, S. D., Madden, E., McCullough, J. E. & Hughes, C. (2014). "A systematic review investigating the effectiveness of Complementary and Alternative Medicine (CAM) for the management of low back and/or pelvic pain (LBPP) in pregnancy," *Journal of Advance Nursing*, 70(8): 1702–1716.

18. Yuan, J., Kerr, D., Park, J. , Liu, X. H. & McDonough, S. (2008). "Treatment regimens of acupuncture for low back pain-a systematic review," *Complementary Therapies in Medicine*, 16(5): 295–304.
19. Huang, C. Y., Choong, M. Y. & Li, T. S. (2013). "Effectiveness of cupping therapy for low back pain: A systematic review," *Acupuncture in Medicine*, 31(3): 336–337. doi: 10.1136/acupmed-2013-010385.
20. Evers, J. L. (2002). "Female subfertility," *Lancet*, 360, pp. 151–159.
21. Centers for Disease Control and Prevention. (2011). *Assisted Reproductive Technology Success Rates: National Summary and Fertility Clinic Reports 2009* (US Department of Health and Human Services, Centers for Disease Control and Prevention, Atlanta, GA, USA).
22. Smith, J. F., Eisenberg, M. L., Millstein, S. G. & Nachtigall, R. D., Shindel, A. W., Wing, H., Cedars, M., Pasch, L. & Katz P. P. (2010). "The use of complementary and alternative fertility treatment in couples seeking fertility care: Data from a prospective cohort in the United States," *Fertility and Sterility*, 93: 2169–2174.
23. Domar, A. D., Conboy, L., Denardo-Roney, J. & Rooney, K. L. (2012). "Lifestyle behaviors in women undergoing *in vitro* fertilization: A prospective study," *Fertility and Sterility*, 97: 697–701.
24. Hopton, A. K., Curnoe, S., Kanaan, M. & MacPherson, H. (2012). "Acupuncture in practice: Mapping the providers, the patients and the settings in a national cross-sectional survey," *BMJ Open*, 2: e000456.
25. de Lacey, S,, Smith, C. A. & Paterson, C. (2009). "Building resilience: A preliminary exploration of women's perceptions of the use of acupuncture as an adjunct to *in vitro* fertilisation," *BMC Complementary and Alternative Medicine*, 9: 50.
26. Isoyama, D., Cordts, E. B., de Souza van Niewegen, A. M., de Almeida Pereira de Carvalho, W., Matsumura, S. T. & Barbosa, C. P. (2012). "Effect of acupuncture on symptoms of anxiety in women undergoing *in vitro* fertilisation: A prospective randomised controlled study," *Acupuncture in Medicine*, 30: 85–88.
27. Nedeljković, M., Bouzas-Ammann, G., Zimmermann, L., Stute, P. & Ausfeld-Hafter, B. "Modalities of acupuncture treatments in assisted reproductive technology-a comparison of treatment practice in Swiss, German, and Austrian fertility centers with findings from randomized controlled trials," *Forsch Komplementmed*, 20(2): 112–118. doi: 10.1159/000350717.
28. Zheng, C. H., Huang, G. Y., Zhang, M. M. & Wang, W. (2012). "Effects of acupuncture on pregnancy rates in women undergoing *in vitro* fertilization: A systematic review and meta-analysis," *Fertility and Sterility*, 97: 599–611.

29. Manheimer, E. (2011). "Selecting a control for *in vitro* fertilization and acupuncture randomized controlled trials (RCTs): How sham controls may unnecessarily complicate the RCT evidence base," *Fertility and Sterility*, 95: 2456–2461.
30. Qian, Y., Xia, X. R., Ochin, H., Huang, C., Gao, C., Gao, L., Cui, Y. G., Liu, J. Y. & Meng, Y. (2017). "Therapeutic effect of acupuncture on the outcomes of *in vitro* fertilization: A systematic review and meta-analysis," *Archives of Gynecology and Obstetrics*, 295(3): 543–558.
31. Humaidan, P. & Stener-Victorin, E. (2004). "Pain relief during oocyte retrieval with a new short duration electro-acupuncture technique-an alternative to conventional analgesic methods," *Human Reproduction*, 19(6): 1367–1372.
32. Dohle, G. R., Colpi, G. M., Hargreave, T. B., Papp, G. K., Jungwirth, A. & Weidner, W. (2005). "EAU Working Group on Male Infertility. EAU guidelines on male infertility," *European Urology*, 48(5): 703–711.
33. Sharlip, I. D., Jarow, J. P., Belker, A. M. *et al.* (2002). "Best practice policies for male infertility," *Fertility and Sterility*, 77(5): 873–882.
34. Jerng, U. M., Jo, J. Y., Lee, S., Lee, J. M. & Kwon, O. (2014). "The effectiveness and safety of acupuncture for poor semen quality in infertile males: A systematic review and meta-analysis," *Asian Journal of Andrology*, 16(6): 884–891.
35. Dieterle, S., Li, C., Greb, R., Bartzsch, F., Hatzmann, W. & Huang, D. A. (2009). "Prospective randomized placebo-controlled study of the effect of acupuncture in infertile patients with severe oligoasthenozoospermia," *Fertility and* Sterility, 92(4): 1340–1343.
36. Pei, J., Strehler, E., Noss, U. *et al.* (2005). "Quantitative evaluation of spermatozoa ultrastructure after acupuncture treatment for idiopathic male infertility," *Fertility and Sterility*, 84(1): 141–147.

Chapter 23

Scientific Evidences in Acupuncture

Umberto Mazzanti and Maria Letizia Barbanera

1. INTRODUCTION

Acupuncture has a long history that began as intuitive healing method in the East. The mystical base has resisted for a while, but in recent centuries, it has been supplanted by the need to prove its effectiveness through scientific methods, in order to be accepted by the modern medical world. Research in acupuncture has greatly developed, considering that about 26,000 studies have been published, and that research output in this sector has quadrupled in the last 10 years. The problem with acupuncture research lies in the fact that it is not possible to apply some sort of standardization to the experimental protocols, so there are always studies with a high risk of bias, higher than every experimental study on drugs. An example is the need to use sham acupuncture that has been proven not to be inert, as we will see later, or the need to use a standardized protocol to be repeatable and comparable. Standardization is not always possible and Chinese Medicine is very subjective because, for every disease, several organs and tissues can be involved, requiring different treatments even with the same problem at the base. However, with the research carried out until now, many effects of acupuncture have been highlighted, such as the promotion of homeostasis, improvement in cerebral blood flow and microcirculation, pain control, and neuromodulatory function in the central nervous system, inducing measurable effects, with changes in hormonal, immune, blood, and nervous systems. The following section provides an overview of some research studies to understand the evidences obtained so far.

2. SCIENTIFIC EVIDENCES IN RESEARCH

Recent research studies demonstrate that acupuncture is a traumatic physical stimulation. A study found that the acupuncture needle could cause muscle fiber fracture in the acupoint after inserting the needle into the acupoint, with a large number of red blood cells and fracture fragments in the muscle fiber gap and inflammatory cells infiltration, explaining the mechanism of interaction of acupuncture with cells and tissues where needles are inserted. Also, with the traumatic stimulus, acupuncture can activate the neuroendocrine–immune network, producing regulating effects.[1] A systematic review[2] about acupuncture and immune modulation analyzed studies published in the last two decades, affirming that acupuncture enhances the natural killer cell activity through increased levels of IFN-γ, β-endorphin, protein tyrosine kinase (PTK) secretion, and protein tyrosine phosphatase-1 (SHP-1) inhibition. Furthermore, the review shows the effects of acupuncture on Th1/Th2 balance. However, this review fails in the details of the studies it takes into consideration, such as the type of intervention or the protocol used. With regard to the effectiveness of acupuncture and endocrine system, a review[3] published in China on type-2 diabetes mellitus compared acupuncture and usual care versus usual care only. The results show that the clinical diagnosis and treatment of diabetes with integrative medicine based on the three-typed syndrome differentiation (TTSD) method was significantly better than that of Western medicine (WM) alone, and, beyond the efficacy of WM, could continue to significantly reduce the fasting plasma glucose concentration and the 2-hour postprandial glucose level. A review[4] on the use of acupuncture for insulin resistance suggests that acupuncture at body points or/and ear points results in regulation of fat metabolism (decreases in total cholesterol, triglyceride, low densitylipoprotein (LDL), lipoprotein A, and apolipoprotein B levels); increase in IgG, insulin, and C-peptide levels; and decrease in glucose levels in patients with obesity. Furthermore, acupuncture is reported in the review to change the levels of blood pressure modulators such as endothelin-1, renin, aldosterone, and angiotensin II in hypertensive patients, and also that Electroacupuncture (EA) restores the expression of a multitude of adipose tissue genes such as leptin, interleukin-6 (IL-6), uncoupling protein 2 (UCP2), and peroxisome proliferator-activated receptor gamma (PPAR-γ). A study[5] observed the impact of acupuncture at Taichong (LR3) point on blood flow velocity in patients with vertebrobasilar insufficiency, discovering that acupuncture improves blood supply in vertebral artery in the mode of dual regulation and rectifies the disturbance of vertebral artery blood flow in dynamics. A recent study[6] valued the neuroimmunomodulation function induced by electro-acupuncture; based on the fact that the severe stress induced by a surgical trauma causes immunosuppression and disturbance of the neuroendocrine system, making the host vulnerable to infections and diseases, the study was designed to evaluate electro-acupuncture administration on cellularity and apoptosis in the spleen of stressed rats. In fact, after the surgical trauma stress, it was observed that the surgical procedure dramatically affected splenic cellularity. These rats showed a 25–30% reduction in their number of splenocytes compared with the control group, but the reduction was abolished when EA was applied (on Zusanli ST 36 and Lanwei Extra 37 acupoints), while there were no changes in number of splenocytes if EA was applied on normal rats. The possible explanation is that stress-induced reduction in splenocytes was due to the induction of apoptosis mediated by lymphocytes, and EA stimulation suppressed the increase of apoptosis via modulating Fas protein expression, consequently preventing deleterious immunological changes in the postoperative state. The same author[7] discovered also that in the case of surgical trauma stress, when there are complicated immune alterations, EA produces anti-inflammatory effects through inhibiting TLR2 and TLR4 expression, downregulating the mRNA expression of IL-1, IL-6, and TNF-α, thereby reducing the inflammatory cytokine expression in the spleen. Other evidences of acupuncture are linked to the synaptic plasticity it induces, as stated in She *et al.*'s study[8] which investigated the effects and mechanisms of electro-acupuncture on depression. It is thought that neural plasticity, especially hippocampal syn aptic plasticity, contributes to learning and memory and is impaired during depression, leading to cognitive deficits and memory loss. EA intervention modulates hippocampal galanin and dopamine and enhances the expression of GluN2B, which plays a critical role in the improvement of long term potentiation (LTP) in the CA1 region, promoting the learning and memory performance and alleviating depression-like behavior. In addition, acupuncture has a role in inflammation: in this study,[9] the authors examined the effects of electro-acupuncture at ipsilateral or contralateral ST36 and ST37 acupoints on inflammatory pain, evaluating the transient receptor potential vanilloid 1 (TRPV1) and associated signaling pathways that are always increased in inflammation. They discovered that EA can reduce inflammatory pain and also alleviate nociceptive Nav sodium currents in dorsal root ganglion (DRG) neurons. EA also attenuated the overexpression of TRPV1 and associated signaling pathways. A recent study indicated that the amount of TRPV1 is higher in acupoints than it is in tissue along the meridian and non-acupoints. An acupoint such as ST36 is TRPV1 rich, and this may be the reason why some acupoints are used for pain control. There is an increasing number of new molecular and neurophysiological research reports on stress effect studies. Some neuroimaging-based studies, such as that by Cho *et al.*[10] explored the effectiveness of acupuncture in the brain for pain using fMRI. In this study, the pain stimuli activated most of the known pain-processing brain centers, such as the dorsal anterior cingulate cortex (ACC), caudal ACC, rostral ACC, supplementary and premotor areas, primary motor areas, and thalamic areas. With acupuncture, administered on the traditionally described acupoints, the activation changed, demonstrating the desensitization of the pain-processing areas. It is interesting that the same experiment with sham-acupuncture points showed similarities in fMRI results, suggesting that the pain relief from acupuncture is effective, regardless the choice of point; therefore, sham acupuncture surely is not inert. Furthermore, it explores the molecular and neurophysiological bases of acupuncture regarding immune, endocrinal, and neural stimulation using electro-acupuncture. The results showed a decrease in proinflammatory cytokines caused by the modulation of hypothalamus — pituitary–adrenal axis, which was also involved in the increase in endogenous opioid levels. In fact, the neurogenic stimuli of acupuncture produced an increased release of endogenous opioids, more specifically via the periventricular structures including the arcuate nucleus of the hypothalamus, thereby increasing the endogenous opioids at specific areas where pain signal processing is believed to occur. The hypothalamus–pituitary–adrenal axis was probably involved in the anti-inflammatory mechanism in conjunction with the neuroimmune pathways and the cholinergic anti-inflammatory mechanism.

3. THE "FURTHER STUDIES ARE NEEDED" PROBLEM

As mentioned earlier, the real problem, which is well known but without a solution yet, is the quality of research methodology. First of all, the inclusion criteria, which are often largely unspecific, increase the risk of bias; then there is the concept of sham acupuncture, which has found to be not inert, because any type of skin stimulation which also involves non-penetration, elicits central and peripheral reactions, hindering the correct blinding of the patients. Furthermore, the tests are not truly double blind, because the doctor is aware which treatment is real and could unwittingly be passing on information to the patient, creating a real risk of bias even in the best research study.[11] Other problems include the lack of use of the standards (e.g., STRICTA, China National Standard GB/T123462006 describing point selection, point location, needling techniques, treatment protocols, and so on), the heterogeneous training of the acupuncturists, the brevity of the follow up (also in the cost-effectiveness research, wherein the long duration of acupuncture results in lower costs compared to usual care), and language, because most of the systematic reviews do not include randomized controlled trials in Eastern languages.

4. CONCLUSIONS

Placebo control and appropriate blinding methods are needed to investigate the efficacy of acupuncture; otherwise, the specific effects cannot be validated. Attention must be given to correct treatment. It is vitally important that competent professionals, both clinically skilled and trained in research, work together with trained acupuncturists because it is necessary for needling to be precise not only in the localization of the acupoints but also in the correct manipulation. Moreover, research should be enhanced on the synergistic effect of acupuncture together with drug therapy, because this would allow a complete integration of medicine. Certain diseases can benefit from an exclusive therapy with acupuncture, but others do not have this possibility, and acupuncture can be an additional tool for the appropriate management of the problem to improve the quality of life.

REFERENCES

1. Ding, S,, Hong, S., Wang, C. *et al.* (2013). "Acupuncture Modulates the Neuro–Endocrine–Immune Network" *GJM: An International Journal of Medicine*, 107(5): 341–345.
2. Sun, K. & Hyunsu, B. (2010). "Acupuncture and immune modulation." *Autonomic Neuroscience*, 157(1): 38–41.
3. Yan, X-f. *et al.* (2014). "A systematic review and meta-analysis of type 2 diabetes mellitus treatment based on the "three-typed syndrome differentiation" theory in Chinese medicine," *Chinese Journal of Integrative Medicine*, 20: 633–640.
4. Liang, F. & Koya, D. (2010). "Acupuncture: Is it effective for treatment of insulin resistance?" *Diabetes, Obesity and Metabolism*, 12(7): 555–569.
5. Wang, G. M., Li, L. X., Wen, F. Y. *et al.* (2011). "Impacts of acupuncture at Taichong (LR3) point on blood flow velocity in patients with vertebrobasilar insufficiency," *Zhongguo Zhen Jiu*, 31(3): 216–218.
6. Wang, J., Wang, Y. Q., Yu, J. *et al.* (2005). "Electroacupuncture suppresses surgical trauma stress-induced lymphocyte apoptosis in rats," *Neuroscience Letters*, 383: 68–72.
7. Wang, J., Zhao, H., Qi, M. Y. *et al.* (2009). "Electroacupuncture downregulates TLR2/4 and pro-inflammatory cytokine expression after surgical trauma stress without adrenal glands involvement," *Brain Research Bulletin*, 80: 89–94.
8. She, Y., Xu, J., Duan, Y. *et al.* (2015). "Possible antidepressant effects and mechanism of electroacupuncture in behaviors and hippocampal synaptic

plasticity in a depression rat model." http://dx.doi.org/10.1016/j.brainres.2015.10.033.

9. Lu, K. W., Hsu, C. K., Hsieh, C. L. *et al.* (2016). "Probing the effects and mechanisms of electroacupuncture at ipsilateral or contralateral ST36–ST37 acupoints on CFA-induced inflammatory pain," *Scientific Reports*, 6: 22123. doi: 10.1038/srep22123.
10. Cho, Z. H., Hwang, S. C., Wong, E. K. *et al.* (2006). "Neural substrates, experimental evidences and functional hypothesis of acupuncture mechanisms," *Acta Neurologica Scandinavia*, 11: 370–377. doi: 10.1111/j.1600–0404.2006.00600.x.
11. Derbyshire, D. (2013). "Why acupuncture is giving scientists the needle." *The Guardian*, 26 July. Available at: https://www.theguardian.com/science/2013/jul/26/acupuncture-sceptics-proof-effective-nhs. Accessed 7 July 2017.

Chapter 24

A Correct Methodology of Research in Acupuncture: The Problem of the Sham Procedures

Carlo Maria Giovanardi, Alessandra Pavesi and Alessandra Poini

1. INTRODUCTION

The nature of the non-pharmaceutical therapy and the complexity of the intervention pose many challenges for research on acupuncture. Even if sham acupuncture is commonly used as control to compare with "real acupuncture" and detect the efficacy of the stimulation by needling, it is found to have a remarkable effect and act as more than just a placebo in many target diseases. In this chapter, we will examine the challenges facing acupuncture research in the light of the nature of the technique (non-pharmacological therapy) and the complexity of the intervention. Evidence-based medicine (EBM), though still controversial, is one of the dominant paradigms within medicine. By integrating individual clinical expertise with the best available clinical evidence from systematic research and patient preferences, it has been established as the standard of modern medical practice worldwide.

However, in a recent article by Greenhalgh *et al.*,[1] it is interesting to note that some criticism on EBM has began to emerge in Western medicine, in particular:

- Statistically significant benefits may be marginal in clinical practice;
- Inflexible rules and technology-driven prompts may produce care that is management-driven rather than patient-centered;
- Evidence-based guidelines often poorly map complex multimorbidity.

These assumptions are essential to define the standards of acupuncture research and apply EBM to acupuncture trials and reviews. Indeed every choice should consider the balance between the proof of evidence and the clinical value of a result.

With this regard, determining an appropriate control for use in acupuncture research remains one of the major methodological challenges acupuncture researchers have to face.[2]

We think it is important to mention the International Symposium on Research in Acupuncture, held in Bologna, Italy, in October 2015 and organized by Association of Medical Acupuncturists of Bologna (A.M.A.B), and Istituto Superiore di Sanità (ISS): this symposium, among the first in Europe, was crucial to the writing of this chapter.

2. RESEARCH METHODOLOGY IN ACUPUNCTURE

2.1. *Challenges of acupuncture researches*

As a non-pharmaceutical therapy, the effect of acupuncture may be related to the distinctive mechanisms of the tehnique (i.e., meridians, depth of the insertion, stimulation, etc.).[3] Also some external components may affect the results of the acupuncture treatment, such as doctor–patient relationship. All of the above-mentioned factors would play a role in the acupuncture's effect during the treatment, thus we define the acupuncture treatment as a complex intervention that offers challenges for the research.[4] First, there is no ideal placebo control for acupuncture treatment even if sham acupuncture is commonly used as control to compare with "real acupuncture".[5] Nevertheless, sham acupuncture cannot be defined as inert:[6] in fact, any type of skin stimulation, not necessarily involving penetration of the skin, elicits central and peripheral reactions. In addition, sham acupuncture with needles penetrating the skin induces an important physiologic activation and so must be avoided: this is the essential point to conduct a correct clinical trial on acupuncture. Penetrating needles have important physiologic activity, even when inserted superficially away from true acupuncture points. In fact when sham control trials use penetrating needles, the effect and size for acupunture is lower than trials that use non-penetrating needles. This suggests that penetrating needles have important physiologic activity, even when inserted superficially away from true acupuncture points.[7] So we can say that for pain, the "research question" remains the primary determinant on choice of control: a useful distinction has been drawn between efficacy trials and effectiveness trials (see Sec. 2.2). When the outcome is totally objective (like pregnancy in fertility studies), the use of a placebo control is not necessary.[8]

2.2. *Questions of interest and types of design*

To address all the above-mentioned challenges, researchers need to be aware of their research purpose. Thus, they should define the research question at the beginning of the study as the first and most important step. At least five factors should be considered for a quality clinical study, including study design, the participants, the intervention, controls, and outcomes. A right research question should come from clinical practice and must be patient-relevant. Therefore, future clinical trials on acupuncture should look at this issue by observing a spectrum between *effectiveness and efficacy*. *Efficacy* is the specific effects which are due to the active ingredient of the treatment, while *effectiveness* involves both specific and non-specific effects, the latter caused by psychological or psycho-physiological effects associated with the act of treatment (such as the placebo effect).[9] Efficacy trials seek to determine whether there are specific effects beyond the placebo in an ideal treatment environment, whereas effectiveness trials seek to determine the overall impact of acupuncture in which specific and non-specific effects are combined. "Blinding" in acupuncture research is a problem because, real blinding in this type of technique is almost impossible. The problem could be solved through specific study designs such as comparative effectiveness research (CER). CER is a type of study which focuses on the comparison of the effectiveness between different interventions, including pragmatic randomized controlled trials (RCTs), qualitative study (survey and interview), most of the observational studies (cohort study, case-control study, cross-sectional study, case series study, and case report), and research synthesis (systematic review and meta-analysis).[10] Attention must be paid to the correct treatment, keeping in mind the differences between Chinese and Western methods with regard to the timing and retention of needles. Importance should be given to the follow up. In particular, patients with moderate and severe pain would use several kinds of treatments, including conventional medicines, during a long study period. Mild-to-moderate benefit of acupuncture compared with sham acupuncture would be diluted under complex treatments. As a consequence, a small sample study is powerless to identify mild or moderate effective difference and achieve statistical significant between two groups.[11] For example, pragmatic trials or large-scale observational studies might be close to the real-world situation, whereas qualitative methods could be used to study the components of therapeutic effect within a trial setting.

2.3. *Appropriateness for meta-analysis of acupuncture*

2.3.1. *Current evidence for acupuncture*

Acupuncture is accepted in many countries for treating pain conditions.[12] However, the clinical practice guidelines for acupuncture still lack high-level evidence such as RCTs and systematic reviews. It is known that systematic reviews of high-quality RCTs are crucial to EBM.[13] Findings from 30 Cochrane reviews related to acupuncture showed insufficient evidence to support and, at the same time, to refute the intervention due to either poor methodology quality of trials or scarce evidence.[14] From these findings we can draw some conclusions. For future research, it is important frame the correct research questions with regard to Traditional Chinese Medicine. It is also important to design clinical trials correctly to raise the quality of the output.

Another important issue in systematic reviews is the adequate preparation of reviewers: Chai *et al.*[15] investigated the characteristics of the authors of acupuncture Cochrane systematic reviews and showed that authors of 25 (64%) reviews have no acupuncture-related education or practice background, whereas 6 (15%) first authors published 15 (38%) reviews.

2.3.2. *Challenges for meta-analysis of acupuncture*

The quality of the evidence from a systematic review/meta-analysis relies on the quality of the trials included. For the primary clinical studies, we have two basic quality considerations: study quality and treatment quality. For study quality, we may use risk of bias[16] to evaluate the methodological quality for a study. Besides, we can use CONSORT Statement[17] plus STRICTA[18] for evaluating the reporting quality of a trial for acupuncture assessment. As there is a large amount of acupuncture research undertaken in non-English-speaking countries, e.g., in China, Japan, Korea, and Germany, it may be feasible to develop a global network of STRICTA research centers.[19] For meta-analysis, another challenge in research methodology is the appropriateness to pool all data to get an overall effect from heterogeneous studies. Heterogeneity among trials included clinical heterogeneity in terms of difference between participants, acupuncture treatment.[20] Another issue is the insufficient numbers of trials included in the meta-analysis. Though the sample size of a systematic review is not required to be calculated, the statistical power could be estimated according to trial sequential analysis (TSA) to determine whether the number of trials included in the meta-analysis is enough to draw a confidential conclusion based on the synthesized results.[21] Also, the publication bias due to incomplete evidence (from incomprehensive literature searching) and the the high rate of appearance of studies with positive results should be detected and discussed in the review.[22] Results of the meta-analysis may exaggerate the effect of the intervention due to the small studies effect and the publication bias. A problem arises from the study's language inclusion: systematic reviews should, by definition, include studies published in all languages

A recent study shows that in Cochrane reviews concerning acupuncture, there is a large heterogeneity in the databases searched and the incorporation of Chinese language expertise in Cochrane acupuncture reviews (among such reviews, only 40% searched Chinese databases). This is concerning as the neglect of Chinese language literature introduces a bias into the systematic reviews. Searching English language databases only may limit the number of trials retrieved for inclusion in systematic reviews. The limitations of this study must be acknowledged.[23] Finally, the research findings should be incorporated and integrated with personal experience and expertise and patient's preference and value. Another point of discussion is the internal and external validity in RCT and meta-analysis. The evidence hierarchy of EBM focuses only on internal validity, the methodological rigor, or a study. Thereby, the external validity, i.e., the question of generalizability and applicability, is neglected with the idea that it is secondary and can be fixed along the way. However, this is not true. Walach[24] suggests that one potential solution is to adopt a circular view, in which various study types complement each other in their strengths and weaknesses to yield a full picture.

3. SHAM PROCEDURES IN ACUPUNCTURE: A PROBLEM TO SOLVE

Considering the common view of modern research, the most concrete evidence of efficacy is due to systematic reviews of double-blind trials. So, acupuncture need to be compared to a sham procedure to be included in clinical guidelines. Various procedures are used as acupuncture placebo controls, but it is a mistake to consider them all inert and equal to each other. A review[25] confronted the problem of sham acupuncture by listing the characteristics and differences of every kind of sham procedure commonly used. The paper listed four characteristics of sham acupuncture controls:

3.1. *Shallow needling*

The needles are inserted in a shallow way theoretically in points that do not reach the meridian. This typology of sham is not inert, because the depth of needling differs between different styles of acupuncture, e.g., in Japanese acupuncture, which practices very superficial needling. Furthermore, the depth of insertion may vary depending on the case. A Japanese trial that tested a shallow needling technique with 0.6 mm depth showed a clinical effect.[26]

3.2. *Non-penetrating needles*

There are different kinds of needles that are able to apply pressure without penetrating the skin. Physical contact with the surface of the skin may provide sensory stimulation, indicating that even blunted needle devices are not entirely inert and may elicit a therapeutic effect of their own. For instance, Lund *et al.*[27] noted that the sensation produced by a needle tip "touch" was substantial and it may activate parts of the peripheral nervous system. The Streitberger, Park, and Japanese devices are three of the most commonly used placebo needle devices in acupuncture research. All three of these devices are used in a similar manner: a blunted needle is inserted, touches the skin, and is retracted. These three devices, while standardized and validated, have physical limitations with regard to their ability to facilitate a range of manipulation methods, such as shallow or horizontal insertion. They are also not effective for all acupoint types and acupuncture positions.[28]

3.3. *Acupuncture in non-acupuncture points*

The needles are inserted far from the traditional acupuncture points. In the tradition of Chinese Medicine, there are active points out of the meridian named as Ashi points (i.e., trigger points). Moreover, the traditional medicine considers all the space occupied by the body as a dense beam of meridians and therefore suitable for needling. Also the accuracy of point location could lead to bias: a study showed the correct needling of a point of acupuncture covers an elliptical area of about 8 cm, so it is possible that in some studies the sham points used fall within the area of a meridian.[29]

3.4. *Acupuncture in points not indicated for the specific condition*

This type of sham is the most questionable, because in traditional practice, one specific point in isolation is not used, it is a combination of points that evokes the response. A real-as-sham acupuncture evoked peripheral and central effects in health and disease conditions.[25] In healthy subjects, sham acupuncture activates mechanoreceptors as the peripheral effect, transmitting the information of mechanical stimulus to the brain by A-beta and C afferents. In pain conditions, sham acupuncture activates the same mechanoreceptors, but the response is stronger and involves different sensory neurons because there is a peripheral and central sensitization. Considering the central effects, sham acupuncture evokes a light activity in various areas of the brain, suggesting a limbic "touch" that causes emotional and hormonal reactions common in the reaction to caress, and if there is pain, the central effect can cause an increase or decrease in pain, depending on the degree of central sensitization. We known that there is a statistically significant difference between the sham procedures and real acupuncture, but the effect size is too small due to the physiological effects of sham devices to provide the evidence required to include acupuncture in the guidelines. Some systematic reviews' findings, failed to demonstrate that acupuncture is statistically superior of sham acupuncture, but at the same time both are better than usual care, with lower side effects.[30] With regard to nononcological chronic pain, more evidence supports the use of acupuncture.[31,32] The judgment of what constitute a clinically significant effect size should not be based on the comparison between acupuncture and inert procedures, because it demonstrates a lack of knowledge of acupuncture. The problem of placebo could be solved without provoking an incompatibility with EBM because sham controls are not a necessary part of the EBM hierarchy. This type of intervention is more similar to surgery: some placebo-controlled surgery trials have been conducted (for ambiguity of the particular kind of surgery), and the result demonstrated that some or all the benefits of the procedures could be attributed to non-specific and placebo effects. Furthermore, acupuncture is a complex intervention.[33] A recent Cochrane review on placebo interventions for all kinds of conditions found that "physical placebos" (which included sham acupuncture) were associated with larger effects over no-treatment control groups than "pharmacological placebos".[34] MacPherson[35] proposed to focus on two fundamental questions:

- Is acupuncture more effective than sham acupuncture?
- Is acupuncture more effective than standard usual care?

With these two questions in mind, he collected data from 29 studies about chronic pain from almost 18,000 patients. Of the 29 studies examined, 20 used sham control, involving 5,230 patients, but the sham methods used were too heterogeneous to compare. Eighteen studies used usual care for the control group. The results showed that acupuncture is a statistically significant effective treatment ($p < 0.001$) for chronic pain with a clinically relevant effect size of 0.5. The difference between acupuncture and sham acupuncture was small (effect size 0.2), and so was that between acupuncture and NSAIDs (effect size 0.3). Despite these results, it is important to consider the almost total absence of adverse effects of acupuncture, which has a better safety profile than usual care.[35] In conclusion, placebo-controlled trials for acupuncture should avoid sham procedures used until now. It is necessary to establish a clinical research method for acupuncture that respects the theory of TCM, to discover the real advantages of the effect of acupuncture and promote it to mainstream medicine.

REFERENCES

1. Greenhalgh, T. (2014). "Evidence based medicine: A movement in crisis?" *BMJ*, 348: 3725.
2. Giovanardi, C. M. *et al.* (2015). "Toward a definition of the standards for research in acupuncture: The Bologna International Symposium," *European Journal of Integrative Medicine*, 7(4): 429–431.
3. Cao, H., Liu, J., Farella, M. G., Barbanera, M. L., Poini, A., Mazzanti, U. & Giovanardi, C. M. (2015). *Methodology of Research and EBM in Acupuncture* (Manuscript).
4. Campbell, M. *et al.* (2000). "Framework for design and evaluation of complex interventions to improve health," *BMJ: British Medical Journal*, 321(7262): 694–696.

5. Zhang, C. S. *et al.* (2015). "Placebo devices as effective control methods in acupuncture clinical trials: A systematic review," *PloS one*, 10(11): e0140825.
6. Birch, S. (2006). "A review and analysis of placebo treatments, placebo effects, and placebo controls in trials of medical procedures when sham is not inert," *J Altern Complement Med*, 12: 303–310.
7. MacPherson, H. *et al.* & Acupuncture Trialists' Collaboration. (2014). "Influence of control group on effect size in trials of acupuncture for chronic pain: A secondary analysis of an individual patient data meta-analysis," *PloS one*, 9(4): e93739.
8. Manheimer, E. (2011). "Selecting a control in IVF and acupuncture RCTs: How sham controls may unnecessarily complicate the RCT evidence base," *Fertility and Sterility*, 95(8): 2456.
9. Witt, C. M. & Linde, K. (2012). *Clinical Research in Complementary and Integrative Medicine: A Practical Training Book* (Urban and Fischer, Hackerbrucke).
10. Schneeweiss, S. *et al.* (2013). "Methods for comparative effectiveness research/patient-centered outcomes research: From efficacy to effectiveness," *Journal of Clinical Epidemiology*, 66(8): S1–S4.
11. Junhua Zhang & Yuhong Huang (2015). "Why the clinical effect of acupuncture is controversial?" *European Journal of Integrative Medicine*, 7(4): 434–435. Paper presented at International Symposium on Research in Acupuncture Bologna-Italy, October 3, 2015.
12. Chou, R. *et al.* (2007). "Diagnosis and treatment of low back pain: A joint clinical practice guideline from the American College of Physicians and the American Pain Society," *Annals of Internal Medicine*, 147(7): 478–491.
13. Centre for Evidence Based Medicine. "What is EBM?" Available at: http://ktclearinghouse.ca/cebm/intro/whatisebm Accessed on 12 December 2015.
14. Manheimer, E. *et al.* (2009). "Evidence from the Cochrane Collaboration for traditional Chinese medicine therapies," *The Journal of Alternative and Complementary Medicine*, 15(9): 1001–1014.
15. Chai, Q. *et al.* (2014). "Characteristics of the authors and intervention heterogeneity in acupuncture Cochrane Systematic Reviews," *The Journal of Alternative and Complementary Medicine*, 20(5): A40–A40.
16. Higgins, J. P. T. & Green, S. (eds.) (2011). *Cochrane Handbook for Systematic Reviews of Interventions*, Version 5.1.0. The Cochrane Collaboration. Available at: www.cochrane-handbook.org (updated March 2011).
17. Moher, D. *et al.* (2010). "CONSORT 2010 explanation and elaboration: Updated guidelines for reporting parallel group randomised trials," *BMJ*, 340(1): c869–c869.

18. MacPherson, H. *et al.* (2010). "Revised standards for reporting interventions in clinical trials of acupuncture (STRICTA): Extending the CONSORT statement," *Journal of Evidence-Based Medicine*, 3(3): 140–155.
19. Liu, L. *et al.* (2015). "STRICTA: Is it time to do more?" *BMC Complementary and Alternative Medicine*, 15(1): 190.
20. Song, F. (2001). "Methods for exploring heterogeneity in meta-analysis," *Evaluation & The Health Professions*, 24(2): 126–151.
21. Brok, J. *et al.* (2008). "Trial sequential analysis reveals insufficient information size and potentially false positive results in many meta-analyses," *Journal of Clinical Epidemiology*, 61(8): 763–769.
22. Parekh-Bhurke, S. *et al.* (2011). "Uptake of methods to deal with publication bias in systematic reviews has increased over time, but there is still much scope for improvement," *Journal of Clinical Epidemiology*, 64(4): 349–357.
23. Lui, S. *et al.* (2010). "Heterogeneity in search strategies among Cochrane acupuncture reviews: Is there room for improvement?" *Acupuncture in Medicine*, 28(3): 149–153.
24. Walach, H. (2015). "The incompatibility of external and internal validity invalidates the evidence hierarchy–Theoretical and practical consequences," *European Journal of Integrative Medicine*, 7(4): 434.
25. Appleyard, I. *et al.* (2014). "Should systematic reviews assess the risk of bias from sham–placebo acupuncture control procedures?" *European Journal of Integrative Medicine*, 6(2): 234–243.
26. Kaneko, Y. *et al.* (2009). "The effects of press-tack needle treatment on muscle soreness after triathlon race–sham controlled study," *JAM*, 5(1): 22–30.
27. Lund, I. *et al.* (2009). "Minimal acupuncture is not a valid placebo control in randomised controlled trials of acupuncture: A physiologist's perspective," *Chinese Medicine*, 4(1): 1.
28. Zhu, D. *et al.* (2013). "Placebo acupuncture devices: considerations for acupuncture research," *Evidence-Based Complementary and Alternative Medicine*, 2013: 628907.
29. Molsberger, A. F. *et al.* (2012). "Acupuncture points are large fields: The fuzziness of acupuncture point localization by doctors in practice," *European Journal of Pain*, 16(9): 1264–1270.
30. Paley, C. A., *et al.* (2011). "Acupuncture for cancer pain in adults," *Cochrane Database of Systematic Reviews*, 1(10).
31. Manyanga, T. *et al.* (2014). "Pain management with acupuncture in osteoarthritis: A systematic review and meta-analysis," *BMC Complementary and Alternative Medicine*, 14(1): 312.

32. Zeng, Y. *et al.* (2015). "Acupuncture for chronic non-specific low back pain: An overview of systematic reviews," *European Journal of Integrative Medicine*, 7(2): 94–107.
33. Guttman, J. (2015). Can complementary and alternative medicine be evaluated within the framework of evidence-based medicine? Dissertation, University of Pittsburgh.
34. Linde, K. *et al.* (2010). "Are sham acupuncture interventions more effective than (other) placebos? A re-analysis of data from the Cochrane review on placebo effects," *Forschende Komplementärmedizin/Research in Complementary Medicine*, 17(5): 259–264.
35. MacPherson, H. (2015). "Acupuncture for chronic pain: Definitive results on treatment and placebo effects," *European Journal of Integrative Medicine*, 4(7): 436.

Chapter 25

Safety of Acupuncture

Umberto Mazzanti and Maria Letizia Barbanera

1. INTRODUCTION

One of the main reasons for the growing success of non-conventional medicine is linked to the safety of the practice, because it considers the individual to be at the center, different from traditional medicine that observes and cures only the diseased organ. Modern medicine has the advantage of being extremely effective in case of need, especially in acute conditions that require rapid assistance, but it is used also to manage chronic conditions. Therefore, frequently, people who suffer from chronic illnesses are obliged to take several medicines every day, increasing the risk of side effects. Polypharmacy is common in older adults: Maher[1] wrote that nearly 50% of older adults take one or more medications that are not medically necessary, and that polypharmacy is associated with an increased risk of adverse drug events (ADEs), drug-interactions, outpatient visits, and hospitalization, with an approximate 30% increase in medical costs. In a prospective cohort study of older hospitalized adults taking five or more medications, the prevalence of a potential hepatic cytochrome enzyme-mediated, drug–drug interaction was 80%. The probability of a drug–drug interaction increased with the number of medications. Specifically, a patient taking five to nine medications had a 50% probability, whereas the risk increased to 100% when a patient was found to be taking 20 or more medications. Based on this, it is clear that the modern medicine needs an alternative therapy to reduce the need of medication.

In the field of non-conventional medicine, acupuncture is perfect for this purpose, in fact, it is the only safely accepted treatment recommended by specialists in the field of oncology, who must always take into account the possible drug interactions that they are obliged to report if the patient is also using other drugs such as herbs or ayurvedic medicines during the chemotherapy protocols.

A 2015 study showed the safety profile of acupuncture in cancer patients who developed thrombocytopenia as side effect of chemotherapy or radiation, showing that acupuncture can be used safely within an integrated model of care because no adverse events of increased bruising or bleeding were noted after the treatment.[2]

2. RESEARCH ABOUT SAFETY OF ACUPUNCTURE

Various authors have carried out research studies to evaluate the safety profile of acupuncture. In 2009,[3] a German study interviewed 13,579 physicians practicing acupuncture; all had at least 140 hours of acupuncture training and on average 6.9 years of acupuncture practice. With them, the researchers reached out to 229,230 patients treated with a total of 2.2 million acupuncture sessions. About 8.6% of the patients reported at least one adverse effect, with a total of 24,377 adverse events. The most common were minor bleeding and hematomas, followed by pain and vegetative symptoms. Two cases of pneumothorax occurred. The longest duration of a side effect was 180 days (nerve lesion of the lower limb). There were no acupuncture-associated deaths or permanent injuries associated with the acupuncture treatments. The study states that many of these events may have been caused by malpractice or negligence and concludes that acupuncture provided by physicians is a relatively safe treatment (the highest risk of experiencing an adverse effect due to acupuncture is seen in about 1 in 76,000 patients, with 95% probability) but severe complications should not be over- or underestimated by physicians.

Another review[4] reported very heterogeneous results: the most common adverse events were needle pain (1–45%), tiredness (2–41%), and bleeding (0.03–38%), with faintness and syncope only in 0–0.3%, while infections and other life-threatening complications were not reported. Pneumothorax occurred only twice, estimating that a pneumothorax would be expected to occur once in every 41 years of full-time practice. Two retrospective studies also considered the indirect adverse events of treatment by practitioners who are not trained in orthodox medicine, particularly failure to detect underlying pathology or recommend conventional treatment of known effectiveness. MacPherson *et al.*[5] conducted a study on the adverse events of acupuncture contacting the patients directly with a questionnaire: 682 patients (10.7%) reported a total of 1,044 adverse events, where the most common events reported were severe tiredness and exhaustion, pain at the site of needling and headache. Only three cases required admission to the hospital but not for life-threatening conditions. Only 40 out of 6,348 patients said they would not be willing to have acupuncture again. MacPherson *et al.* affirmed that adverse events related to advice about medication and delayed conventional treatment were infrequent, and in their study, there was no evidence that patients seeking treatment outside the NHS (i.e., not defined training) were at greater risk of adverse events. Another survey[6] collected data from 78 acupuncturists in Britain (61% doctors and 39% physiotherapists); out of 31,822 treatments, 2,135 minor adverse events (like bleeding, pain in the site of needling, etc.) have been reported, and 42 significant events cleared within one week, except for one incident of pain that lasted two weeks and a sensory symptom that lasted several weeks. None of these events was serious. Bensoussan *et al.*[7] examined the adverse events reported by medical and non-medical acupuncturists in Australia, obtaining no significant differences in the proportion of practitioners reporting adverse events (63.6% of medical practitioners and 60.1% of non-medical practitioners). However, he noted that reports from medical practitioners resulted in a higher rate of adverse events, probably because of an increased willingness by medical practitioners to indicate adverse events and because patients suffering an adverse reaction were more likely to return to the practitioner responsible for the reaction if the practitioner were medically qualified. A 2014 study[8] explored the situation in China, collecting data on the frequency and severity of adverse complications and events in acupuncture treatment reported from 1980 to 2013. Over the 33 years, 182 incidents were identified in 133 relevant papers. Some adverse events were mild, such as hematomas, pain in the site of needling, cold during the treatment, headache, syncope, or somnolence, but others were serious, like pneumothorax and injury to internal organs, tissues, nerves, and the central nervous system. Based on this research, the major cause of injuries was the lack of knowledge about anatomy and other systems. In fact, the cases of 1980s were from Chinese rural areas (remember that acupuncture was born as a medicine for the poor who could not afford the drugs), so the deficient knowledge on anatomy led to many cases of pneumothorax and subarachnoid hemorrhage, as well as injuries to abdomen organs, heart, and peripheral nerves. In fact, with the increasing requirement for acupuncturists, these accidents decreased from the 1990s, as we can see in Fig. 1.

Figure 1. Cases of Pneumothorax and Central Nervous System Injury from 1980 till 2013.

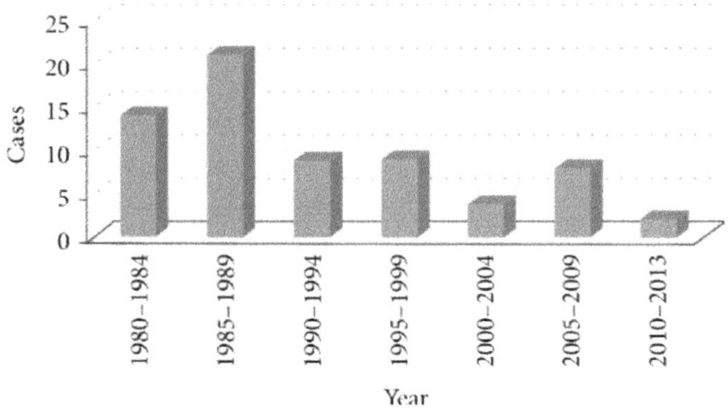

Source: From Ref. 8.

In addition, the study reports that some effects were actually indirectly related to acupuncture, such as a case that had a gastric abscess caused by perforation of a gastric ulcer treated with electroacupuncture at Zusanli (ST36). The acupoint was located without violation, but the acupuncturist underestimated the patient's ulcer that evolved to perforation. This point highlights how important is the preparation of the therapist, who needs to be able not only to not cause harm to the patient but also to understand the situation that faces and to act accordingly, also advising the patient to a specialist. This kind of mindset is a prerogative of a medical doctor, so it is important that an acupuncturist is also prepared in medicine, to know the limitation of the profession.

3. THE DRY NEEDLING PROBLEM

This important topic of preparation for the profession of acupuncturist links to a new problem we actually have to face: the dry needling. Dry needling is a method generally used by physiotherapists to treat dysfunctions in skeletal muscle, fascia, and connective tissue; diminish persistent peripheral nociceptive (pain) inputs; and reduce or restore impairments of body structure and function leading to improved movement and function.[9]

In March 2016, US Senator Randi Becker, Chair of the Senate Health Care Committee requested the Department of Health conduct a sunrise review of a proposal to add dry needling to the physical therapist scope of practice. The issues being considered include whether dry needling is acupuncture, whether it is in the physical therapy scope of practice, and whether physical therapists have sufficient training to safely add it to their statutory scope of practice. This debate has been contentious and has been resolved in many different ways across the states. In the US, out of 3,666 liability claims filed against physical therapists between 2009 and 2014, 20 were for dry needling. There has been a nationwide debate about whether physical therapists should be practicing dry needling. More than half the states in the US permit physical therapists to dry needle. Nine states, including California, prohibit it, while others such as Washington are grappling with which way to move the needle.

The result of the sunrise review process (an evaluation of a proposal to change the laws regulating health profession in Washington was the following:

"The department does not support the applicant's proposal as submitted to add dry needling to the physical therapy scope of practice. It does not meet the sunrise criteria for increasing a profession's scope of practice".

However it says also that "with adequate training that includes a clinical component, dry needling may fit within the physical therapist's scope of practice in treating neuro-musculoskeletal pain and movement impairments," so "the legislature may wish to consider adding dry needling to the physical therapist scope of practice through proposed legislation that includes additional safety requirements such as specific education".[10]

The problem of dry needling has been perceived also in this side of the ocean: the Pan-European Federation of Traditional Chinese Medicine Societies (PEFOTS), which represents Traditional Chinese Medicine (TCM) organizations in European countries, organized the First Meeting of Experts of Regulation on TCM on September 24, 2016, with participants from 14 European countries producing a declaration about the practice of dry needling (see Appendix).

4. CONCLUSIONS

Based on the results of the studies, it is clear that acupuncture can be defined as safe because the number of serious adverse events is extremely rare, while mild ones are self-limiting conditions without sequelae. Undoubtedly the side effects are not comparable to those due to medications that interfere each other and increase the risks with every drug added. However, the acupuncturist's training is an essential element for the success of the treatment. The medical training of an acupuncturist ensures the ability to discriminate between adverse events and recognize the cases that need to be addressed to other specialists.

REFERENCES

1. Maher, R., Hanlon, J. & Hajjar, E. (2014). "Clinical consequences of polypharmacy in elderly," *Expert Opinion on Drug Safety*, 13(1): 1–11. doi: 10.1517/14740338.2013.827660.

2. Esteban, M. (2016). "Acupuncturists, therapists battling over so-called 'dry needling technique.'" Available at: http://komonews.com/news/komo-4-investigators/acupucnturists-therapists-battling-over-so-called-dry-needling-technique. Accessed 8 July 2017.
3. Witt, C., Pach, D. & Brinkhaus, B. *et al.* (2009). "Safety of acupuncture: Results of a prospective observational study with 229,230 patients and introduction of a medical information and consent form," *Forschende Komplementärmedizin*, 16(2): 91–97. doi: 10.1159/000209315.
4. Ernst, E. & White, A. R. (2001). "Prospective studies of the safety of acupuncture: A systematic review," *American Journal of Medicine*, 110(6): 481–485.
5. MacPherson, H., Scullion, A., Thomas, K. J. *et al.* (2004). "Patient reports of adverse events associated with acupuncture treatment: A prospective national survey," *Quality & Safety in Health Care*, 13(5): 349–355.
6. MacPherson, H., Thomas, K., Walters, S. *et al.* (2001). "The York Acupuncture Safety Study: Prospective survey of 34,000 treatments by traditional acupuncturists," *BMJ*, 323(7311): 486–487.
7. Bensoussan, A., Myers, S. P. & Carlton, A. L. (2000). "Risks associated with the practice of traditional Chinese medicine: An Australian study," *Archives of Family Medicine*, 9(10): 1071–1080.
8. Wu, J., Hu, Y., Zhu, Y. *et al.* (2015). "Systematic review of adverse effects: A further step towards modernization of acupuncture in China," *Evidence-Based Complementary and Alternative Medicine*, Art. ID 432467, 19. Available at: http://dx.doi.org/10.1155/2015/432467.
9. Cybularz, P., Brothers, K., Singh, G. *et al.* (2015). "The safety of acupuncture in patients with cancer therapy–related thrombocytopenia." *Medical Acupuncture*, 27(3): 224–229. doi: 10.1089/acu.2015.1099.
10. Washington State Department of Health (2016). *Physical Therapy Dry Needling Sunrise Review*. Publication Number 631-063.

APPENDIX

DECLARATION OF MADRID ABOUT THE PRACTISE OF THE DENOMINATED DRY NEEDLING

The participants in the First Meeting of Experts of Regulation on TCM, from 14 european countries, reunited in Madrid the 24th september 2016, states that:

a) Dry needling is an invasive therapeutic practice, commonly used for rehabilitation and pain therapy, by traditional chinese acupuncture, in which "Ashi" points or painful points or trigger points are used as stimulation points.

b) The therapeutic practise of painful points by acupuncture is inherent in the practice of Chinese medicine. "Trigger points" were being described for the first time (trigger points, TRP), also often called trigger myofascial points (PGM), in Steinbrocker and Travell theories, that assume that the curative effect of the "bite" could be due to the physical action of the needle and the evocation of the "TwitchResponse local" (LTR). Travell was, as far as we understand, who used for the first time in 1968 the term "dry needle".

c) This therapeutic practise has extended recently as an evolution of the "anaesthetic blockade of "trigger points", practice proposed in 1949 by J. Travell. The practice consists on the insertion of acupuncture points in "painful points", beyond the skin and sometimes reaching the muscle layer. Once inserted, it stimulates the needle. This therapeutic practice it's being used by professionals with lack of preparation, who are not acupuncturists.

d) In acupuncture this practice, described thousands of years ago, is used as a "dispersion vertical handling practice". Gunn et al, described in 1980 this practise, as the development of the old chinese practise. The dry needling can not be understood out of the therapeutic context of acupuncture.

e) There is considerable research published in many systematic reviews on this subject. One of the first, Ernst E. And A. White, published in 1997 in the Pain magazine, supports this position. An analysis in a series of publications is carried out (case reports, series of cases, clinical trials or bibliographical reviews), in a period of time between 1969 and 1996 further supports the necessity of sufficient training as acupuncturists for anyone practising dry needling therapy.

f) Physiotherapists, in accordance to their professional profile, within their faculties, can practice their patients attention, through "physical therapies, manual, massage therapy and of use", but they are not independently trained as acupuncturists and should not use acupuncture as adjunctive treatment.

g) To conclude "dry needling" should be practiced only by properly trained acupuncturists and not by other health and non-health professionals without adequate theoretical and practical training.

BIBLIOGRAPHY

Vasapollo D, Monti M, Rocca L, Pieraccini L."Il Dry Needling: Note "A Prima Lettura" Del Disegno Di Legge N. 1461/2014". Rivista Italiana di Medicina Legale (e del Diritto in campo sanitario) gennaio 2016 Travell J. "Basis for the multiple uses of local block of somatic trigger areas; procaine infiltration and ethyl chloride spray"Miss Valley Med J. 1949 Jan;71(1):13-21. American Association of Acupuncture and Oriental Medicine (AAAOM) (2013). Position Statement on Trigger Point Dry Needling (TPDN) and Intramuscular Manual Therapy (IMT).
Disponibile su https://www.aaaomonline.org/?page=Governance,visitato il 16.11.2015)

Dunning, James, et al. "Dry needling: a literature review with implications for clinical practice guidelines." Physical Therapy Reviews 19.4 (2014): 252-265. Ernst, E., and A. White. "Life-threatening adverse reactions after acupuncture? A systematic review." Pain 71.2 (1997): 123-126.

Mutrie T. Torin under pressure. X Games. 2014 Jan 13.http://xgames.espn.go.com/xgames/skiing/article/10269254/torin-yater-wallace-ski-halfpipe-favorite-winter-olympics

Axon R. TorinYater-Wallace bounces back from collapsed lung with top run. USA Today. 2013 Dec 14
http://www.usatoday.com/story/sports/olympics/sochi/2013/12/13/torin-yater-wallace-dew-tour-ion-mountain-championship-halfpipe-qualifying/4019707/

Giamberardino MA "Referred muscle pain/hyperalgesia and central sensitisation". J Rehabil Med. 2003 May;(41 Suppl):85-8.

Lewit K, Simons DG. "Myofascial pain: relief by post-isometric relaxation". Arch Phys Med Rehabil. 1984 Aug;65(8):452-6. PubMed PMID: 6466075

Sohns S, Schnieder K, Licht G, von Piekartz H. "Manual trigger point therapyof shoulder pain : Randomized controlled study of effectiveness". Schmerz. 2016Jun 13. [Epub ahead of print] German. PubMed PMID: 27295296

Rodríguez-Fuentes I, De Toro FJ, Rodríguez-Fuentes G, de Oliveira IM,Meijide-Faílde R, Fuentes-Boquete IM. "Myofascial Release Therapy in the Treatmentof Occupational Mechanical Neck Pain: A Randomized Parallel Group Study" .Am JPhys Med Rehabil. 2016 Jul;95(7):507-15.

Ajimsha MS, Al-Mudahka NR, Al-Madzhar JA. "Effectiveness of myofascialrelease:systematic review of randomized controlled trials". J Body MovTher. 2015Jan;19(1):102-12. Renan-Ordine R, Alburquerque-Sendín F, de Souza DP, Cleland JA,Fernández-de-Las-Peñas C. "Effectiveness of myofascial trigger point manualtherapy combined with a self-stretching protocol for the management of plantarheel pain: a randomized controlled trial".J Orthop Sports PhysTher. 2011Feb;41(2):43-50.

Bron C, de Gast A, Dommerholt J, Stegenga B, Wensing M, Oostendorp RA. "Treatment of myofascial trigger points in patients with chronic shoulder pain: a randomized, controlled trial". BMC Med. 2011 Jan 24;9:8.

La Touche R, Fernández-de-las-Peñas C, Fernández-Carnero J, Escalante K,Angulo-Díaz-Parreño S, Paris-Alemany A, Cleland JA,"The effects of manual therapyand exercise directed at the cervical spine on pain and pressure pain sensitivityin patients with myofascialtemporomandibular disorders". J Oral Rehabil. 2009Sep;36(9):644-52.

Hong CZ. "Treatment of myofascial pain syndrome".Curr Pain Headache Rep. 2006Oct;10(5):345-9. http://www.ama-assn.org/ama/pub/news/news/2016/2016-06-15-new-policies-annual-meeting.page

Addendum: Dommerholt J, "Dry-needling – peripheral and central considerations" Journal of Manual and Manipulative Therapy. 2011 19(4) 223-237

Chapter 26

A Window on Acupuncture Research in China: Systematic Review of Clinical Trials in Treating Low Back Pain, Headache, and Infertility*

Federico Marmori, Yang Shuo, Zhang Huamin, Li Zongyou, Tong Yuanyuan, Liu Yang, He Wei, Yin Renfang, Yang Kunjie, Zhang Lei, Claudia Skopalik and Carlos Llopis

* Federico Marmori is from European Foundation of Chinese Traditional Medicine and the Acupuncture Department, Vithas Medimar Hospital; Yang Shuo, Zhang Huamin, Li Zongyou, Tong Yuanyuan, Liu Yang, He Wei, Yin Renfang, Yang Kunjie, and Zhang Lei are from Chinese Academy of Traditional Chinese Medicine Information Institute, China Academy of Chinese Medical Sciences; Claudia Skopalik and Carlos Llopis are from European Foundation of Chinese Traditional Medicine, and they have collaborated in presenting this work on acupuncture treatment of low back pain, headache, and infertility in China, within the scope of the CHETCH project. Review and analysis of 11,237 papers, including 3,938 on headache, 6,723 on low back pain, and 576 on infertility, have been carried out to assess the efficacy of acupuncture treatment. Data information has been extracted from major scientific and academic databases such as CNKI, CBM, and PubMed.

1. EVIDENCE-BASED EVALUATION OF ACUPUNCTURE TREATMENT FOR LOW BACK PAIN

1.1. *Data collection and establishment of database*

1.1.1. *Data sources*

Database: In order to identify Chinese language articles, we searched Traditional Chinese Medical Database System (TCMD), the new platform of China National Knowledge Infrastructure (CNKI), Chinese Science and Technology Journal Database (VIP), Chinese Biomedical Literature Database (CBM), and Wan Fang Data Knowledge Service Platform. For English language articles, we searched PubMed, and altogether, six databases.

Time range: From 2005 to 2015, a total of 11 years.

Data extraction method: Computerized extraction and manual extraction.

1.1.2. *Search strategy*

English literature search: We searched PubMed using the following keywords: (Acupuncture OR Acupuncture-Moxibustion OR Electroacupuncture) AND (Back ache OR Back pain/lumbar disc herniation/prolapse of intervertebral disc/ Lumbago).

Chinese literature search: We searched the Traditional Chinese Medical Database System (TCMD), China National Knowledge Infrastructure (CNKI), China Excellent Doctoral Dissertation Full Text Database, and Wan Fang Data Knowledge Service Platform. For instance, we searched CNKI using the following keywords: (1) SU = acupuncture and moxibustion + acupuncture + electroacupuncture + point + needle + ear needle + warm needle + laser needle + electrical stimulation + eye needle + head needle + wrist ankle needle + skin needle + fire needle + electric hot needle + electromagnetic needle + bleeding + triangular needle + bee needle + floating needle + elongated needle + penetration needling + round needling; (2) SU = lumbago + back pain + lumbago and back pain + low back pain + lumbosacral pain + lumbar muscle pain + lumbar sprain +

third lumbar transverse process syndrome + ankylosing spondylitis + lumbago and leg pain + lumbar intervertebral disc; (3) SU = random + control + blind + single blind + double blind + clinical trials + clinical efficacy + clinical observation + meta + systematic review + systematic assessment + comparative study + multicenter + case + clinical + observation + efficacy + treatment.

1.1.3. *Search results*

Extracted data: 6,723 clinical trials of acupuncture for low back pain from CNKI, CBM, and PubMed databases.

1.2. *Inclusion and exclusion procedure for eligible trials and articles*

1.2.1. *Criteria for clinical trials*

1.2.1.1. Inclusion and exclusion criteria

(1) Inclusion criteria:

i. Research design: Randomized controlled trials or semi-randomized controlled trials.
ii. Object of research: Patients with low back pain as a main symptom.
iii. Interventions: Acupuncture (including acupuncture, head acupuncture, body acupuncture, Mang needle (long needle), electroacupuncture, ear seeds, fire needle, plum blossom needle, etc.)

(2) Exclusion criteria:

i. Non-trial studies, such as review, theoretical research;
ii. Biological experiments or cell tissue research;
iii. Acupuncture combined with other therapies (including moxibustion, cupping, Tuina, traction, manipulation, acupressure, acupoint injection, needle-knife, acupoint catgut embedding, etc.);
iv. Medical records, experience case studies;
v. Studies with less than ten subjects.

1.2.1.2. Diagnostic criteria

Based on the *People's Republic of China Chinese Medicine Industry Standards· Orthopedics in Chinese Medicine. Diagnostic and efficacy criteria*[1]:

(1) Congestive pain or soreness in the lower back, reduced when resting, aggravated by fatigue, decreased with movement and frequent changes in position, aggravated by extended period of lumbar flexion and bad weather.
(2) Pain is present in the morning, with evident lumbar soreness when getting up. Pain is relieved when moving, with significant reduction of symptoms after a few hours. In severe cases, the patient is awakened by pain in the early morning or cannot sleep, but pain decreases when getting up.

The diagnosis is performed according to Modern Chinese Medicine Clinical Diagnosis.[2] The patient has an history of lumbar trauma, lumbar chronic strain, or invasion of cold dampness. Low back pain can irradiate to the buttock, leg, and foot; pain is aggravated with increased abdominal pressure. Scoliosis, disappearance of the physiological lumbar curvature, limitation of lumbar movements, and paraspinal tenderness in the affected area is present, with pain irradiating to the lower limbs. Hypersensitivity or hyposensitivity of the lower limb corresponding to the innervation territory is present. CT scan shows lumbar disc herniation.

1.2.1.3. Efficacy criteria

Based on the *Chinese Medicine Diagnostic and Efficacy Criteria*[3]:
Total recovery: Disappearance of lumbar and leg pain; Lasègue's test is negative, with the patient raising his leg at an angle of 70°, the patient can go back to work and can walk more than 2 km.
Improvement: Reduction of lumbar and leg pain and improvement of lumbar movements.
No improvement: No improvement in symptoms and clinical signs.

1.2.1.4. Intervention procedure

(1) Acupuncture therapy in treatment group with low back pain.
(2) **Control drug**: Medication, placebo, or other medication for symptomatic treatment.
(3) **Outcome indicators**: Symptomatology improvement is the main efficacy indicator. Clinical signs are secondary efficacy indicators.
(4) **Safety**: Includes physical and chemical examination (routine blood test, liver function, renal function, electrocardiogram, etc.), and adverse events.

1.2.2. *Literature exclusion criteria*

(1) Articles where the treatment protocol used combined Chinese medicine treatment and Western medication, and in addition those where the treatment protocol and control protocol used different medication.
(2) When the same author and basically similar content appeared in conference paper as well as in journal articles, the conference paper was excluded.
(3) When the same author and basically similar content appeared in two or more papers, the latest published papers were excluded.

1.2.3. *Literature screening and database building*

A total of 6,723 articles in Chinese and English were retrieved from January 2005 to December 2015, of which 442 articles were selected after literature screening (i.e., reading title and abstract). The database was built according to the extraction test method, number of groups, intervention measures, statistical methods, treatment results, follow-up, adverse events, and other related information. Concurrently, 111 clinical trials with evidence-based evaluation were screened for evidence-based study.

1.3. *Analysis and discussion of test results*

1.3.1. *Comprehensive analysis*

1.3.1.1. Publication time range statistics

According to data analysis, 2010 and 2014 emerged as the peak periods for paper publication about low back pain with acupuncture treatment (Fig. 1).

1.3.1.2. Related disease analysis

According to data analysis, lumbar disc herniation, intervertebral disc displacement, acute lumbar sprain, low back pain and sciatica stand as most frequent lumbar-pain–related diseases (Table 1).

1.3.1.3. Statistical analysis of case numbers

According to data analysis, the patient total was within 200 cases in most clinical trials on acupuncture treatment of low back pain, with a higher incidence of trials with patient range between 60–100.

Figure 1. Clinical Trials Related to Acupuncture Treatment of Low Back Pain During 2005–2015.

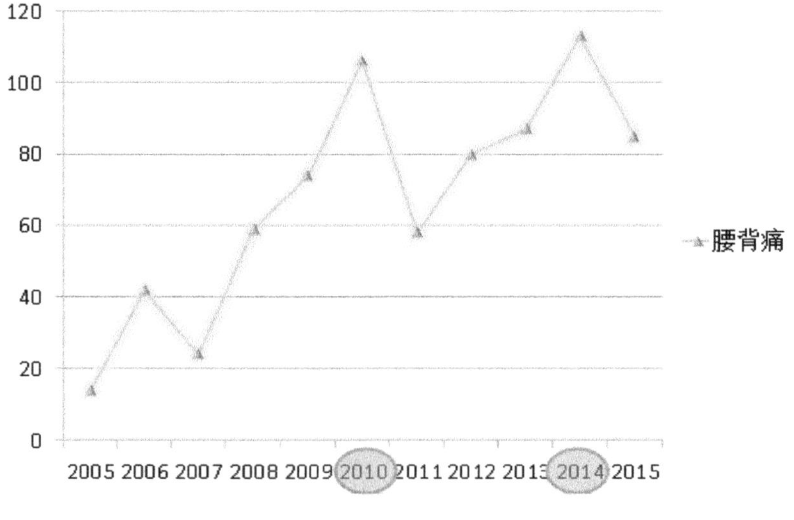

Table 1. Clinical Trials Related to Acupuncture Treatment of Low Back Pain and Related Diseases During 2005–2015.

Disease Name	Related Disease	Frequency
Lumbar pain	Lumbar disc herniation	260 articles
	Intervertebral disc displacement	43 articles
	Acute lumbar sprain	31 articles
	Low back pain	24 articles
	Sciatica	11 articles
	Cervical, shoulder, back, and leg pain	9 articles
	Lumbar muscle strain	8 articles

1.3.1.4. Meridians and acupuncture points involved in acupuncture treatment of low back pain

According to data analysis, meridians involved in acupuncture treatment of low back pain clinical trials involved a total of 11 meridians and 222 common acupoints (Table 2).

1.3.2. *Evidence-based analysis*

The forest plot shows that clinical efficacy for the acupuncture treatment group is 3.04 times superior compared to the control group (Fig. 2). Heterogeneity test I2 = 22%, thus less than 50%, indicates that the heterogeneity of the study is small, so the fixed effect model was used when merged.

The funnel plot including all studies shows clear symmetry indicating that there is no obvious publication bias (Fig. 3). It indicates an evident clinical efficacy of acupuncture in the treatment of low back pain.

Table 2. Meridians Involved in Acupuncture Treatment of Low Back Pain Clinical Trials (2005–2015).

Meridians Standard Names	Meridians Additional Names
Ren Mai	
Foot Yangming Stomach Meridian	Foot Yangming Meridian and its points
Foot Jueyin Liver Meridian	Jueyin Meridian of Foot and its points
Foot Taiyin Spleen Meridian	Foot Taiyin Meridian and its points
Foot Shaoyin Kidney Meridian	Foot Shaoyin Meridian and its points
Chong Mai	
Du Mai	
Foot Shaoyang Gall Bladder Meridian	Foot Shaoyang Meridian and its points
Hand Shaoyang Sanjiao Meridian	Hand Shaoyang Meridian and its points
Foot Taiyang Bladder Meridian	Foot Taiyang Meridian and its points
Hand Taiyang Small Intestine Meridian	Hand Taiyang Meridian and its points

2. EVIDENCE-BASED EVALUATION OF ACUPUNCTURE TREATMENT FOR HEADACHE

Headache is a condition where the patient experiences pain in the head. Its etiology is complex, and headache can appear with brain, eye, mouth, and nose pathologies as well as several systemic diseases. The most common types of primary headaches are migraines, trigeminal neuralgia, cervical headaches, tension-type headaches, and vascular headaches. At present, medication is still the main treatment for headache, but despite the treatment, many patients still experience a downgrade in their quality of life. Drugs adverse reaction and unknown long-term effects of drugs make it difficult for the patient to comply with the treatment. In recent years, non-drug therapy in headache management is emerging, showing different degrees of efficacy.[4]

Acupuncture treatment for headache in China has a history of more than a millennium, bringing wide clinical experience in treating headache with various etiologies.

Figure 2. Forest Plot Evidence-based Analysis of Acupuncture Treatment in 111 Trials of Low Back Pain.

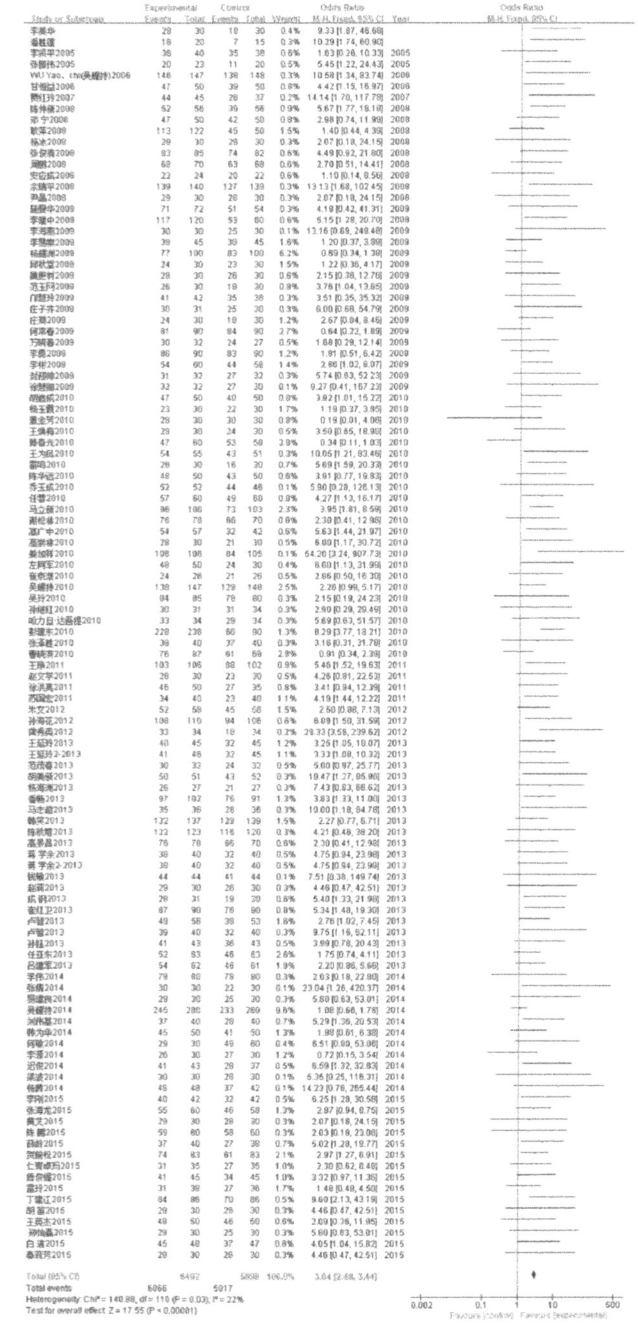

Figure 3. Funnel Plot Evidence-based Analysis of Acupuncture Treatment in 111 Trials of Low Back Pain.

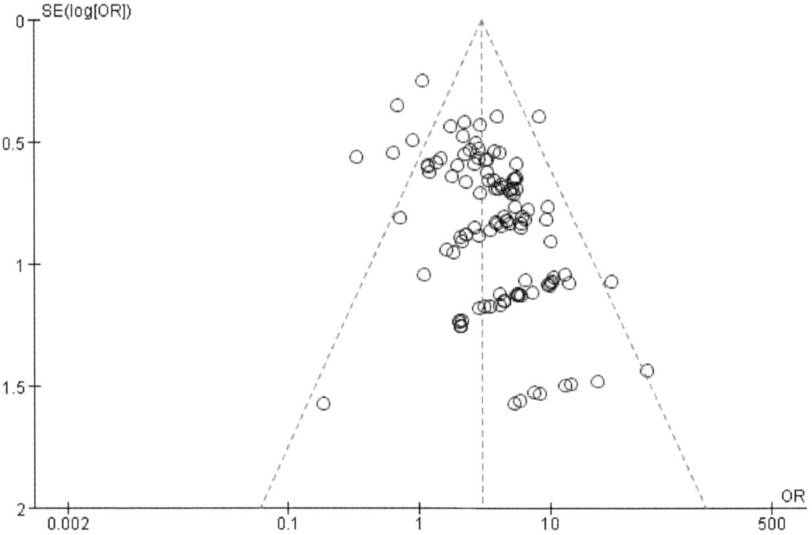

In 1998, experts from the US National Institutes of Health (NIH) reached a consensus on integrating acupuncture as one of the possible interventions in headache treatment. However, the still unknown mechanism of action of acupuncture has brought many foreign researchers to discard its efficacy or dismiss it as having a placebo effect. Several rigorous randomized controlled studies of acupuncture in the treatment of headache have been published.

We collected the related literature published from 2005 to 2015, with data analysis of clinical research on single acupuncture for headache treatment, stating specifically "randomized controlled" in the text, in order to explore the clinical efficacy of acupuncture on headache and its remaining shortcomings.

2.1. *Data collection and establishment of database*

2.1.1. *Data sources*

Database: In order to identify Chinese language articles, we searched Traditional Chinese Medical Database System (TCMD), the new platform of China National Knowledge Infrastructure (CNKI), Chinese Science and Technology Journal Database (VIP), Chinese Biomedical Literature Database (CBM), and Wan Fang Data Knowledge Service Platform. For English language articles, we searched PubMed, and altogether, six databases.

Time range: From 2005 to 2015, a total of 11 years.

Data extraction method: Computerized extraction and manual extraction.

2.1.2. *Search strategy*

English literature search: We searched PubMed using the following keywords — (Acupuncture OR Acupuncture-Moxibustion OR Electro-acupuncture) AND (Headache OR Migraine OR Paroxysmal Migraine OR Trigeminal Autonomic Cephalalgias/Trigeminal neuralgia).

Chinese literature search: We searched the Traditional Chinese Medical Database System (TCMD), China National Knowledge Infrastructure (CNKI), China Excellent Doctoral Dissertation Full Text Database, and Wan Fang Data Knowledge Service Platform. For instance, we searched CNKI using the following keywords: (1) SU = acupuncture and moxibustion + acupuncture + electroacupuncture + point + needle + ear needle + warm needle + laser needle + electrical stimulation + eye needle + head needle + wrist ankle needle + skin needle + fire needle + electric hot needle + electromagnetic needle + bleeding + triangular needle + bee needle + floating needle + elongated needle + penetration needling + round needling; (2) SU = headache + migraine + trigeminal neuralgia; (3) SU = random + control + blind + single blind + double blind + clinical trials + clinical efficacy + clinical observation + meta + systematic review + systematic assessment + comparative study + multicenter + case + clinical + observation + efficacy+ treatment.

2.1.3. *Search results*

Extracted data: 3,938 clinical trials of acupuncture for headache from CNKI, CBM and PubMed databases.

2.2. *Inclusion and exclusion procedure for eligible trials and articles*

2.2.1. *Criteria for clinical trials*

2.2.1.1. Inclusion and exclusion criteria

(1) Inclusion criteria

i. Research design: Randomized controlled trials or semi-randomized controlled trials.
ii. Object of research: Patients with headache as a main symptom.
iii. Interventions: Acupuncture (including acupuncture, head acupuncture, body acupuncture, Mang needle (long needle), eletroacupuncture, ear seeds, fire needle, plum blossom needle, etc.).

(2) Exclusion criteria

i. Non-trial studies, such as reviews, theoretical research;
ii. Biological experiments or cell tissue research;
iii. Acupuncture combined with other therapies (including moxibustion, cupping, tuina, traction, manipulation, acupressure, acupoint injection, needle-knife, acupoint catgut embedding, etc.);
iv. Medical records, experience case studies:
v. Studies with less than ten subjects.

2.2.1.2. Diagnosis criteria

Based on the International Headache Society (IHS) *International Classification of Headache Disorders*,[4] *Emergency Diagnosis and Treatment of Neurology*,[5] and *Guiding Principles for Clinical Study of New Chinese Medicines*,[6] the criteria were formulated as follows: (1) long history of relapsing attacks; (2) moderate or severe headache; (3) mostly unilateral throbbing pain; (4) headache often accompanied by nausea, vomiting, photophobia, and phonophobia; (5) physical examination, neurological examination, and complementary exams are all showing negative results.

2.2.1.3. Efficacy criteria

The evaluation of clinical efficacy was based on the *Chinese Medicine Diagnostic and Efficacy Criteria.*[7]

Total recovery: No migraine attack within one month after the end of the treatment.

Effectiveness: Headache score decreased by more than 50% after treatment.

Improvement: Headache score decreased by 21–50% after treatment.

No improvement: Headache score decreased by less than 20% after treatment. Headache score reduction rate = [(pre-treatment headache score − post-treatment headache score)/Pre-treatment headache score]×100%.

2.2.1.4. Intervention procedure

(1) Acupuncture therapy in treatment group with headache.
(2) **Control drug**: Medication, placebo, or other medication for symptomatic treatment.
(3) **Outcome indicators**: Symptomatology improvement is the main efficacy indicator. Clinical signs are secondary efficacy indicators.
(4) **Safety**: Includes physical and chemical examination (blood, liver function, renal function, electrocardiogram, etc.), and adverse events.

2.2.2. *Literature exclusion criteria*

(1) Articles where the treatment protocol used combined Chinese Medicine treatment and Western medication, and in addition those where the treatment protocol and control protocol used different medication.
(2) When the same author and basically similar content appeared in conference papers as well as in journal articles, the conference paper was excluded.
(3) When the same author and basically similar content appeared in two or more papers, the latest published papers were excluded.

2.2.3. *Literature screening and database building*

A total of 3,938 articles in Chinese and English were retrieved from January 2005 to December 2015, of which 279 articles were included after literature screening (i.e., reading titles and abstracts). The database was compiled according to the extraction test method, number of groups, intervention measures, statistical methods, treatment results, follow-up, adverse events, and other related information. Concurrently, 83 clinical trials with evidence-based evaluation were screened for evidence-based study.

2.3. *Analysis and discussion of test results*

2.3.1. *Comprehensive analysis*

2.3.1.1. Publication time range statistics

According to data analysis, 2010, 2012, and 2014 emerged as the peak periods for paper publication about acupuncture treatment of headache (Fig. 4).

Figure 4. Chart of Clinical Trials of Acupuncture Treatment of Headache During 2005–2015.

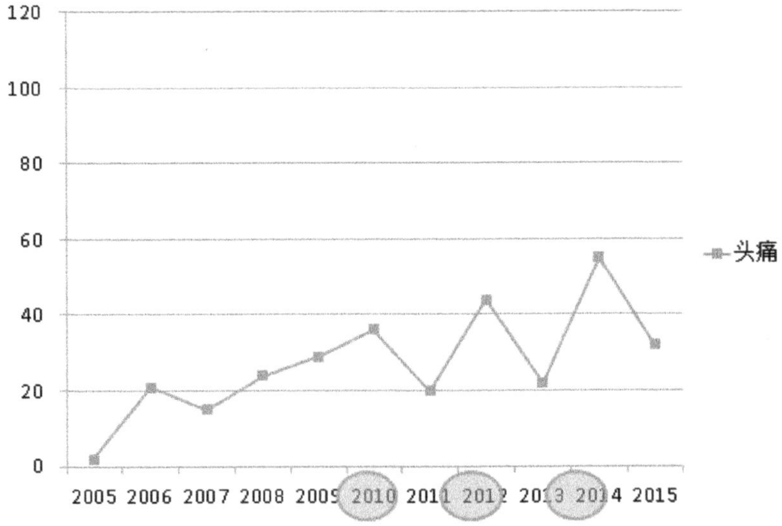

2.3.1.2. Related disease analysis

According to data analysis, migraine, trigeminal neuralgia, cervical headache, tension-type headache, and cervical spondylosis stand as most frequent headache-related diseases (Table 3).

2.3.1.3. Statistical analysis of case numbers

According to data analysis, the patient total was within 200 cases in most clinical trials of acupuncture treatment of headache, with a higher incidence of trials including a patient number range of 60–100.

2.3.1.4. Meridians and acupuncture points involved in acupuncture treatment of headache

According to the data analysis, the clinical trials of the acupuncture treatment of headache involved a total of 11 meridians and 212 common acupoints (Table 4).

Table 3. Clinical Trials Related to Acupuncture Treatment of Headache and Related Diseases During 2005–2015.

Disease Name	Related Disease	Frequency
Headache	Migraine	119 articles
	Trigeminal neuralgia	36 articles
	Cervical headache	19 articles
	Tension-type headache	9 articles
	Cervical spondylosis	8 articles
	Menstrual headache	7 articles
	Vascular headache	5 articles

Table 4. Meridians Involved in Acupuncture Treatment of Headache Clinical Trials (2005–2015).

Meridians Standard Names	Meridians Additional Names
Ren Mai	
Foot Yangming Stomach meridian	Foot Yangming meridian and its points
Foot Jueyin Liver meridian	Foot Jueyin meridian and its points
Foot Taiyin Spleen Meridian	Foot Taiyin Meridian and its points
Foot Shaoyin Kidney Meridian	Foot Shaoyin Meridian and its points
Chong Mai	
Du Mai	
Foot Shaoyang Gall Bladder Meridian	Foot Shaoyang Meridian and its points
Hand Shaoyang Sanjiao Meridian	Hand Shaoyang Meridian and its points
Foot Taiyang Bladder Meridian	Foot Taiyang Meridian and its points
Hand Taiyang Small Intestine Meridian	Hand Taiyang Meridian and its points

2.3.2. *Evidence-based analysis*

2.3.2.1. Study of the clinical evaluation of the acupuncture treatment for headache

The forest plot shows that clinical efficacy for the acupuncture treatment group is 3.04 times superior compared to the control group (Fig. 5).

The heterogeneity test indicates with I2 = 22%, thus less than 50%, that the heterogeneity of the study is small, so the fixed effect model was used when merged.

The funnel plot including all studies shows clear symmetry indicating that there is no obvious publication bias (Fig. 6). It indicates an evident clinical efficacy of acupuncture in the treatment of headache.

2.3.2.2. Long-term efficacy evaluation

The forest plot shows that the long-term clinical efficacy for the acupuncture treatment group is 3.76 times superior compared to the control group (Fig. 7). The combined data show a 24% heterogeneity, implying a mild

Figure 5. Forest Plot Evidence-based Analysis of Acupuncture Treatment in 83 Trials of Headache.

	Experimental		Control			Odds Ratio	
Study or Subgroup	Events	Total	Events	Total	Weight	M-H, Fixed, 95% CI	Year
刘国良2006	27	30	25	30	1.3%	1.80 [0.39, 8.32]	2006
刘波2006	51	58	27	57	1.8%	8.10 [3.14, 20.84]	2006
杨传崇2006	39	42	36	48	1.3%	4.33 [1.13, 16.61]	2006
李丽霞2006	73	79	59	77	2.4%	3.71 [1.39, 9.95]	2006
宋旦旨2006	36	40	29	40	1.6%	3.41 [0.98, 11.85]	2006
贾春生2007	97	138	80	137	12.9%	1.69 [1.02, 2.78]	2007
石云琼2007	45	45	15	45	0.1%	179.06 [10.32, 3105.76]	2007
郑士立2008	44	45	37	45	0.4%	9.51 [1.14, 79.60]	2008
林汉芳2008	48	50	23	30	0.6%	7.30 [1.41, 37.97]	2008
求小恩2008	29	31	26	30	0.9%	2.23 [0.38, 13.20]	2008
韩林2008	37	40	24	31	1.1%	3.60 [0.85, 15.29]	2008
马新平2008	39	40	37	40	0.5%	3.16 [0.31, 31.78]	2008
付有春2008	50	54	38	54	1.5%	5.26 [1.63, 17.03]	2008
徐碧林2008	32	35	25	35	1.2%	4.27 [1.06, 17.17]	2008
孙舟红2008	36	42	32	42	2.5%	1.88 [0.61, 5.74]	2008
吕慧玲2008	35	38	33	38	1.4%	1.77 [0.39, 7.99]	2008
古英2008	97	97	32	33	0.1%	9.00 [0.36, 226.41]	2008
冶尕西2009	26	28	24	28	0.9%	2.17 [0.36, 12.92]	2009
彭建民2009	59	63	55	63	1.9%	2.15 [0.61, 7.53]	2009
张路2009	18	26	7	20	1.3%	4.18 [1.21, 14.44]	2009
邵立原2010	48	50	40	50	0.9%	6.00 [1.24, 28.99]	2010
金英爱2010	92	96	41	48	1.2%	3.93 [1.09, 14.16]	2010
王国建2010	99	100	20	30	0.2%	49.50 [6.00, 408.71]	2010
耿连岐2010	27	30	22	30	1.2%	3.27 [0.77, 13.83]	2010
韩励兵2010	31	31	16	28	0.1%	47.73 [2.66, 857.72]	2010
彭东2010	84	84	77	84	0.2%	16.35 [0.92, 291.13]	2010
李滋平2010	37	40	32	40	1.3%	3.08 [0.75, 12.61]	2010
李桂敏2010	65	68	62	69	1.5%	2.45 [0.61, 9.89]	2010
李悦2010	31	32	24	30	0.4%	7.75 [0.87, 68.77]	2010
朱耀華2010	16	15	13	15		Not estimable	2010
廖志山2010	56	60	48	60	1.7%	3.50 [1.06, 11.57]	2010
邵素菊2011	24	26	22	26	0.9%	2.18 [0.36, 13.11]	2011
郑英2011	31	33	27	33	0.9%	3.44 [0.64, 18.51]	2011
苏圣博2011	26	30	25	30	1.8%	1.30 [0.31, 5.40]	2011
苏春荀2011	31	31	20	27	0.2%	23.05 [1.25, 425.75]	2011
林锦长2011	31	34	25	34	1.2%	3.72 [0.91, 15.22]	2011
潘炎顺2011	27	30	25	30	1.3%	1.80 [0.39, 8.32]	2011
齐鹏宇2011	33	35	20	35	0.6%	12.38 [2.56, 59.87]	2011
马玉丹2011	28	30	26	30	0.9%	2.15 [0.36, 12.76]	2011
刘疆2011	39	39	39	39		Not estimable	2011
刘香君2011	27	30	22	30	1.2%	3.27 [0.77, 13.83]	2011
刘广霞2011	30	32	26	35	0.8%	5.19 [1.03, 26.23]	2011
张训浩2011	28	30	23	30	0.8%	4.26 [0.81, 22.53]	2011
张定隆2011	30	30	30	30		Not estimable	2011
钟惠如2012	28	30	23	30	0.8%	4.26 [0.81, 22.53]	2012
闵冬梅2012	29	31	54	59	1.3%	1.34 [0.25, 7.35]	2012
闵冬梅 2012	25	30	9	30	0.8%	11.67 [3.38, 40.22]	2012
赵丽2012	30	35	26	35	2.0%	2.08 [0.62, 6.98]	2012
邓竹青2012	29	31	54	59	1.3%	1.34 [0.25, 7.35]	2012
翟春梅2012	78	86	59	86	3.0%	4.46 [1.89, 10.53]	2012
武洪魁2012	88	90	76	90	0.9%	8.11 [1.79, 36.80]	2012
陈逢伟2012	22	26	20	26	1.7%	1.65 [0.41, 6.71]	2012
陈平2012	30	31	28	31	0.5%	3.21 [0.32, 32.74]	2012
魏丹2012	28	30	25	30	0.9%	2.80 [0.50, 15.73]	2012
马志伟2012	44	45	38	45	0.5%	8.11 [0.95, 68.87]	2012
刘芳2012	100	100	96	96		Not estimable	2012
刘薇2012	63	69	40	51	2.2%	2.89 [0.99, 8.42]	2012
文胜2012	29	30	24	30	0.4%	7.25 [0.82, 64.46]	2012
吴文飞2012	92	100	54	80	2.6%	5.54 [2.34, 13.09]	2012
司晓华2012	30	30	29	30	0.3%	3.10 [0.12, 79.23]	2012
张林华2012	39	43	20	42	1.0%	10.72 [3.25, 35.39]	2012
宋玉芳2012	29	30	19	30	0.3%	16.79 [2.00, 140.90]	2012
焦洋2013	28	31	26	33	1.3%	2.51 [0.59, 10.76]	2013
朱晓蕾2013	27	30	19	30	1.0%	5.21 [1.28, 21.24]	2013
李甘2013	31	32	46	61	0.5%	10.11 [1.27, 80.50]	2013
李勇华2013	23	25	19	25	0.8%	3.63 [0.66, 20.11]	2013
赵云霞2014	49	54	41	54	2.0%	3.11 [1.02, 9.44]	2014
赵宗仙2014	49	50	37	50	0.4%	17.22 [2.15, 137.57]	2014
王 乐2014	26	28	19	28	0.7%	6.16 [1.19, 31.82]	2014
王慧珍2014	31	35	25	35	1.5%	3.10 [0.87, 11.08]	2014
王婉芳2014	17	19	14	19	0.8%	3.04 [0.51, 18.11]	2014
王新春2014	22	25	23	25	1.5%	0.64 [0.10, 4.19]	2014
梁玉磊2014	41	43	34	42	0.9%	4.82 [0.96, 24.25]	2014
毛亮2014	47	50	36	50	1.2%	6.09 [1.63, 22.82]	2014
刘丹2014	28	30	26	30	0.9%	2.15 [0.36, 12.76]	2014
孙立明2014	41	43	34	42	0.9%	4.82 [0.96, 24.25]	2014
卢金荣2014	44	48	30	48	1.3%	6.60 [2.03, 21.45]	2014
张建华2014	37	42	29	42	1.9%	3.32 [1.06, 10.37]	2014
谢丹2015	24	28	16	27	1.3%	4.13 [1.12, 15.25]	2015
彭易雨2015	47	50	40	50	1.3%	3.92 [1.01, 15.22]	2015
周立华 2015	28	30	22	30	0.8%	5.09 [0.98, 26.43]	2015
张炳冉2015	27	30	24	30	1.3%	2.25 [0.51, 9.99]	2015
张慧2015	48	55	29	55	2.0%	6.15 [2.37, 15.95]	2015
Total (95% CI)		3682		3502	100.0%	4.11 [3.54, 4.78]	
Total events	3417		2672				

Heterogeneity: $Chi^2 = 73.70$, $df = 78$ ($P = 0.62$); $I^2 = 0\%$

Test for overall effect: $Z = 18.43$ ($P < 0.00001$)

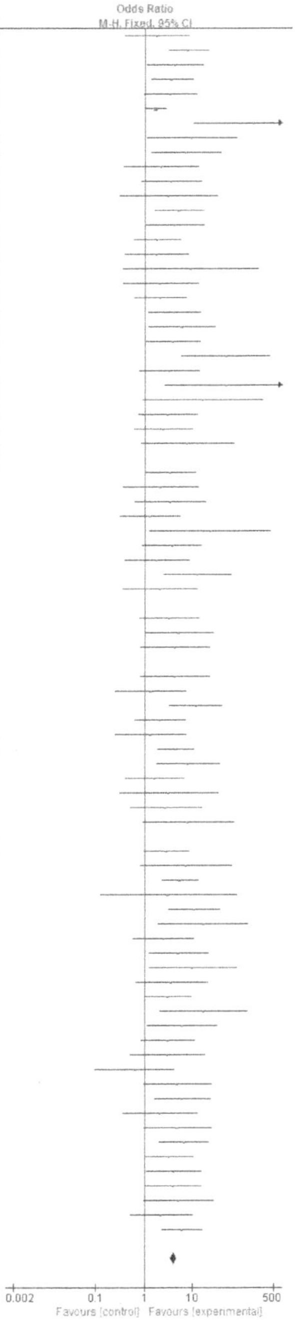

Figure 6. Funnel Plot Evidence-based Analysis of Acupuncture Treatment in 83 Trials of Headache.

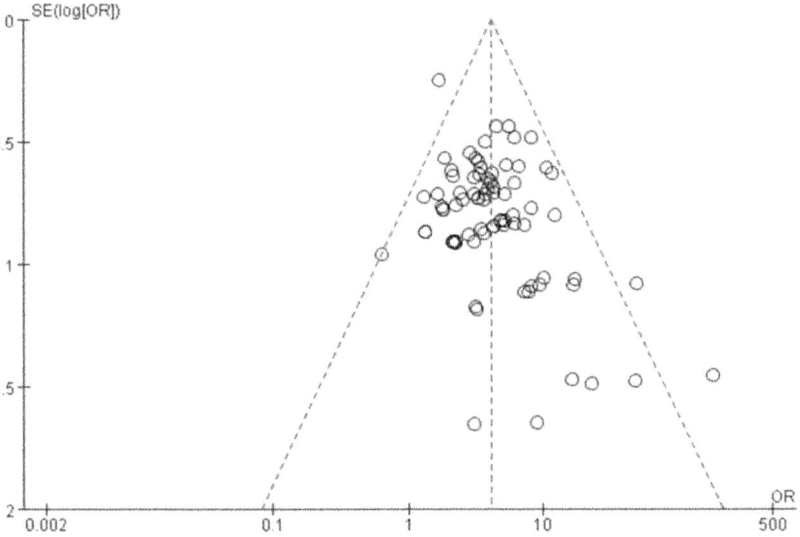

Figure 7. Forest Plot Evidence-based Analysis of Long-term Efficacy of Acupuncture Treatment in 11 Trials of Headache.

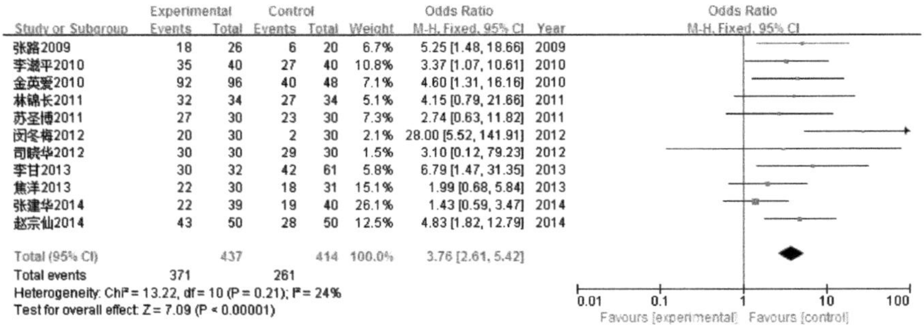

heterogeneity, Z = 7.09, $p < 0.00001$, which indicates an overall statistical significance.

The funnel plot indicates obvious publication bias in the 11 studies (Fig. 8).

Figure 8. Funnel Plot Evidence-based Analysis of Long-term Efficacy of Acupuncture Treatment in 11 Trials of Headache.

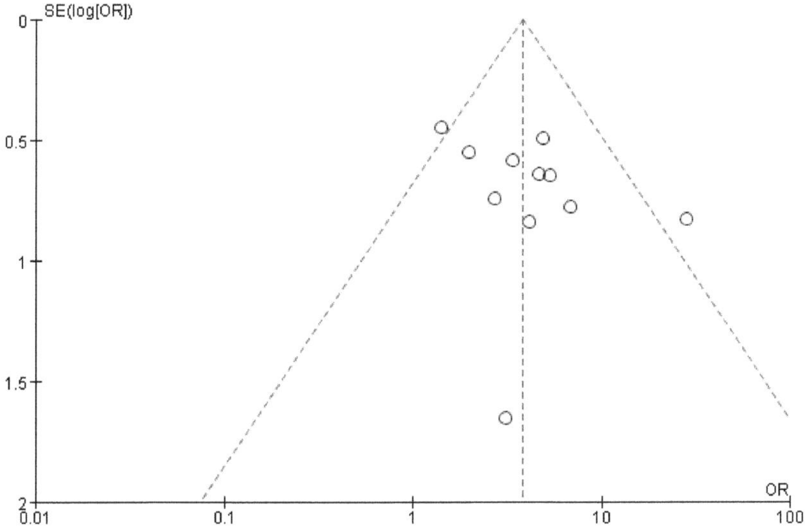

2.3.3. *Discussion*

This study was designed to evaluate the clinical efficacy of single acupuncture in the treatment of headache. Consequently, only studies which used single acupuncture in the treatment group compared to Chinese medicine treatment or Western medical treatment were selected.

A wide range of studies were selected, from rigorous controlled clinical studies to randomized controlled studies, with the intention to investigate the reliability of the clinical efficacy of acupuncture in the treatment of headache.

Our study shows that the expansion of clinical research in acupuncture treatment of headache became critical from 2010 onward. The overall upward trend does not show a straight line which could be influenced by funding or project issues.

The studies include several meridians, as well as a significant large number of acupuncture points.

The data analysis shows that acupuncture has a significant efficacy in the treatment of headache with evidence in reliability. On the other hand, there is no indication of long-term efficacy.

3. EVIDENCE-BASED EVALUATION OF ACUPUNCTURE TREATMENT FOR INFERTILITY

Infertility is defined as not being able to get pregnant after one year of unprotected sex, excluding male sexual dysfunction. Primary infertility refers to the absence of pregnancy in women who have not used any contraceptives and without previous pregnancy. Secondary infertility refers to women with previous pregnancy not having used any contraceptives during a year's time without being able to get pregnant. Absolute infertility indicates that pregnancy cannot be achieved due to congenital or acquired anatomical or physiological anomalies that cannot be corrected in either the male or female partner. Relative infertility stands for a condition where pregnancy disorders can be corrected and fertility restored.

The *WHO Manual for the Standardized Investigation and Diagnosis of the Infertile Couple* sets the clinical criteria for infertility within one year. The psychological impact and trauma of infertility can have negative repercussions on everyday life and work; therefore, it should be given proper attention.

3.1. *Data collection and establishment of database*

3.1.1. *Data sources*

Database: In order to identify Chinese language articles, we searched Traditional Chinese Medical Database System (TCMD), the new platform of China National Knowledge Infrastructure (CNKI), Chinese Science and Technology Journal Database (VIP), Chinese Biomedical Literature Database (CBM), and Wan Fang Data Knowledge Service Platform. For English language articles, we searched PubMed, altogether six databases.

Time range: From 2005 to 2015, a total of 11 years.

Data extraction method: Computerized extraction and manual extraction.

3.1.2. *Search strategy*

English literature search: We searched PubMed using the following keywords: (Acupuncture OR Acupuncture-Moxibustion OR Electro-acupuncture) AND Infertility/sterility.

Chinese literature search: We searched Traditional Chinese Medical Database System (TCMD), China National Knowledge Infrastructure (CNKI), China Excellent Doctoral Dissertation Full text Database, and Wan Fang Data Knowledge Service Platform. For instance, we searched CNKI using the following keyword:

(1) SU = acupuncture and moxibustion + acupuncture + electroacupuncture + point + needle + ear needle + warm needle + laser needle + electrical stimulation + eye needle + head needle + wrist ankle needle + skin needle + fire needle + electric hot needle + electromagnetic needle + bleeding + triangular needle + bee needle + floating needle + elongated needle + penetration needling + round needling; (2) SU = infertility + anovulation; (3) SU = random + control + blind + single blind + double blind + clinical trials + clinical efficacy + clinical observation + meta + systematic review + systematic assessment + comparative study + multi-center + case + clinical + observation + efficacy + treatment.

3.1.3. *Search results*

Extracted data: 576 clinical trials of acupuncture for infertility from CNKI, CBM, and PubMed databases.

3.2. *Inclusion and exclusion procedure for eligible trials and articles*

3.2.1. *Criteria for clinical trials*

3.2.1.1. Inclusion and exclusion criteria

(1) Inclusion criteria:

i. **Research design**: Randomized controlled trials or semi-randomized controlled trials.

ii. **Object of research**: Patients with infertility as a main symptom.
iii. **Interventions**: Acupuncture (including acupuncture, head acupuncture, body acupuncture, Mang needle (long needle), electroacupuncture, ear seeds, fire needle, plum blossom needle, etc.)

(2) Exclusion criteria:

i. Non-trial studies, such as review, theoretical research;
ii. Biological experiments or cell tissue research;
iii. Acupuncture combined with other therapies (including Chinese herbal treatment, moxibustion, cupping, Tuina, traction, manipulation, acupressure, acupoint injection, needle-knife, acupoint catgut embedding, etc.);
iv. Medical records, experience case studies;
v. Studies with less than ten subjects.

3.2.1.2. Diagnosis criteria

Based on *Infertility*[8] and *Practical Obstetrics and Gynecology in Integrated Chinese and Western Medicine*[9] for Western medical diagnosis and based on *Chinese New Herbal Medicine Clinical Research Guidelines*[10] for Chinese medicine diagnosis.

(1) Married women aged between 22 and 40 years, married for more than one year, or with history of marriage, with failure to achieve pregnancy after 12 months or more of regular unprotected sexual intercourse.
(2) Presence of reproductive immune antibodies in the patient serum, such as antisperm antibodies (AsAb) or (and) anti-endometrial antibodies (EMAb). Additional diagnosis criteria were based on *Obstetrics and Gynecology*[11] and *Practical Gynecology in Chinese Medicine*.[12] Main symptoms: irregular menstrual cycle, polymenorrhea or oligomenorrhea, menorrhagia, or hypomenorrhea. Secondary symptoms: lumbar soreness with weak legs or pain in the heel, dizziness, tinnitus, abulia; pollakiuria or post-micturition incontinence; insomnia, memory disorders; tongue with pale and red color, thin and white

tongue fur, sunken and fine pulse or sunken and weak pulse. At least two main symptoms should be present and one or two secondary symptoms.

3.2.1.3. Intervention procedure

(1) Acupuncture therapy in treatment group with infertility.
(2) Control drug: Medication, placebo, or other medication for symptomatic treatment.
(3) Outcome indicators: The main indicators of efficacy were endometrial thickness, dominant follicle diameter, serum progesterone hormone level improvement, and pregnancy situation after treatment.
(4) Safety: Includes physical and chemical examination (blood, liver function, renal function, electrocardiogram, etc.) and adverse events.

3.2.2. *Literature exclusion criteria*

(1) Articles where the treatment protocol used combined Chinese medicine treatment and Western medication, and in addition those where the treatment protocol and control protocol used different medication.
(2) When the same author and basically similar content appeared in conference papers as well as in journal articles, the conference paper was excluded.
(3) When the same author and basically similar content appeared in two or more papers, the latest published papers were excluded.

3.2.3. *Literature screening and database building*

A total of 576 articles in Chinese and English were retrieved from January 2005 to December 2015, of which 26 articles were obtained after literature screening (i.e., reading title and abstract). The database was compiled according to extraction test method, number of groups, intervention measures, statistical methods, treatment results, follow-up, adverse events, and other related information. Concurrently, eight clinical trials with evidence-based evaluation were screened for evidence-based study.

3.3. *Analysis and discussion of test results*

3.3.1. *Comprehensive analysis*

3.3.1.1. Publication time range statistics

According to data analysis, 2006, 2012, and 2015 emerge as peak periods for paper publication about treatment of infertility with acupuncture (Fig. 9).

3.3.1.2. Related disease analysis

According to data analysis, luteinized unruptured follicle syndrome, infertility with endocrine disorders, and endometriosis are the most frequent infertility-related diseases (Table 5).

3.3.1.3. Statistical analysis of case numbers

According to data analysis, the patient total was within 60 cases in most acupuncture treatment of infertility clinical trials with a higher incidence

Figure 9. Clinical Trial Chart of Acupuncture Treatment of Infertility During 2005–2015.

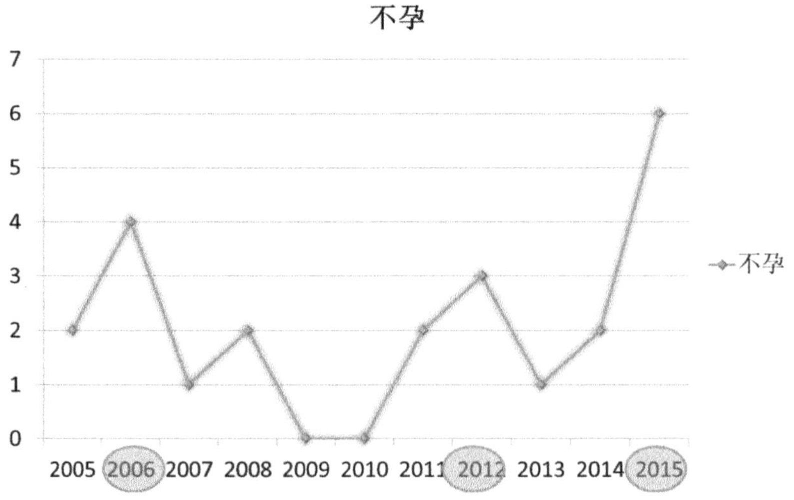

Table 5. Clinical Trials Related to Acupuncture Treatment of Infertility and Related Diseases During 2005–2015.

Disease Name	Related Disease	Frequency
Infertility	Luteinized unruptured follicle syndrome	5 articles
	Infertility with endocrine disorders	4 articles
	Endometriosis	2 articles
	Polycystic ovary syndrome	2 articles
	Infertility due to poor ovarian response	2 articles
	Infertility due to ovulation disorders	1 articles

of trials with patient range between 10 and 50 and no trial involving more than 100 cases.

3.3.1.4. Meridians and acupuncture points involved in acupuncture treatment of infertility

According to the data analysis, the clinical trials of acupuncture treatment of infertility involved 11 meridians (Table 6). Common needle techniques included warm needling, sparrow pecking, raising up needling (Yang needle-technique), balanced needling, ear needle, contralateral needling, combination of Shu-Mu points, etc.

3.3.2. *Evidence-based analysis*

The study included 8 articles with a total of 1,309 patients, of whom 704 patients assigned to the treatment group obtained 404 successful pregnancies, and 605 assigned to the control group obtained 281 successful pregnancies (Fig. 10).

The forest plot shows that the pregnancy rate for the acupuncture treatment group is 1.69 times superior compared to the control group.

The heterogeneity test 95% CI = [1.33, 2.14], I2 = 43%, thus less than 50%, indicates that the heterogeneity of the study is moderate, so the fixed

Table 6. Meridians Involved in Acupuncture Treatment of Infertility Clinical Trials (2005–2015).

Meridians Standard Names	Meridians Additional Names
Ren Mai	
Foot Yangming Stomach Meridian	Foot Yangming Meridian and its points
Foot Jueyin Liver Meridian	Foot Jueyin Meridian and its points
Foot Taiyin Spleen Meridian	Foot Taiyin Meridian and its points
Foot Shaoyin Kidney Meridian	Foot Shaoyin Meridian and its points
Chong Mai	
Du Mai	
Foot Shaoyang Gall Bladder Meridian	Foot Shaoyang Meridian and its points
Hand Shaoyang Sanjiao Meridian	Hand Shaoyang Meridian and its points
Foot Taiyang Bladder Meridian	Foot Taiyang Meridian and its points
Hand Taiyang Small Intestine Meridian	Hand Taiyang Meridian and its points

Figure 10. Forest Plot Evidence-based Analysis of Acupuncture Treatment in Eight Trials of Infertility.

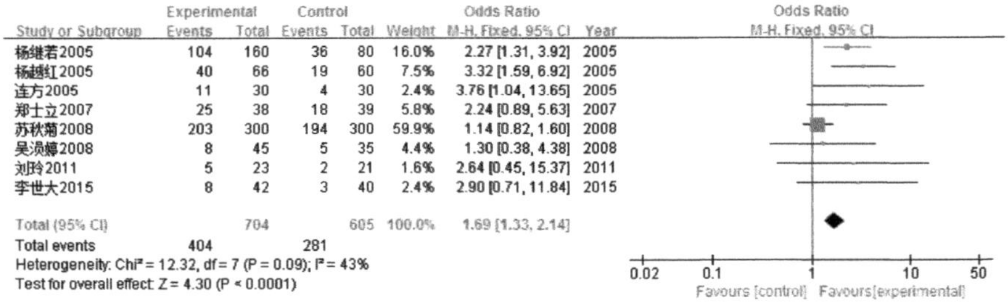

effect model was used when merged; Z = 4.30, $p < 0.0001$, hence the overall result is statistically significant.

The funnel plot including all studies shows clear symmetry indicating that there is no obvious publication bias (Fig. 11). It indicates an evident clinical efficacy of acupuncture in the treatment of infertility.

Figure 11. Funnel Plot Evidence-based Analysis of Acupuncture Treatment in Eight Trials of Infertility.

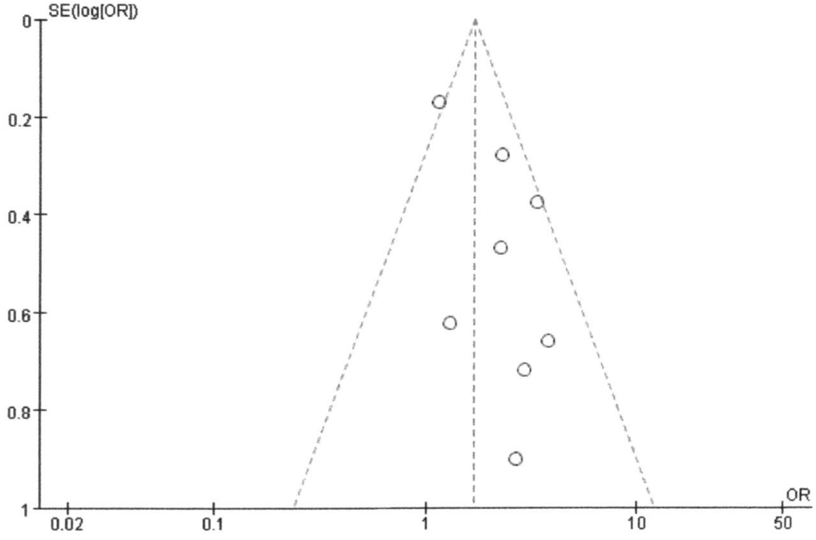

3.3.3. *Discussion*

This study was designed to evaluate the clinical efficacy of acupuncture in the treatment of infertility. Only studies which used single acupuncture in the treatment group compared to Chinese medicine treatment or Western medical treatment were selected, hence the scarce amount of papers compiled. The studies were selected from rigorous clinical controlled studies to randomized controlled studies with the intention to investigate the reliability of acupuncture clinical efficacy in the treatment of infertility.

Our study shows that expansion of clinical research in acupuncture treatment of infertility became critical from 2006 onward. The overall upward trend is inconsistent, which could be influenced by patients' opinion about the reliability of single acupuncture in infertility treatment and funding or other project issues. The data analysis shows that acupuncture has a significant efficacy in the treatment of infertility with evidence in reliability. On the other hand, the scarce literature amount limits the impact of clinical guidance.

REFERENCES

1. Ministry of Health (1994). *People's Republic of China Chinese Medicine Industry Standards: Diagnostic and Efficacy Criteria for Orthopedics in Chinese Medicine* (People's Health Publishing House, Beijing), p. 197.
2. Zhu, W. Q. & He, Q. H. (2003). *Modern Chinese Medicine Clinical Diagnosis* (People's Health Publishing House, Beijing), p. 921.
3. State Administration of Traditional Chinese Medicine (1994). *Chinese Medicine Diagnostic and Efficacy Criteria* (Nanjing University Press, Nanjing), p. 7.
4. Olesen, J. (2005). "The International Classification of Headache Disorders, 2nd Edn. (ICHD-II)," *Revue Neurologique (Paris)*, 161(6–7), pp. 689–691.
5. Yang, M. S. (1995). *Emergency Diagnosis and Treatment of Neurology* (Hubei Science and Technology Press, Wuhan), p. 482.
6. Zheng, X. Y. & Ren, D. Q. (2002). *Guiding Principles for Clinical Study of New Chinese Medicines* (China Medical Science and Technology Press, Beijing), pp. 108–109.
7. State Administration of Traditional Chinese Medicine. (1994). *Chinese Medicine Diagnostic and Efficacy Criteria* (Nanjing University Press, Nanjing), p. 7.
8. Luo, L. L. (1998). *Infertility* (People's Medical Publishing House, Beijing), p. 281.
9. Yu, J. (1997). *Practical Obstetrics and Gynecology in Integrated Chinese and Western Medicine* (Beijing Medical University, China Union Medical College Joint Publishing House, Beijing), p. 123.
10. *Chinese Ministry of Health.* Chinese New Herbal Medicine Clinical Research Guidelines (China Medical Science and Technology Press, Beijing), p. 276.
11. Feng, Y. J. & Shen, K. (2001). *Obstetrics and Gynecology* (People's Medical Publishing House, Beijing), p. 394.
12. Luo, Y. K. (1996). *Practical Gynecology in Chinese Medicine* (Shanghai Science and Technology Press, Shanghai), p. 287.

Chapter 27

Regenerative Medicine Approaches: Different Cultural Backgrounds but Similar Strategies

Monica Mattioli-Belmonte, Monia Orciani,
Giulia Sorgentoni, Miriam Caffarini
and Roberto Di Primio

1. BACKGROUND

Regenerative medicine (RM) is a branch of translational research in tissue engineering (TE) and molecular biology. It deals with the "procedure of replacing, regenerating or engineering human cells, tissues or organs to restore or establish normal function." RM holds the potential of engineering damaged tissues and organs by stimulating the body's own repair apparatuses to heal functionally previously irreparable tissues or organs.[1] RM medicine also includes the possibility to grow tissues and organs in the laboratory and then implanting them into the body that cannot heal itself.

Some of the biomedical approaches within the field of regenerative medicine may include the use of stem cells,[2] and stem cell biology is one of the fastest growing areas of biomedical research worldwide. Examples of RM approaches include (i) the inoculation of progenitor or stem cells obtained through directed differentiation (cell therapies); (ii) the induction of regeneration by biologically active molecules administered alone or as result of infused cell secretion (immunomodulation therapy); and (iii) transplantation of *in vitro*-grown tissues and organs (tissue engineering).[3,4]

China is becoming an important contributor in RM research, including tissue engineering, stem cell research, and gene therapy. Because of policy support, China has made considerable progress in basic research of stem cells and attracted the most patients for stem cell treatment worldwide. Since 2002, for rapid and effective development, the Chinese government has provided abundant research funding, such as that from the National Basic Research Program of China, National High Technology Research and Development Program of China, and National Natural Science Foundation of China (NSFC), to support related research on stem cell.[5]

Starting from that data, major foreign media has paid much attention to the progress of RM in China,[6,7] noting the significant progress in China, and construing China's policies on stem cells, TE, and related areas. Some reports also indicated that the Chinese government has been active in recruiting well-trained researchers in the 21st century and that China is leading the area in some aspects. However, China still faces challenges in innovation, translational application, regulation, governance, and management.

2. CHINESE PROGRESS IN THE FIELDS OF STEM CELLS

Chinese researchers started to pay much consideration to stem cells during the 1980s. In China, it is forbidden to perform reproductive cloning, use a human embryo beyond day 14, fuse human and nonhuman gametes, and implant research embryos into a human or animal uterus.

In 2001, the Chinese Academy of Sciences (CAS) founded a key laboratory of stem cell biology, which was followed by the establishment of a stem cell research network composed of different biological and zoological research institutes and medical universities as scientific partners for the biomedical translation of base researches.[8] By means of these structures, research activities focused on the creation of embryonic stem cell lines and/or the isolation of tissue stem cells, studying their stemness and differentiation potential and stem cell immunology. The regulation of stem cells differentiation capability aims to solve several major complications in their clinical application, whilst the development of protocols for the obtainment of inducible pluripotent stem cells (iPS) helps a further understanding of stem cells roles in disease development. A further focus has been on stem cell three-dimensional (3D) culture and self-renewal regulatory network as well as stem cell and biomedical materials, tissue regeneration and wound healing, and stem cell translational medicine. Thus, at present, China is close to the global advanced-research level of embryo and other stem cells.[8,9]

In 2007, the Ministry of Science and Technology (MST) founded four stem cell banks, supporting each other with their own technological advantages, which covered the north, south, and east of China. These banks are expected to create a platform for the key technologies of stem cells as well as take charge of the National Stem Cell bank websites and databases and stem cell bank management and coordination.

As far as research topic is concerned, before 2007, basic stem cell studies in China were concentrated on bone-marrow and embryo stem cells.[10] Since then, China was gradually moving toward the top position in basic stem cell research.[11] For instance, researchers reported the first iPS cell line from rhesus monkey,[12] with the isolation of reproductive stem cells and the assessment of their long-term self-renewal capability.[13,14] Moreover, *The Times* elected the proof of iPS cell totipotency[15] as one of the Global Top 10 Biomedicine Advances and, in 2012, *Cell* published a special "Spotlight on China,"[a] stressing the rapid development of immunological studies in China in view of their use for clinical treatment.

---

[a] See: http://www.cell.com/spotlightonchina.

The practice of stem cell clinical trials in China goes back to the 1960s, with the transplantation of stem cells in bone marrow. It must be stressed that China stated the legality of stem cell treatments as a medical procedure immediately after the UK and the US. Different therapeutic applications were reported, including the use of neural stem cells[16] and bone-marrow mesenchymal stem cells (MSCs)[17] for the restoration of different tissues/organs. The latter has been used in more than 30 cases, with follow-up longer than three years. In 2013, a randomized study with umbilical-cord MSC transplantation was started in 40 patients with post-traumatic brain syndrome, demonstrating an improvement of the neurological function in the patients. However, prospective, randomized, multicenter, large clinical studies are necessary to confirm these results.[18]

Indeed, China had no stem cell therapies and/or clinical trials registered at ClinicalTrials.gov before 2005.[b] From then on, the projects registered by Ministry of Health (MH) increase annually (Fig. 1)

3. COMPARISON WITH STEM CELL RESEARCH-ADVANCED IN OTHER COUNTRIES

The US maintains a leading position in stem cell research, with the difference with China being the strict management in the US since 1998, whilst China (CAS, MST, and MH) started to make laws and policies on stem cells in 2003. Thereafter, China has improved a variety of policies for effective enforcement. In European countries, such as the UK and Sweden, the collection of human embryonic stem cells for application is relatively free but it is more stringent in other countries (e.g., Italy). In all countries, human cloning and destruction of human embryos are forbidden.

In 2009, the US Food and Drug Administration (FDA) allowed a biotech company in California to perform the world's first clinical trial on human embryonic stem cells, which was a milestone in the history of

[b] ClinicalTrials.gov. (2012). "Safety study of GRNOPC1 in spinal cord injury." Available at: http://clinicaltrials.gov/ct2/show/NCT01217008. Accessed 12 April 2012.

Figure 1. (a) Clinical Trials on Stem Cells Factors in China, European Countries, and the US from 2006 to 2016 (www.clinicaltrials.gov/). (b) Relative Relevance of Clinical Trials Performed in China, European Countries, and the US.

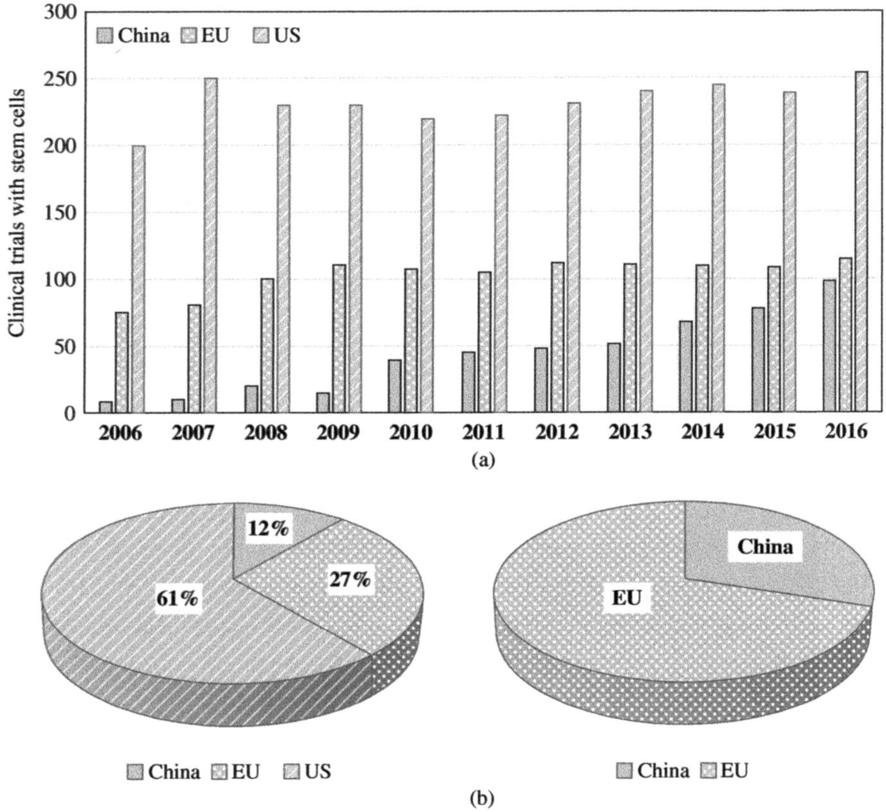

medicine.[19,20] In 2010, the UK approved its first stem cell trial in humans. Then, stem cell therapeutic agents have been approved in South Korea, Canada, and Australia, and more than 2,000 clinical trials (phases I to II) of stem cell therapy are ongoing at present, mainly performed in the US and Europe.

In China, stem cell therapy is limited, and the hospitals need to file with the regulatory authorities to perform studies. The first clinical trial was started in 2012. China lagged behind other countries with regard to strong stem cell research capability and also because of the lack of detailed rules in laws that reveal concern about the safety of stem cell therapy in the country.[21] Therefore, in China, the number of stem cell clinical trials is significantly smaller compared to the leading countries in the area of stem cell research.

4. CHINESE PROGRESS IN THE FIELDS OF TISSUE-ENGINEERING

Tissue-engineering (TE) research in China started in 1994, when the Shanghai Science and Technology Committee recognized TE research as a priority. In 1997, the first TE laboratory (Shanghai Key Laboratory of Tissue Engineering Research) was founded and, in 1998, TE was recognized as one of the research topics. In 2001, the Shanghai Research and Development Center of Tissue Engineering was established. Then, in 2012, 39 representative Colleges and Universities in the field of TE and RM founded BIOTECH,[c] a collaborative innovation center for TE and RM.

Starting from 2007, TE studies lead to the development and approval, by State Food and Drug Administration (SFDA), of TE products such as *ActivSkinã* that made China the second country in the world possessing the technology of artificial skin after the US. China continued to develop tissue-engineered decellularized dermal matrix, skin containing adipose layers, skin containing pigmentation, skin containing capillary-like network, skin containing hair follicles, and dermal equivalents. In 2010, the SFDA approved bone-repair scaffolds. This product, used in more than 30,000 patients, was endorsed in other countries worldwide. Other products approved by SFDA include tissue-engineered tendons, cartilage/bone, and neural tubes.[22]

5. COMPARISON WITH OTHER RESEARCH-ADVANCED COUNTRIES

The US National Science Foundation formally proposed the concept of TE in 1987, and research projects for TE were sponsored starting

---

[c] See: http://www.biotech.org.cn/.

from 1988. Institutions involved in this item are research institutes (i.e., NASA, the US Department of Energy, and NIH), universities (e.g., MIT, Harvard Medical School, Georgia Institute of Technology, and University of California at San Diego), and enterprises.

In China, tissue-engineered skin has been approved, which marked the beginning of the industry for TE products. The technical level of China in TE is superimposable to international standards, but a delay in TE research and translational application in China is still present and is mainly related to regulations and product standards.

6. RESEARCH DATA DISSEMINATION

As stated before, China is becoming an important contributor in RM research.[23,24] To deepen China's role in this field, an analysis on the role of China in the field of RM scientific literature in the last 10 years (2006–2016) was performed. In particular, the comparison of the number and type of publications with data from Europe were analyzed. Data analysis was generated using keyword searches in the Elsevier's Scopus,[d] which is the largest abstract and citation database of peer-reviewed literature. "Regenerative medicine" was used as a topic search term, and results were segmented by author's country as listed by the index. Note that China included only mainland China and not Hong Kong. As far as Europe (EU) is concerned, the UK was composed of publications for England, Scotland, Wales, and Northern Ireland, and for Other EU, we intended all countries of the European Community with less than 400 publications in the examined period. Country names were not used as an address search term to diminish false-cases in which a country name was part of the address other than as the country (e.g., as part of the institute name). Then, the papers generated for each country were segmented across publication years.

This analysis evidenced that overall 17,000 publications were performed in the last 10 years (2006–2016) on RM. Among these, 5,767 research papers were from the US, as expected, while Japan came at the second place with 1,665 publications. In Europe, 6,069 papers were published during this period, with the major role of three countries

---

[d] See: www.scopus.com.

Figure 2. Documents on RM and Stem Cells Published from 2006 to 2016 in China, European Countries, and the US.

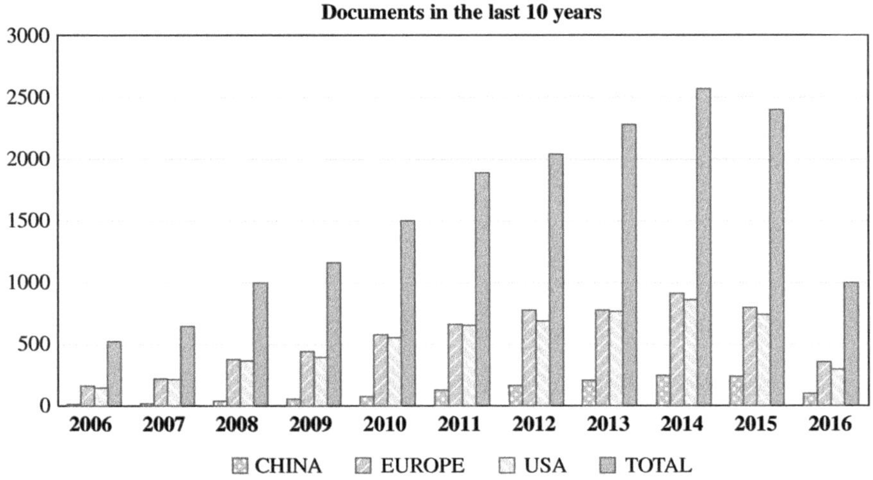

(UK, Germany, and Italy) that published more than 1,000 papers each. It is worthy of mention that the increase in China's visibility in the scientific world was evident in 2008 when Chinese publications overtook the level of almost every single European Country, except for UK, Germany, and Italy (Figs. 2 and 3)

This trend was maintained in the following years, and from 2013, China also surpassed these countries. Comparing the kind of publications, China published more research articles in international peer-reviewed journals (67.4%) in comparison with the whole world and Europe's production (53.7% and 54.1%, respectively). This difference could be attributable both to the less number of review articles from China (23.8%) compared to total world and Europe's production (25.8% and 27.5%, respectively) and to the scarce presence of book chapter from Chinese authors.

From 2006 to 2016, China published most frequently in *Biomaterials* (42 papers), *Chinese Journal of Tissue Engineering* (41 papers), *PlosOne* (33 papers), *Journal of Cellular and Molecular Medicine* (20 papers), *Journal of Clinical Rehabilitative Tissue Engineering Research* (20 papers), and *Acta Biomaterialia* (16 papers). Indeed a large part of these publications is in Chinese journals, without international indexing (i.e., Impact

Figure 3. Relative Relevance of Documents Published from 2006 to 2016 in China and European Countries.

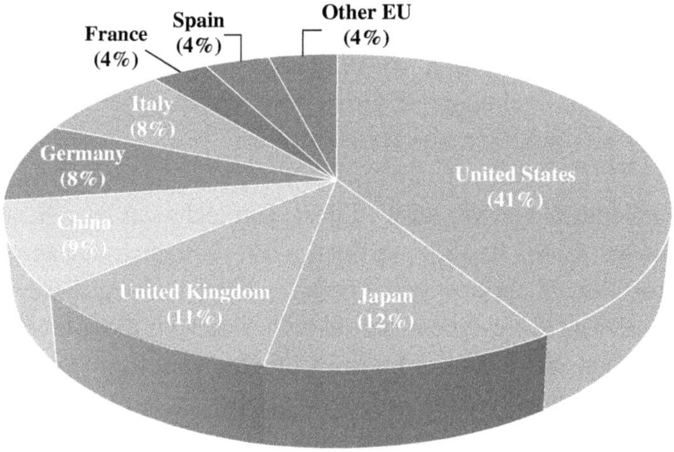

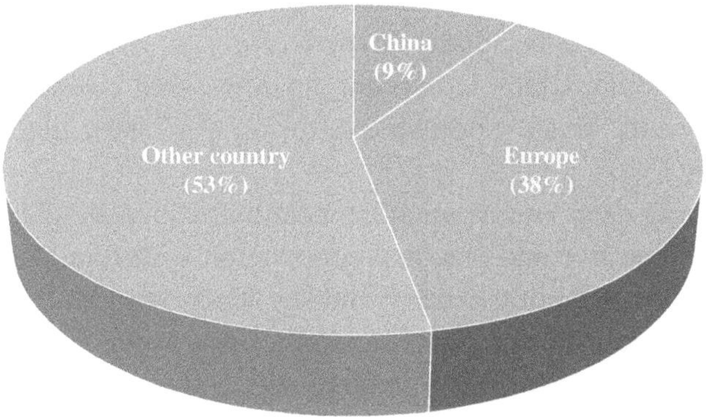

Factor) and with a limited scientific diffusion. In the same time interval, the European Scientific Community published in more important journals with a wide international distribution (*Stem Cells, PlosOne, Regenerative Medicine, Biomaterials, Stem Cells and Development, Acta Biomaterialia, Tissue Engineering Nature*, and *Nanomedicine*).

Another difference between Chinese and European scientific production is related to the subject area of interest, which was mainly biochemistry for the former (59.7%) and Medicine for the latter (55%).

7. CONCLUSIONS

In 2012, a special edition of *Science* (sponsored supplement for *Regenerative Medicine in China*) gave a wide-ranging snapshot of the development of RM in China, with particular emphasis on stem cells, TE, and trauma.[25] Even though successes are outstanding and impressive, China needs to strengthen aspects relative to:

(1) Administrative system, laws, ethical, and technical specifications and guidelines: China has not yet fixed a truly effective management system for clinical application of cells, and detailed regulatory rules are not clear. The achievement should be in line with the rules released by the International Society of Stem Cell Research for stem cell clinical translation. Ethical norms and legal supplies should be firmly followed to compel the application and clinical trials of stem cells. Attention should be also paid on the protection of intellectual property.
(2) Lack of originality: China lacks worldwide significant scientists in the area of tissue regeneration (including stem cell and TE) and coordination among multidisciplinary experts.
(3) Dissemination: China is building an active RM scientific literature. However, the actual worldwide diffusion of Chinese literature is still lacking.
(4) Broad and deep international cooperation: China should continue to stress exhaustive and practical cooperation with foreign well-known universities, scientific centers, and key laboratories.
(5) Diversification of investment and other new technologies: Stem cell technology is attracting scientists and entrepreneurs from various countries with its huge market potential and has tremendous business opportunities for stem cell industry. Some new technologies may bring breakthrough developments for RM, such as the effect of 3D biological printing technology on RM.

REFERENCES

1. Mason, C. & Dunnill, P. (2008). "A brief definition of regenerative medicine," *Regenerative Medicine*, 3(1): 1–5.

2. Riazi, A. M., Kwon, S. Y. & Stanford, W. L. (2009). "Stem Cell Sources for Regenerative Medicine," In *Methods in Molecular Biology*, Audet J. and Stanford W. L. (eds.) (Humana Press), 482, pp. 55–90.
3. Stoick-Cooper, C. L., Moon, R. T. & Weidinger, G. (2007). "Advances in signaling in vertebrate regeneration as a prelude to regenerative medicine," *Genes & Development*, 21(11): 1292–1315.
4. Muneoka, K., Allan, C. H., Yang, X., Lee, J. & Han, M. (2008). "Mammalian regeneration and regenerative medicine," *Birth Defects Research. Part C, Embryo Today*, 84(4): 265–280.
5. Cheng, B., Lu, S. L. & Fu, X. (2016). "Regenerative medicine in China: Demands, capacity, and regulation," *Burns & Trauma*, 2, pp. 24–.
6. Dennis, C. (2002). "Stem cells rise in the East," *Nature*, 419(6905): 334–336.
7. Cheng, B., Lu, S. L. & Fu, X. B. (2016). "Regenerative medicine in China: Main progress in different fields," *Military Medical Research*, 3: 24. doi: 10.1186/s40779-016-0096-z. eCollection 2016.
8. Zhou, Q., Ren, X., Yang, X., Yao, Y., Yang, W. & Xia, Y. (2015). "Confronting coming medical renovation — Progress on stem cell and regenerative medicine research," *Bulletin of the Chinese Academy of Sciences*, 30(2): 262–271.
9. Tang, X., Qin, H., Gu, X. & Fu, X. (2017). "China's landscape in regenerative medicine," *Biomaterials*, 124(4): 78–94.
10. Liao, L., Li, L. & Zhao, R. C. (2007). "Stem cell research in China," *Philosophical Transactions of the Royal Society of London B: Biological Sciences*, 362: 1107–1112.
11. Salter, B. & Qiu, R. Z. (2009). "Bioethical governance and basic stem cell science: China and the global biomedicine economy," *Science and Public Policy*, 36: 47–59.
12. Liu, H., Zhu, F., Yong, J., Zhang, P., Hou, P., Li, H., Jiang, W., Cai, J., Liu, M., Cui, K., Qu, X., Xiang, T., Lu, D., Chi, X., Gao, G., Ji,W., Ding, M. & Deng, H. (2008). "Generation of induced pluripotent stem cells from adult rhesus monkey fibroblasts," *Cell Stem Cell*, 3(6): 587–590.
13. Zou, K., Yuan, Z., Yang, Z., Luo, H., Sun, K., Zhou, L., Xiang, J., Shi, L., Yu, Q., Zhang, Y., Hou, R. & Wu, J. (2009). "Production of offspring from a germline stem cell line derived from neonatal ovaries," *Nature Cell Biology*, 11(4): 631–636.
14. Yang, H., Shi, L., Wang, B.A., Liang, D., Zhong, C., Liu, W., Nie, Y., Liu, J., Zhao, J., Gao, X., Li, D., Xu, G. L. & Li J. (2012). "Generation of genetically

modified mice by oocyte injection of androgenetic haploid embryonic stem cells," *Cell*, 149(3): 605–617.

15. Li, W., Shuai, L., Wan, H., Dong, M., Wang, M., Sang, L., Feng, C., Luo, G. Z., Li, T., Li, X., Wang, L., Zheng, Q. Y., Sheng, C., Wu, H. J., Liu, Z., Liu, L., Wang, L., Wang, X. J., Zhao, X. Y. & Zhou, Q. (2012). "Androgenetic haploid embryonic stem cells produce live transgenic mice," *Nature*, 490(7420): 407–411.
16. Zhu, J., Zhou, L. & Xing Wu, F. (2006). "Tracking neural stem cells in patients with brain trauma," *New England Journal of Medicine*, 355(2): 2376–2378.
17. Sheng, Z., Fu, X., Cai, S, Lei, Y., Sun, T., Bai, X. & Chen, M. (2009). "Regeneration of functional sweat gland-like structures by transplanted differentiated bone marrow mesenchymal stem cells," *Wound Repair & Regeneration,* 17(3): 427–435.
18. Wang, S., Cheng, H., Dai, G., Wang, X., Hua, R., Liu, X., Wang, P., Chen, G., Yue, W. & An, Y. (2013). "Umbilical cord mesenchymal stem cell transplantation significantly improves neurological function in patients with sequelae of traumatic brain injury," *Brain Research*, 1352(9): 76–84.
19. Geron. (2011). "GRNOPC1." Available at: http://cell-therapies.geron.com/grnopc1_pipeline. Accessed 12 April 2012.
20. Stein, R. (2011). "First Human Embryonic Stem Cell Therapy in People Discontinued." *Washington Post*, November 14.
21. Cyranoski, D. (2009). "Stem-cell therapy faces more scrutiny in China," *Nature,* 459(7244): 146–147.
22. Hvistendahl, M. (2012). "China's push in tissue engineering," *Science*, 388(6109): 900–902.
23. Huang, S. & Fu, X. (2014). "Stem cell therapies and regenerative medicine in China," *Science China Life Sciences*, 57(2): 157–161.
24. Jin, X., Zheng, L., Zheng, R. H. & Li, Y. M. (2009). "China's policies on stem cell research: an opportunity for international collaborations," *Nature Reviews Molecular Cell Biology*, 10(4): 286.
25. Fu, X., Leshner, A., Shi T. Z. *et al.* (2012). "Regenerative medicine in China," *Science*, 336: 497–573.

Chapter 28

Endometriosis Treatment Opportunities: Western Conventional Medicine, Chinese Alternative Medicine, and Novel Strategies

Andrea Ciavattini, Nina Montik,
Alessandra Biagini and Matteo Serri

1. INTRODUCTION

Endometriosis, first described in 1860[1] is a common gynecological disease, which affects approximately 10% of reproductive-aged women and 20–50% of infertile women.[2] Endometriosis is a chronic, estrogen-dependent disorder characterized by the presence of tissue that is morphologically and biologically similar to normal endometrium in ectopic locations outside the uterine cavity. The exact pathogenic mechanisms of endometriosis remain unknown, although recently, researchers proposed several theories, including implantation theory, coelomic epithelium metaplasia theory, and induction theory. Recent evidence supports the presence of endometrial stem/progenitor cells and their possible involvement in endometrial regeneration and differentiation. The stem cell theory is a new hypothesis which may clarify the underlying pathophysiologic mechanisms of endometriosis. However, this theory could not only account for an alternative pathogenic mechanism of endometriosis but also be involved in all conventional theories.

In combination with the observations that the endometrium basalis contains endometrial stem cells and that women have retrograde menstrual efflux, we posit that stem cells are present in the blood that achieves the peritoneal cavity. Endometrium-derived stem cells residing in the basalis layer can be shed through the fallopian tube to the peritoneal cavity during menses and establish endometriotic implants.[3] It is possible that abnormal endometrial stem cells increase their capacity to implant and establish themselves as an ectopic tissue, or that normal stem cells find an abnormal peritoneum a proper implantation site.

Research continues to examine other risk factors that may be potentially involved in the formation of endometriosis, including genetics,[4] immune factors,[5] inflammatory factors,[6] eutopic endometrium specificity, and environmental toxins.[7] Hormonally stimulated cyclical bleeding from the endometriotic deposit appears to contribute to the induction of a local inflammatory reaction and fibrous adhesion and, in the case of deep implants in the ovary, leads to the formation of an endometrioma or chocolate cyst.

Endometriosis classically presents with severe dysmenorrhea, pelvic pain, dyspareunia, menstrual irregularities, and infertility. Systemic symptoms may also occur, such as fatigue, increased incidence of allergies, and autoimmune disease.[8] The diagnosis of endometriosis is based on the women's history, symptoms, and signs, and the diagnosis is corroborated by physical examination and imaging techniques, and finally proven by histology. The visual recognition of endometriosis during laparoscopy alone is of limited value as it has a high false-positive rate. On the other hand, diagnosis during laparoscopy is dependent on the ability of the surgeon to recognize peritoneal disease in all its different appearances.[9]

Recently, the World Endometriosis Research Foundation's[10] EndoCost study has shown that the costs arising from women with endometriosis treated in referral centers are substantial, resulting in an economic burden that is at least comparable to the burden associated with other chronic diseases like diabetes mellitus. Apart from the economic burden, endometriosis has a significant effect on the various aspects of women's life, including their social and sexual relationships, work, and study.[11] Therefore, there is a significant need to optimize the management of women with endometriosis to improve diagnosis and endometriosis care and reduce both the personal and societal costs of this disease.

2. WESTERN CONVENTIONAL MEDICINE

The conventional treatment of endometriosis can be broadly divided into medical and surgical management. Medical treatment ranges from symptomatic control with nonsteroidal anti-inflammatory drugs (NSAIDs) and analgesics to treatments suppressing normal ovarian production of estrogen with continuous oral contraceptives (COCs), progestins, or inducing a temporary similar-menopausal condition (Danazol and gonadotropin-releasing hormone agonists (GnRH-a)). Surgical intervention can be either "conservative," involving the removal of endometrial lesions or "definitive," involving the removal of the uterus and ovaries.

Danazol, progestins, GnRH-a, and the COCs have comparable short-term rates of success in alleviating the symptoms of endometriosis and in partially reducing the size of endometriosis-related lesions[12] but with a high rate of recurrence of the symptoms at six months post-treatment. Furthermore, short-term benefits of conventional medical treatment have to be balanced against the unpleasant and sometimes dangerous side effects resulting from these therapies.

COCs have been associated with increased thromboembolic risks,[13] is unsuitable for women over the age of 35 years who smoke or who have a history of cardiovascular disease, and is obviously inappropriate for women trying to conceive. Patients using progestin therapy reported a higher incidence of acne, fluid retention, bloating, and spotting. In addition, progestins are known to unfavorably reduce the level of high-density lipoproteins (HDLs), which could potentially increase the risk of cardiovascular side effects such as thrombosis.

Danazol is associated with androgenic changes, such as acne and weight gain, and menopausal symptoms such as flushing and fatigue. Moreover, there are increasing evidences of its potential role in raising low-density lipoprotein (LDL) cholesterol levels[14] and in possibly contributing to ovarian cancer.[15] GnRH-a tends to produce a more hypoestrogenic state than Danazol, with more severe menopausal side effects, such as hot flushes, insomnia, reduced libido, and vaginal dryness.[16] Low estrogen levels can also cause serious osteoporosis.

The surgical management of endometriosis is also far from satisfactory. Although several studies demonstrate a significant symptomatic relief after conservative laparoscopic surgery,[17,18] these benefits were relatively short-lived, with up to 44% of women experiencing a return of symptoms after one year.[19] Moreover, surgical treatment of endometriosis is often complicated by bladder and bowel lesions and sexual dysfunctions, which are sometimes irreversible. In addition, especially in deep infiltrating endometriosis, highly complex multivisceral surgical procedures with extensive dissection, such as segmental colorectal resection, is needed. Due to such possible side effects, endometriosis surgery often faces difficulty in being accepted by young women of fertile age presenting a benign disease. Endometriosis recurrence rate ranged between 20% and 40% within five years following conservative surgery, unless patients reached menopause or hysterectomy was performed.

In summary, current treatments all have high rates of recurrence and their short-term benefits have to be balanced with concerns over immediate and longer-term side effects. Consequently, it is important to continue looking for other strategies to treat endometriosis that may result at least in a comparable effectiveness but with less adverse side effects.

3. CHINESE ALTERNATIVE MEDICINE

Complementary and alternative medicine (CAM), commonly designated as "other than" conventional medicine, is widely accepted as a type of medical treatment. Most CAM therapies can be considered as part of five broad classes: biological-based approaches, energy therapies, alternative medical systems, muscle and joint manipulation, and mind–body therapies.

CAM is usually suggested as available complementary therapies. Among CAM, the non-pharmacological interventions can reduce pain and concomitant mood disturbance to increase quality of life by employing mind–body interventions.[20] In the western world, CAM is predominantly used to treat or prevent musculoskeletal conditions or other conditions associated with chronic or recurring pain.[21] As endometriosis is typically accompanied by chronic pelvic pain and dysmenorrhea, CAM therapies could be an effective treatment strategy. The CAM therapies for endometriosis in the published literature mainly include herbal products, acupuncture, microwave physiotherapy, Chinese Herbal Medicine (CHM) enema, and psychological interventions.

Herbal products typically involve the use of herbal formulae of between 10 and 20 separate herbal ingredients selected from a Materia Medica of several hundred common herbs that are prepared either as a boiled decoction or dried herbal extracts, or taken as pills or capsules.

In the past 10 years, more than 30 herbal patents have been commonly used to treat endometriosis-affected patients, including capsule, pill, and liquid. These patents are made up of several herbs based on thousands of clinical experiences. Herbal patent is more convenient than the decoction formula due to its modified formulation.

A recent Cochrane review analyzed the effectiveness and safety of CHM in alleviating endometriosis-related pain. The included trials suggest that, following laparoscopic surgery, combined oral and enema administration of CHM has a comparable beneficial effect to Gestrinone but with fewer adverse effects. Oral and enema administration of CHM may be more effective than Danazol in providing extended relief of endometriosis symptoms and in shrinking adnexal masses, with fewer adverse effects. However, this review included only two very small trials and it may not be possible to generalize the results.

Further research, with larger numbers of participants, is required to substantiate these results and to explore the role of CHM as a standalone medical option or as a post-surgical adjuvant in the treatment of endometriosis.[22]

Acupuncture is one of the main forms of Traditional Chinese Medicine (TCM) and has been practiced within the Chinese healthcare system for thousands of years.[23] Since the late 20th century, the demand for acupuncture has been growing steadily in many Western nations.[24,25]

In China, acupuncture is currently used in public hospitals for the treatment of endometriosis.[26] Practitioners of acupuncture and moxibustion regard the human body as a whole based on the theories of meridian, viscera, and qi-blood.

Chinese medicine believes that qi (vital energy) is the most basic form of human material foundation, human life, and activities. Qi and blood have different roles but are interdependent with each other, supplying nutrients for the organs and tissues to maintain life activities. The term "meridian" in TCM refers to the pathways of qi and blood, which are interconnected with each other.

There are several different forms of acupuncture, including body acupuncture, electroacupuncture, auricular acupuncture, and scalp acupuncture.[27] Even if endometriosis was not recorded in the classical text as a defined entity, its symptoms are treated under the categories of dysmenorrhea, irregular menstruation, abdominal mass, and infertility.[28]

In TCM, endometriosis is caused by impeded flow of qi and blood, resulting in obstruction of the Chong and Ren channels.[29] The principle behind the application of acupuncture is to rectify the imbalance and unblock the obstruction in the related channels.

The mechanism of action of acupuncture in the treatment of endometriosis remains largely unclear. However, emerging literature demonstrates acupuncture-mediated analgesia and alteration of specific hormone levels. The influence of acupuncture on the body's naturally occurring pain mediators (endogenous opioids such as *ß*-endorphin) has been established since the 1970s.[30]

Cabýoglu *et al.*[31] summarized the findings from several studies which propose that increases of endogenous opioids and the neurotransmitters serotonin and dopamine cause analgesia, sedation, and recovery of motor function. It is also reported that acupuncture may induce visceral and somatic signals that are transmitted to the central nervous system to induce an anti-inflammatory signal through both humoral and neural mechanisms.[32]

Lin *et al.*[33] found that the therapeutic effect of acupuncture for dysmenorrhea may be through its influence on prostaglandin F2α (PGF2α) levels in menstrual fluid. Studies of auricular acupuncture suggest that its main therapeutic actions may be through elevation of plasma β-endorphin levels and coordination of uterine activity.[34]

A recent Cochrane review[35] regarding the role of acupuncture in endometriosis treatment strategies concluded that there is not enough evidence to support the effectiveness of acupuncture to alleviate pain due to endometriosis. Xiang *et al.*[26] found that auricular acupuncture decreased pain from endometriosis in comparison to CHM, but the overall low quality of methodology and the small sample of women make its clinical use difficult to determine. Therefore, there is currently a lack of high-quality trials to determine the effectiveness of acupuncture versus conventional therapies or placebo. Actually, acupuncture may be a treatment option for women who do not satisfactorily respond to conventional interventions or who seek an alternative for managing pain from endometriosis.

Moxibustion is a technique which applies heat to acupoints by burning compressed powdered herbal material at the acupoints to stimulate them. Moxibustion includes moxibustion with moxa cone, moxa stick, and herbal medicine cake; burning rush moxibustion; and crude herb moxibustion. Chinese medicine believes that moxibustion could warm meridians, relieve pain, and promote blood circulation. Combined with acupuncture, moxibustion treatment can effectively arouse the regulating function of meridian, thereby improving the body's immune function to relieve endometriosis symptoms.

Chinese herbal enema consists of pouring Chinese herbal medicine into the rectum where it remains for four to five hours to allow the Chinese herbal medicine to be fully absorbed through the intestinal mucosa. Chinese herbal enema can improve the bioavailability of the drug and reduce liver damage. There were several observations about endometriosis treatment using Chinese herbal enema which found that Chinese herbal enema has significant therapeutic effects, especially in reducing endometriotic lesions.[36] Chinese herbal enemas combined with oral Chinese herbal medicine are the most commonly utilized treatment for endometriosis-affected patients who are treated in the hospital, with the total effective rate in reducing pelvic pain varying between 83.8% and 93.88%.[37,38]

Microwave physiotherapy is a safe therapy that functions by absorbing the surrounding material and producing a heating effect, without changing the chemical nature of the surrounding substance.[39] Microwaves produce non-ionizing radiation and ultrahigh frequency electromagnetic waves with frequencies between 300 and 300,000 MHz.

Sharma *et al.*[40] found that microwave physiotherapy could adjust menorrhagia and inhibit uterus enlargement caused by adenomyosis . As an adjuvant treatment for endometriosis, microwave physiotherapy shows a synergistic effect which increases the absorption rate of Chinese herbal products. Microwave physiotherapy should be used only in the non-acute phase of endometriosis. Microwave physiotherapy is often combined with Chinese herbal enema for the treatment of endometriosis as adjuvant therapy which can produce a heating effect to promote the increased absorption of Chinese herbal enema via rectum mucosa.

4. NOVEL THERAPEUTIC STRATEGIES

Since some authors have theorized that endometriosis should be considered a multifactorial disease, involving genetic, hormonal, immunological, and environmental factors,[41,42] the development of new medical treatments is of prime importance.

Researchers are studying novel treatment strategies that ideally fulfill several requisites such as an acceptable side-effect profile, growth inhibition of existing endometriotic lesion and prevention of *de novo* lesions and their recurrence after surgery. Preferably, they should not interfere with ovulation in order to be administered to young women who are trying to conceive.

Most new medical treatments being developed also have hormonal targets such as GnRH antagonists, aromatase inhibitors (AIs), selective progesterone receptor modulators (SPRMs), and selective estrogen receptor modulators (SERMs). Non-hormonal treatments with targets such as angiogenesis, immune system, and inflammation are also being tested in women with endometriosis.

4.1. *Hormonal targets*

There are only scarce data on the use of GnRH antagonists for the treatment of endometriosis-associated pain. Their oral administration in healthy premenopausal women has been shown to immediately suppress luteinizing hormone (LH) and follicle-stimulating hormone (FSH) levels associated with a dose-related suppression in estrogen levels.[43] This property could permit the inhibition of endometriotic cell growth, while maintaining sufficient estradiol production to avoid bone loss and other side effects related to hypoestrogenism.

The GnRH antagonist analogues may be superior to GnRH agonists because they produce immediate suppression of LH and FSH secretion and avoid the agonist phase of GnRH agonist therapy. In premenopausal women, the use of aromatase inhibitors (AIs) as a sole therapy induces central hypoestrogenism in the hypothalamus and pituitary gland, resulting in elevation of FSH levels and follicular growth.[44] AIs can, therefore, not be used as a sole therapy in the treatment of premenopausal endometriosis and should be combined to treatments that block the hypothalamo–pituitary–ovarian axis such as the COC pill or GnRH-a.[45] In theory, central blockage induces hypoestrogenism in the pelvic cavity by inhibiting ovarian activity, whereas AIs inhibit the production of estrogens in endometriotic lesions themselves, thus stopping the stimulatory feedback loop between local estrogens and inflammation.[46]

A number of studies in nonhuman primates have shown certain SPRMs (e.g., onapristone, ulipristal) inhibit endometrial proliferation, leading to endometrial atrophy,[47,48] while information regarding its use in humans for endometriosis disease are scarce. They have the potential to induce reversible amenorrhea through selective inhibition of endometrial proliferation, a direct effect on endometrial blood vessels, and the potential to suppress endometrial prostaglandin production in a tissue-specific manner without the systemic effects of estrogen deprivation, providing a rationale for the treatment of endometriosis-related pain.[49] No serious drug-related adverse events were reported during the treatment or follow-up period.

There is emerging data indicating that SERMs, specifically agonists toward the b-subunit, may be able to be used to treat endometriosis. The b-unit is felt to act on different targets than classic a-SERMs, such as bone, mammary, and endometrium.[50] SERMs directed toward the b-subunit have been found to have anti-inflammatory action in several rat models toward other inflammatory-mediated diseases, such as inflammatory bowel disease and rheumatoid arthritis.[51] One study demonstrated that SERMS resolved endometriosis in 40–75% of mice treated with a SERM directed toward the b-subunit.[50]

4.2. *Angiogenesis inhibitors*

Retrograde menstruation with peritoneal attachment is believed to lead to the development of endometriotic lesions. However, this shed endometrial tissue requires the establishment of a new blood supply in order to survive in the peritoneal cavity.[52] The endometrium has angiogenic potential, and endometriotic lesions grow in areas with a rich

vascularization, suggesting that angiogenesis is a prerequisite for endometriosis development. Therefore, inhibition of proangiogenic factors (e.g., VEGF and MMPs) may offer new therapeutic opportunities.[53]

Antiangiogenic agents tested so far have proven effective for preventing neovascularization of endometriotic lesions and are likely to be efficient for early-stage disease. However, antiangiogenic treatments may alter reproductive function by impairing physiological angiogenesis, the greatest concern being the potential risk of teratogenicity. The initial promise of vascular therapy has not yet been fulfilled, mainly due to the limited selectivity of the vascular therapies available.

Even if the administration of antiangiogenic drugs has been proved to reduce the establishment, maintenance and progression of endometriotic lesions in different animal models, further investigations are required before clinical trials can be planned in humans.

4.3. *5-Fluorouracil*

A recent study investigated the effects of antiproliferative drugs (anastrozole, methotrexate, and 5-fluorouracil (5-FU)) on the proliferation of endometriotic cells *in vitro* and *in vivo*.[54] Although anastrozole, methotrexate, and progesterone were ineffective, 5-FU significantly decreased the proliferation of endometriotic cells *in vitro* and controlled the growth of both cells from ovarian endometrioma and deep infiltrating endometriosis. Considering common features between endometriotic cells and tumor cells, the use of 5-FU could be an option in the management of severe endometriosis.

4.4. *Immunomodulators*

The mounting evidence shows that altered immune function plays a crucial role in the genesis and development of endometriosis. It has become clear that pelvic inflammation, increased macrophage activation, and invasion of the extracellular matrix are potential targets for endometriosis treatment and/or prevention.[53] This broad group of medications includes loxoribine, IFN-a 2b, and TNF-a inhibitors.

In this context, the potential role of Vitamin D is of increasing interest, since previous studies have demonstrated the role of Vitamin D as a modulator of the immune system.[55] In particular, several *in vitro* studies have demonstrated the anti-inflammatory, antiproliferative, and anti-invasive effects of vitamin D in various pathologies such as rheumatoid arthritis,[56] psoriasis,[57] and cancers.[58]

Only a few *in vivo* studies have investigated the relationship between hypovitaminosis D and endometriosis, with opposing results.[59–61] Some authors suggested a correlation between endometriosis and hypovitaminosis D[59,60] and, recently, it has been observed that higher Vitamin D serum levels seem to be associated with a lower endometriosis risk, while women with endometriosis have lower Vitamin D serum levels than disease-free controls.[60] Indeed, in women with endometriosis, an altered immune surveillance with depressed cell mediated immunity and heightened humoral immune response has been described.[62] Hence, Vitamin D might influence the development and progression of endometriosis through its role in the reduction of proinflammatory processes.

In a recent observational study conducted by our department,[63] we focused on Caucasian women with single ovarian endometrioma, and we analyzed a potential correlation between hypovitaminosis D and endometriosis. At inclusion, the mean (±SD) 25-OH-D3 serum level in the initial study cohort was 22.0 (± 8.9) ng/ml. Furthermore, 42 women (85.7%) were diagnosed with hypovitaminosis D while the remaining 7 women had normal 25-OH-D3 serum levels.

In the "hypovitaminosis D women," the mean (± SD) diameter of ovarian endometriomas was 40.2 ± 22.6 mm, while in the "normal Vitamin D serum level women," it was 26.7 ± 12.1 mm ($p = 0.1$). Although the mean diameter of ovarian endometriomas was not different between the two subgroups, a significant linear correlation between 25-OH-D3 serum level and the diameter of ovarian endometriomas emerged ($r = -0.3$, $p = 0.03$).

Also adjusting for confounders (age, BMI, tobacco use, age at menarche, and number of pregnancies) in a stepwise multiple regression, the mean 25-OH-D3 serum level was significantly and independently correlated with the mean diameter of endometriomas ($r = -0.3$, $p = 0.03$).

According to these findings, hypovitaminosis D could play a role in the development of endometriosis and could correlate with the severity of the disease. Thus it is possible to speculate that Vitamin D supplementation in women with hypovitaminosis D might be a novel, safe, and low-cost therapeutic strategy both in the primary prevention and treatment of endometriosis. However, in order to properly evaluate the possible therapeutic role of Vitamin D in women with endometriosis, future studies and well-designed randomized control studies are necessary.

Although hypovitaminosis D deficiency is common worldwide, national data regarding its prevalence in China is severely lacking. Most information about hypovitaminosis D in China concern studies focused on special populations, limited in the number of patients, and with data from specific age groups or a single province that cannot accurately reflect the general vitamin D status of Chinese population. A multicentric study with a large population covering all adult age groups revealed a striking high prevalence of Vitamin D insufficiency (92.5% of women) and deficiency (66.3% of women) in the Chinese population. Moreover, Vitamin D status was much worse among women and younger participants (< 39 years), and the degree of hypovitaminosis D was higher in inland regions than coastal regions.[64]

These findings suggest that Vitamin D status may differ by race and ethnicity and there are various reasons why Vitamin D status might be so different in the Chinese population compared to Caucasian population. First, genetic factors: e.g., variants of Vitamin D–metabolizing enzymes CYP24A1 (24-hydroxylase), CYP2R1 (25-hydroxylase), Vitamin D–binding protein (DBP), and DHCR7 (7- dehydrocholesterol reductase) can contribute to the variation in 25(OH)D concentrations.[65,66] Second, the average dietary calcium intake in the Chinese population is low, leading to secondary hyperparathyroidism and increased turnover of Vitamin D metabolites. In addition, some lifestyle factors (e.g., behavior in the sun) may differ between races as, e.g., the Chinese population tends to have a sun-avoiding behavior due to smog levels and professional pressure.

To date, there are no studies regarding the relationship between hypovitaminosis D and endometriosis in the Chinese population. In our opinion, because of the high prevalence of hypovitaminosis D among Chinese women, analyzing the potential role of Vitamin D supplementation in the primary prevention and treatment of endometriosis in Chinese population could be of great interest.

In conclusion, none of these therapies are entirely curative for endometriosis. While current traditional treatments all have high rates of recurrence with several side effects, and most hormonal therapies are useless in young infertile women, researchers are engaged in finding alternative and new treatment strategies for endometriosis. Chinese alternative therapies may effectively modulate the progress of endometriosis by shrinking the lesions, suppressing the symptoms, and decreasing the recurrence rate.

Although CAM therapies have been gradually accepted in some countries, some obstacles, such as the lack of more thorough safety and efficacy studies and the lack of large-sample sizes and randomized controlled trials, still hinder more widespread application of CAM therapies throughout the world.

In summary, the active principle of the CAM therapies has a strong scientific foundation, and researchers are increasing their interest in this area of medical treatment.

Standardizations of the effective CAM therapies are still needed; however, managing the pharmaceutical form of herbal agents and controlling the quality of acupuncture methods need to be included in order to increase the benefits of these alternative medical interventions on patients with endometriosis throughout the world.

Therapeutic research efforts should focus on identifying and testing substances capable of acting locally on the lesions themselves, without interfering with ovulation, in order to be efficacious on both pain symptoms and infertility. Of great interest is the burgeoning role of Vitamin D in pain alleviation in endometriosis affected women as a therapy with no side affects, safe, low cost and usable also by women of childbearing age desiring pregnancy.

REFERENCES

1. Von Rokitansky, C. (1860). "Ueber uterusdrusen-neubildung in uterus and ovarilsarcomen," *Z Ges Aerzte Wein*, 37: 577–593.
2. Taylor, R. N., Lebovic, D. I. & Mueller, M. D. (2002). "Angiogenic factors in endometriosis," *Annals of the New York Academy of Sciences*, 955: 89–100; Discussion, 118: 396–406.
3. Sasson, I. E. & Taylor, H. S. (2008). "Stem cells and the pathogenesis of endometriosis," *Annals of the New York Academy of Sciences,* 1127: 106–115.
4. Fauser, B. C. J. M., Diedrich, K., Bouchard, P. *et al.* (2011). "Contemporary genetic technologies and female reproduction," *Human Reproduction Update*, 17(6): 829–847.
5. Sinaii, N., Cleary, S. D., Ballweg, M. L., Nieman, L. K. & Stratton, P. (2002). "High rates of autoimmune and endocrine disorders, fibromyalgia, chronic fatigue syndrome and atopic diseases among women with endometriosis: A survey analysis," *Human Reproduction*, 17(10): 2715–2724.
6. Wellbery, C. (1999). "Diagnosis and treatment of endometriosis," *American Family Physician*, 60(6): 1753–1762.
7. Guo, S.-W., Simsa, P., Kyama, C. M. *et al.* (2009). "Reassessing the evidence for the link between dioxin and endometriosis: From molecular biology to clinical epidemiology," *Molecular Human Reproduction*, 15(10): 609–624.
8. Ballweg, M. L. (2004). "Impact of endometriosis on women's health: Comparative historical data show that the earlier the onset, the more severe the disease," *Best Practice & Research Clinical Obstetrics and Gynaecology*, 18(2): 201–218.
9. ESHRE (2013). Guideline on the Management of Women with Endometriosis. September.
10. Simoens, S., Dunselman, G., Dirksen, C., *et al.* (2012). The burden of endometriosis: Costs and quality of life of women with endometriosis and treated in referral centres. *Human Reproduction*, 27(5): 1292–1299.
11. De Graaff, A. A., D'Hooghe, T. M., Dunselman, G. A., Dirksen, C. D. & Hummelshoj, L. (2013). "WERF EndoCost Consortium"; Simoens, S. "The significant effect of endometriosis on physical, mental and social well-being: Results from an international cross-sectional survey," *Human Reproduction,* July, p. 11.
12. Selak, V., Farquhar, C., Prentice, A. & Singla, A. (2007). "Danazol for pelvic pain associated with endometriosis," *Cochrane Database of Systematic Reviews*, 17(4): 4.
13. Anderson, G. L., Limacher, M., Assaf, A. R. *et al.* (2004). "Effects of conjugated equine estrogen in postmenopausal women with hysterectomy: The Women's Health Initiative randomized controlled trial," *JAMA*, 291(14): 1701–1712.

14. Hughes, E., Fedorkow, D., Collins, J. & Vandekerchove, P. (2004). "Ovulation suppression for endometriosis," *Cochrane Database of Systematic Reviews*. Chichester: John Wiley & Sons, Ltd.
15. Cottreau, C. M., Ness, R. B., Modugno, F., Allen, G. O. & Goodman, M. T. (2003). "Endometriosis and its treatment with danazol or lupron in relation to ovarian cancer," *Clinical Cancer Research*, 9(14): 5142–5144.
16. Prentice, A., Deary, A. J., Goldbeck-Wood, S., Farquhar, C. & Smith, S.K. (2007). "Gonadotrophin-releasing hormone analogues for pain associated with endometriosis," *Cochrane Database of Systematic Reviews*, 18(2)
17. Abbott, J., Hawe, J., Hunter, D., Holmes, M., Finn, P. & Garry, R. (2004). "Laparoscopic excision of endometriosis: A randomized, placebo-controlled trial," *Fertility and Sterility*, 82(4): 878–884.
18. Fedele, L., Bianchi, S., Zanconato, G., Bettoni, G. & Gotsch, F. (2004). "Long-term follow-up after conservative surgery for rectovaginal endometriosis," *American Journal of Obstetrics and Gynecology*, 190(4): 1020–1024.
19. Lapp, T. (2000). "ACOG issues recommendations for the management of endometriosis. American College of Obstetricians and Gynecologists," *American Family Physician*, 62(6): 1431–1434.
20. Pujol, L. A. & Monti, D. A. (2007). "Managing cancer pain with nonpharmacologic and complementary therapies," *The Journal of the American Osteopathic Association*, 107(12 Suppl 7): ES15–ES21.
21. Barnes, P. M., Powell-Griner, E., McFann, K. & Nahin, R. L. (2004). "Complementary and alternative medicine use among adults: United States, 2002," *Advance Data*, 343: 1–19.
22. Flower, A., Liu, J. P., Lewith, G., Little, P. & Li, Q. (2012). "Chinese herbal medicine for endometriosis," *Cochrane Database of Systematic Reviews*, (5).
23. Qiu, M. L. & Li, L. Y. (1993). *Chinese Acupuncture and Moxibustion*. (Churchill Livingstone, Singapore).
24. Hamilton, J. L., Roemheld-Hamm, B., Young, D. M., Jalba, M. & DiCicco-Bloom, Y. (2008). "Complementary and alternative medicine in US family medicine practices: A pilot qualitative study," *Alternative Therapies in Health & Medicine*, 14(3): 22–27.
25. Harkin, C. & Parker, R. (2007). "A prospective, randomised control trial of acupuncture for select common conditions within the emergency department," *Journal of Chinese Medicine*, 85: 41–48.
26. Xiang, D., Situ, Y., Liang, X., Cheng, L. & Zhang, G. (2002). "Ear acupuncture therapy for 37 cases of dysmenorrhoea due to endometriosis," *Zhong Yi Za Zhi [Journal of Traditional Chinese Medicine]*, 22: 282–285
27. Zhang, Y., Peng, W., Clarke, J. & Liu, Z. (2010). "Acupuncture for uterine fibroids," *Cochrane Database of Systematic Reviews*, (1).

28. Xia, G. C. (2010). *Chinese Medicine Diagnosis and Treatment in the Management of Menstrual Disorders* (People's Press, Beijing).
29. Li, J., Zheng, J. & Wang, D. (1999). "Clinical observation on treatment of endometriosis by tonifying qi and promoting blood circulation to remove stasis and purgation principle," *Zhong Guo Zhong Xi Yi Jie He Za Zhi [China Journal of Integrated Traditional and Western Medicine]*, 19(9): 533–535.
30. Lin, J. G. & Chen, W. L. (2008). "Acupuncture analgesia: A review of its mechanisms of actions," *American Journal of Chinese Medicine*, 36(4): 635–645.
31. Cabýoglu, M. T., Ergene, N. & Tan, U. (2006). "The mechanism of acupuncture and clinical applications," *International Journal of Neurosciences*, 116(2): 115–125.
32. Cho, Z. H., Hwang, S. C., Wong, E. K., *et al.* (2006). "Neural substrates, experimental evidences and functional hypothesis of acupuncture mechanisms," *Acta Neurologica Scandinavica*, 113(6): 370–377.
33. Lin, L. L., Liu, C. Z. & Huang, B. Y. (2008). "Clinical observation on treatment of primary dysmenorrhea with acupuncture and massage," *Zhong Guo Zhong Xi Yi Jie He Za Zhi [China Journal of Integrated Traditional and Western Medicine]*, 28(5): 418–420.
34. Xiang, D. F., Sun, Q. Z. & Liang, X. F. (2011). "Effect of abdominal acupuncture on pain of pelvic cavity in patients with endometriosis," *Zhongguo Zhen Jiu*, 31(2): 113–116.
35. Zhu, X., Hamilton, K. D. & McNicol, E. D. (2011). "Acupuncture for pain in endometriosis," *Cochrane Database of Systematic Reviews*, 9.
36. Zhou, S. Y. (2012). "Treatment of 64 endometriosis patients with enema," *Guide of China Medicine*, 10(4): 226–229.
37. Wu, X. H. & Zhang, C. L. (2011). "The treatment for 49 endometriosis patients with Chinese herbal enema and Chinese medicine," *Guangming Journal of Chinese Medicine*, 26(12): 2467.
38. Yu, B. J. & Zhao, Y. H. (2009). "Clinical observation of endometriosis patients treated with Chinese medicine," *Chinese Journal of Misdiagnostics*, 9(9): 2055.
39. Lei, X. P., Ye, Z. P. & Li, R. (2002). "Introduction of microwave treatment principle," *Progress in Physiological Sciences*, 33(3): 286.
40. Sharma, B., Preston, J. & Ray, C. (2004). "Microwave endometrial ablation for menorrhagia: Outcome at two years — experience of a district general hospital," *Journal of Obstetrics and Gynaecology*, 24(8): 916–919.
41. Christodoulakos, G., Augoulea, A., Lambrinoudaki, I. *et al.* (2007). "Pathogenesis of endometriosis: The role of defective 'immunosurveillance,'" *European Journal of Contraceptive and Reproductive Health Care*, 12(3): 194–202.

42. Anger, D. L. & Foster, W. G. (2008). "The link between environmental toxicant exposure and endometriosis," *Frontiers in Bioscience*, 13: 1578–93.
43. Struthers, R. S., Nicholls, A. J., Grundy, J., *et al.* (2009). "Suppression of gonadotropins and estradiol in premenopausal women by oral administration of the nonpeptide gonadotropin-releasing hormone antagonist elagolix," *Journal of Clinical Endocrinology & Metabolism*, 94(2): 545–551.
44. Colette, S. & Donnez, J. (2011). "Are aromatase inhibitors effective in endometriosis treatment?" *Expert Opinion on Investigational Drugs*, 20(7): 917–931.
45. Lossl, K., Loft, A., Freiesleben, N. L., Bangsbøll, S., *et al.* (2009). "Combined down-regulation by aromatase inhibitor and GnRH-agonist in IVF patients with endometriomas-A pilot study," *European Journal of Obstetrics, Gynecology & Reproductive Biology*, 144(1): 48–53.
46. Bulun, S. E. (2009). "Endometriosis," *New England Journal of Medicine*, 360(3): 268–279.
47. Gopalkrishnan, K., Katkam, R. R., Sachdeva, G. *et al.* (2003). "Effects of an antiprogestin onapristone on the endometrium of bonnet monkeys: Morphometric and ultrastructural studies," *Biology of Reproduction*, 68(6): 1959–1967.
48. Brenner, R. M., Slayden, O. D., Nath, A. *et al.* (2010). "Intrauterine administration of CDB-2914 (Ulipristal) suppresses the endometrium of rhesus macaques," *Contraception*, 81(4): 336–342.
49. Chwalisz, K., Garg, R., Brenner, R. M., Schubert, G. & Elger, W. (2002). "Selective progesterone receptor modulators (SPRMs): A novel therapeutic concept in endometriosis," *Annals of New York Academy of Sciences*, 955: 373–388;
50. Harris, H. A., Bruner-Tran, K. L., Zhang, X., Osteen, K. G. & Lyttle, C. R. (2005). "A selective estrogen receptor-beta agonist causes lesion regression in an experimentally induced model of endometriosis," *Human Reproduction*, 20(4): 936–941.
51. Harris, H. A., Albert, L. M., Leathurby, Y., *et al.* (2003). "Evaluation of an estrogen receptor-beta agonist in animal models of human disease," *Endocrinology*, 144(10): 4241–4249.
52. Novella-Maestre, E., Carda, C., Noguera, I., *et al.* (2009). "Dopamine agonist administration causes a reduction in endometrial implants through modulation of angiogenesis in experimentally induced endometriosis," *Human Reproduction*, 24(5): 1025–1035.
53. Hompes, P. G. & Mijatovic, V. (2007). "Endometriosis: The way forward. *Gynecological Endocrinology*, 23(1): 5–12.
54. Ngo, C., Nicco, C., Leconte, M., Chereau, C., Weill, B., Batteux, F. & Hapron, C. (2010). "Antiproliferative effects of anastrozole, methotrexate,

and 5-fluorouracil on endometriosis *in vitro* and *in vivo*," *Fertility and Sterility*.
55. Holick, M. F. (2004). "Sunlight and vitamin D for bone health and prevention of autoimmune diseases, cancers, and cardiovascular disease," *American Journal of Clinical Nutrition*, 80(6 Suppl): 1678S–1688S.
56. Van Hamburg, J. P., Asmawidjaja, P. S., Davelaar, N., *et al.* (2012). "TNF blockade requires 1,25(OH)2D3 to control human Th17-mediated synovial inflammation," *Annals of Rheumatic Diseases*, 71(4): 606–612.
57. Karthaus, N., van Spriel, A. B., Looman, M. W. G., *et al.* (2014). "Vitamin D controls murine and human plasmacytoid dendritic cell function," *Journal of Investigative Dermatology*, 134(5): 1255–1264.
58. Krishnan, A. V., Swami, S., Peng, L., *et al.* (2010). "Tissue-selective regulation of aromatase expression by calcitriol: Implications for breast cancer therapy," *Endocrinology*, 151(1): 32–42.
59. Grzechocinska, B., Dabrowski, F. A., Cyganek, A. *et al.* (2013). "The role of vitamin D in impaired fertility treatment," *Neuroendocrinology Letters*, 34(8): 756–762.
60. Miyashita, M., Koga, K., Izumi, G. *et al.* (2016). "Effects of 1,25-Dihydroxy Vitamin D3 on endometriosis," *Journal of Clinical Endocrinology & Metabolism*, 101(6): 2371–2379.
61. Somigliana, E., Panina-Bordignon, P., Murone, S. *et al.* (2007). "Vitamin D reserve is higher in women with endometriosis," *Human Reproduction*, 22(8): 2273–2278.
62. Nothnick, W. B. (2001). "Treating endometriosis as an autoimmune disease," *Fertility and Sterility*, 76(2): 223–231.
63. Ciavattini, A., Serri, M., Delli Carpini, G., Morini, S. & Clemente, N. (2017). "Ovarian endometriosis and vitamin D serum levels," *Gynecological Endocrinology*, 33(2): 164–167.
64. Yu, S., Fang, H., Han, J., *et al.* (2015). "The high prevalence of hypovitaminosis D in China: A multicenter vitamin D status survey," *Medicine (Baltimore)*. 94(8): e585.
65. Cheung, C. L., Lau, K. S., Sham, P. C., Tan, K. C. & Kung, A. W. (2013). "Genetic variant in vitamin D binding protein is associated with serum 25-hydroxyvitamin D and vitamin D insufficiency in southern Chinese," *Journal of Human Genetics*, 58: 749–751.
66. Lu, L., Sheng, H., Li, H., Gan, W., Liu, C., Zhu, J., Loos, R. J. & Lin, X. (2012). "Associations between common variants in GC and DHCR7/NADSYN1 and vitamin D concentration in Chinese Hans," *Human Genetics*, 131: 505–512.

Chapter 29

Western Medicine and Traditional Chinese Medicine in Chronic Pelvic Pain Treatment: A Literature Review

Andrea Ciavattini, Nina Montik, Matteo Serri
and Alessandra Biagini

1. INTRODUCTION

Chronic pelvic pain (CPP) is a prevalent and costly condition for which diagnosis and management are often difficult because of the complexities of causative factors and the multitude of involved structures. CPP is defined as nonmalignant continuous or recurrent pain in structures related to the pelvis, lasting at least six months, and often associated with negative cognitive, behavioral, sexual, and emotional consequences. If nonacute and central sensitization pain mechanisms are present, then the condition is considered chronic, regardless of the time frame.[1] The multifactorial etiology of CPP contributes to the challenges of its medical and rehabilitative management and has been described as a medical "nightmare" for clinicians.[2] CPP is not a disease; rather, it is a condition associated with dysfunction in one or usually more of the following body systems: gynecological, urological, gastrointestinal, musculoskeletal, and neurological. The community prevalence of CPP in the US, UK, and New Zealand are estimated to be 14.7%, 24%, and 25%, respectively,[3–5] and an estimated prevalence of CPP in primary care of 3.7% is comparable to those for low back pain (4.1%) and asthma (3.8%).[6] A recent study estimated the annual costs of endometriosis alone in 2002 to be $22 billion.[7] In addition to the economic impact, CPP is costly in terms of emotional and psychological distress. Women with CPP are likely to report depression, anxiety, and sleep disturbances, in addition to limitations in sexual activity and mobility.[8–10]

CPP commonly afflicts about 14% of women at least once in their life, and the global prevalence of CPP for women in their reproductive ages is estimated between 14% and 24%.[11] However, the true CPP incidence and prevalence and the related socioeconomic impact are still unknown. CPP causes are still not well understood but may be associated with gynecologic and non-gynecologic conditions.

CPP's differential diagnosis frequently involves both psychological and organic factors, but it is still a poorly understood condition and there is a lack of understanding of the etiology and pathogenesis; therefore, CPP management often constitutes a major challenge to the clinician.

Gynecologic diseases are the cause of CPP in about 20% of patients. The most common gynecologic CPP causes can be extrauterine or uterine. Common uterine causes include adenomyosis, post-hysterectomy pain, pelvic congestion syndrome, fibroids, vulvodynia, dysmenorrhea or ovulatory pain, cervical stenosis, endometritis, endometrial or cervical polyps, intrauterine contraceptive device, or genital prolapses. Extrauterine causes can be endometriosis, adnexal cysts, endosalpingiosis, ovarian dystrophy or ovulatory pain, pelvic congestion syndrome, residual ovary syndrome, neoplasia of the genital tract, pelvic adhesions, or pelvic inflammatory disease.

Other common causes of CPP in women can be identified in urological (urethral syndrome, chronic urinary-tract infection or interstitial cystitis, bladder neoplasm, lithiasis, detrusor dyssynergia, urethral diverticulum, urethral caruncle), gastrointestinal (irritable bowel syndrome or inflammatory bowel disease, chronic appendicitis, carcinoma of the colon, colitis, diverticula and hernias), and musculoskeletal disorders (myofascial pain, nerve entrapment syndrome, mechanical low back pain, degenerative joint disease, hernias, fibromyositis, spinal cord or sacral nerve neoplasia, pelvic neuralgia or myalgia, piriformis syndrome).

The etiology of CPP is complex and involves not only gynecological, urological, gastrointestinal, musculoskeletal, or nerve-related disorders but also psychosomatic, social, and psychological factors such as depression, physical or sexual abuse, sleep disturbance, psychologic stress, or substance abuse.[12] It has been shown that women with CPP often have co-existing conditions such as depression.

CPP may also cause additional stress and low self- and sexual confidence. There is also a complex relationship between chronic pain and a history of abuse: this may predispose adults to develop chronic pain syndrome rather than having a direct causative effect. Psychosocial circumstances can also complicate CPP diagnosis and treatment: if CPP can produce a psychopathology, it is also true that an existing psychopathology may influence the pain perception.

2. MANAGEMENT

CPP syndrome is a multisystem disorder, so a multidisciplinary approach is frequently recommended. An initial detailed history and clinical examination is needed to relate the possible causes of CPP; patients should be investigated through complete blood and serum analysis, urine microscopy culture and sensitivity, and vaginal and endocervical samples to screen for infections. Pelvic ultrasound scan and magnetic resonance can be useful to investigate and identify gynecologic pathologies (e.g., adenomyosis, hydrosalpinx, endometriosis, adnexal cysts).[13]

CPP is the indication for at least 40% of all gynecologic laparoscopies, and a diagnostic laparoscopy in CPP should be considered in case of high suspicion of adhesive disease or endometriosis that potentially may affect the fertility and require surgical intervention.

Biopsies and histologic confirmation of suspicious areas are recommended because visual diagnoses are incorrect in 10–90% of cases.[14,15]

Conscious pain mapping can be an alternative to diagnostic laparoscopy; it can be performed under local anesthesia to confirm or identifying sources of pain in women with CPP, but nowadays no substantial data confirm improved diagnostic outcomes or accuracy with this technique. Colonoscopy and/or cystoscopy with biopsies may be required in selected cases.

In women with higher levels of anxiety and depression, a psychiatric evaluation should be a part of CPP evaluation, and psychological treatments can be useful in reducing the frequency and severity of chronic pain symptoms.[16,17]

3. WESTERN MEDICINE

The treatment choices currently available for CPP and their effectiveness are still limited.[18] It has been shown that the comparative effectiveness of surgical (e.g., hysterectomy, laparoscopic uterosacral nerve ablation) and non-surgical approaches (e.g., hormonal therapies) for CPP still have insufficient evidence; non-hormonal and non-pharmacologic integrated management approaches seem beneficial but they still have not been adequately studied.[19,20]

3.1. *Medical treatment*

Symptomatic pharmacotherapy can stop or reduce CPP acute exacerbations and can be used as long-term therapy for CPP. An initial treatment should be taken with simple over-the-counter analgesics (e.g., paracetamol, ibuprofen, aspirin, or naproxen).

In CPP, amitriptyline and nortriptyline, two tricyclic antidepressants, frequently used. Selective serotonin reuptake inhibitors (SSRIs) are commonly administered as well, and other antidepressants (e.g., doxepin, desipramine, protriptyline, buspirone) can also be used.

The use of amitriptyline, oxybutinin, solifenacin, and other medication can help with sleep, headaches, persistent pain condition, pelvic muscle pain, and some irritable bowel symptoms;[21] they may also have a direct analgesic effect, as both depressive symptoms and pain are modulated by the neurotransmitters serotonin and norepinephrine.[22] CPP due to endometriosis, dysmenorrhea, or cyclical aggravations may be managed with an estrogen–progestin combination, progestin, danazol, or gonadotropin-releasing hormone (GnRH) agonists, with or without nonsteroidal anti-inflammatory drugs.

With bladder-related symptoms, antibiotics should be avoided unless infection is proven by urine culture. Potential diet triggers (citrus fruits, fizzy drinks, caffeine, cranberries, artificial sweeteners, or tomatoes) must be excluded and a correct hydration is mandatory (1.5–2 L fluid/day).

The management of vulvovaginal irritation depends on the preliminary conditions: first, correct hygienic behavior is recommended, and vaginal candidiasis should be excluded. Low-dose amitriptyline can be administered to give pain relief, and vulvar dermatological review and pelvic physiotherapy should be considered. Treatment of bowel symptoms includes the exclusion of serious underlying pathology symptoms, including blood or mucus per rectum, bowel incontinence, unexplained weight loss or malabsorption of food, correct diet, and low-dose amitriptyline for patients with bloated feeling.

Pudendal neuralgia is a CPP that causes a burning or sharp pain anywhere from the clitoris back to the anal area, when sitting. It may be uni- or bilateral and may be associated with increased clitoral arousal.[23]

Pudendal neuralgia requires avoiding activities that compress the nerve, pelvic physiotherapy, ceasing strain to the bowels or bladder, and neuropathic medications. Adenomyosis medical treatment options include Danazol and GnRH agonists. A selective progesterone receptor modulator (ulipristal acetate) was proposed as a new option in the pharmacological treatment of uterine fibroids in women.[24]

Interestingly, Vitamin D supplementation seems to reduce uterine fibroids progression and thus the need of conventional surgical or medical therapy.[25]

3.2. *Surgical treatment*

Surgical treatment includes interventions to resolve CPP, and the treatment of choice depends on the pathology: cervical dilatation resolves cervix stenosis, and myofascial pain in the pelvic and abdominal muscles is treated with trigger point injections. To alleviate chronic HPV-induced vulvodynia/vestibulitis, it is possible to resect or vaporize vulvar/vestibular tissues; vaporization of the uterosacral nerve is recommended for dysmenorrhea as well.

Laparotomic or laparoscopic myomectomy is an effective treatment for large intramural or subserosal leiomyomas, and a hysteroscopic resection is practiced for intracavitary submucous myomas or intracavitary polyps. An improvement in the quality of life can be achieved after uterine artery embolization. Adhesiolysis and enterolysis can help resolve pain due to adhesions. Salpingectomy is used for symptomatic hydrosalpinx; in case of endometriosis, resection of endometriosis spots can reduce symptoms. Appendectomy is the surgical treatment for chronic appendicitis symptoms, while uterine suspension is for dyspareunia, pelvic congestion, or severe dysmenorrhea. Hysterectomy is a radical treatment that can give relief if not achieved by organ-preserving surgery.

4. COMPLEMENTARY AND ALTERNATIVE MEDICINE

Complementary and alternative medicine (CAM) is a term used in the US to refer to a broad set of healthcare practices, systems, and products that are not part of the country's own tradition and are not integrated into the dominant healthcare system.[26,27] The boundaries between CAM and conventional medicine are not absolute, and specific CAM practices may, over time, become widely accepted.[27] The 2007 National Health Interview Survey from the US Department of Health showed that 38% of Americans used CAM therapies in the previous.[28] This was an increase from their previous survey in 2002 that showed that 33% of Americans had used CAM therapies in the previous year.[28] In this survey, approximately 32% of adults used CAM to treat different types of pain (back, neck, musculoskeletal).[28] The increase in the utilization of CAM, especially for pain, is observed in European countries and in Italy, even if there are no statistical data available at the moment.

4.1. *Acupuncture in CPP*

Acupuncture is one of the most commonly used complementary treatment for CPP, but still there are controversies on the efficacy of acupuncture and Traditional Chinese Medicine (TCM) in general. Acupuncture is a form of traditional Chinese treatment developed in China over 2,000 years ago and requires the insertion of fine needles into defined points distributed over the body surface to induce a local and systemic healing response. Treatment is usually given once a week, even if its frequency and duration is highly variable (i.e., two to three sessions a week for acute disease till once a month in stable conditions and from two to three sessions to several months in case of most complex conditions). The needles can be manipulated manually with heat or electrical stimulation to help relieve pain. The exact mechanism of how acupuncture produces analgesia is unknown but it has been thought to be mediated through the central nervous system.[10]

There are several techniques allied to acupuncture such as acupressure (shiatsu) in which appropriate points are massaged by the fingers, thumbs, or knuckles, or electroacupuncture, in which the acupuncture needles are stimulating by battery-powered pulse generators; but even if several scientific studies have been done on the effectiveness of this treatment, still there are no univocal results.

In literature, there are no trials of acupuncture relating specifically to CPP, but there are trials on acupuncture efficacy in relieving pain and symptoms of dysmenorrhoea, pelvic inflammatory disease, and irritating bowel syndrome, all of which are known to contribute to CPP. In their works Witt *et al.*[29] evidenced that acupuncture reduced the severity of dysmenorrhoea when compared to an untreated control group, and Smith *et al.*[30] found that acupuncture significantly reduced menstrual symptoms compared to standard nonsteroidal anti-inflammatory drugs (NSAIDs),[30] showing that acupuncture can be a potentially effective and safe treatment for pain management, without the risk of adverse gastrointestinal effects from NSAIDs.[31] Ozel *et al.*[32] studied acupuncture in the treatment of CPP secondary to pelvic inflammatory disease, and their preliminary results showed that acupuncture may be beneficial for chronic pelvic inflammatory disease symptoms.

A randomized controlled trial showed that the clinical therapeutic effect of superficial needling on primary dysmenorrhea is better than oral administration of indomethacin;[33] Helms[34] found a 41% reduction of analgesic medication after acupuncture treatment series; and Huyou *et al.*,[35] in a recent study, compared the clinical analgesic efficacy of two different acupuncture methods, finding that both methods have immediate and long-term analgesic effect on primary dysmenorrhea.[35]

A Cochrane review of acupuncture for irritable bowel disease reported clinically important improvements with acupuncture treatments, although there was little difference in outcomes between real and sham acupuncture treatments.

Nowadays, studies on the acupuncture effectiveness are still not univocal and scientific review often show skepticism about the effectiveness of this therapeutic approach: in a systematic review was found that traditional acupuncture was statistically significantly superior to pharmacological treatment for reducing dysmenorrhoea pain in five comparisons while in other five studies the same author found no significant difference between the two groups.[33,36–43]

Cochrane reviewers studied the effect of acupuncture versus a control to reduce menstrual pain and symptoms in all women of reproductive ages with primary dysmenorrhoea and in women with endometriosis. Cochrane found insufficient evidences to demonstrate that acupuncture is effective in treating primary dysmenorrhoea as well as poor effectiveness of acupuncture for pain in endometriosis. For both these studies, the main limitations were high risks of bias and poor reporting.

4.2. *Phytotherapy/herbal medicine*

Phytotherapy is also known as herbal medicine. Herbal medicine dates back as far as 5,000 years ago to the time of the Sumerians,[44] and throughout history, herbal medicine has been used in India, China, and Greece. In the US, herbal medicine is one of the most popular forms of CAM.

The 2007 National Health Interview Survey revealed that nonvitamin/nonmineral natural products made up 17.7% of CAM therapies utilized by American adults.[28] A 2008 analysis of the costs of CAM in the US revealed that Americans spent USD 14.8 billion on nonvitamin/nonmineral natural products.[26] Given their popularity, several herbal medicines have been used in CPP.

In China, the treatment of endometriosis using Chinese herbal medicine (CHM) is routine, and considerable research into the role of CHM in alleviating pain, promoting fertility, and preventing relapse has taken place. A review of the effectiveness and safety of CHM in alleviating endometriosis-related pain and infertility has been performed by Cochrane in 2012. The conclusions were that post-surgical administration of CHM may have comparable benefits to Gestrinone, but with fewer side effects. Oral CHM may have a better overall treatment effect than Danazol; it may be more effective in relieving dysmenorrhea and shrinking adnexal masses when used in conjunction with a CHM enema. However, more rigorous research is required to accurately assess the potential role of CHM in treating endometriosis.[45]

Evidence from seven small studies suggested that CHM as an independent intervention or in conjunction with antibiotics may be beneficial for treating recurrent urinary tract infections (UTIs) during the acute phase of infection and may reduce the recurrent UTI incidence for at least six months post-treatment. CHM treatments specifically formulated for recurrent UTI may be more effective than herbal treatments designed to treat acute UTI. However, the small number and poor quality of the included studies meant that it was not possible to formulate robust conclusions on the use of CHM for recurrent UTIs in women either alone or as an adjunct to antibiotics.

4.3. *Mind–body medicine and massage therapy*

Mind and body practices focus on the interactions among the brain, body, and behavior with the intent to use the mind to affect physical functioning and promote health. Many complementary health practices embody this concept, including massage, spinal manipulation, deep-breathing exercises, guided imagery, hypnotherapy, progressive relaxation, qi gong, and tai chi.

The 2007 National Health Interview Survey revealed that mind–body therapies made up 31.8% of CAM therapies utilized by American adults and that 19.9% of Americans had utilized mind–body therapies within the past year.[28] A 2008 analysis of the costs of CAM in the US revealed that Americans spent USD 4.1 billion dollars per year on various mind–body therapies.[26] Myofascial physical therapy (MPT) is another treatment modality that has been studied in CPP. For instance, 23 men and 24 women with either CPP or painful bladder syndrome were randomized to either MPT or global therapeutic massage (GTM) for one hour a week for 10 weeks. Patients randomized to MPT underwent connective tissue manipulation in clinically diagnosed myofascial trigger points along the abdominal wall, back, buttocks, thighs, as well as transvaginally and/or transrectally to release the trigger points. Patients randomized to GTM received weekly one hour massages consisting of effleurage, petrissage, friction, tapotement, vibration, and kneading. The results showed that MPT resulted in decreased symptom scores for both painful bladder syndrome and CPP ($p < 0.05$). GTM did not provide any significant relief of symptom scores for the painful bladder syndrome group, but resulted in improvements in the CPP group in domains of pain and quality of life ($p < 0.05$).[46] In a recent study, six women with CPP due to tender pelvic floor muscles were treated with Thiele massage. Thiele massage is a technique of transvaginal massage of the levator ani, obturator internus, and piriformis muscles. In this study, the patients underwent Thiele massage for five minutes, one time per week for four weeks. The results showed that, in this group of patients, the median tenderness score decreased from 3 at the first evaluation to 0 after one month of follow-up ($p < 0.01$). The patients' mean Visual Analogue Scale and McGill Pain Index scores also decreased from 8.1 and 34, respectively, to 1.5 and 16.6 ($p < 0.01$).[47] Mindful meditation has been shown to be helpful in patients with lower back pain, cancer pain, and migraine headaches. In one study, 22 women with CPP were enrolled in a mindful meditation program for eight weeks. Patients in the study were assessed daily with multiple scores that evaluate pain, mindfulness, and symptoms of depression. Only 12 out of the 22 participants who were enrolled completed the program. Overall, the participants that completed the trial had significant improvement in pain scores ($p = 0.02$), physical function ($p = 0.01$), mental health ($p = 0.01$), social function ($p = 0.02$), and mindfulness scores ($p < 0.01$).[48]

5. CONCLUSION

CPP is a general term that has been used in various parts of the medical literature for pain syndromes that result from different etiologies. Pain grouped in this category can be due to visceral irritation, muscular dysfunction, nerve damage, or genitourinary pain. Ideally, CPP should be studied according to etiology since each condition may respond to different therapeutic modalities. Conversely, it may be argued that despite various etiologies, CPP results from a common pathway; therefore, all or most pain types would respond to similar treatments. Many of the studies reviewed were not blinded or randomized, resulting in data that is harder to replicate. Furthermore, the studies used small sample sizes and need to be further powered to improve external validity. The recent literature for CPP in men is more extensive and focuses on herbal and acupuncture options. The literature in female patients is more centered on mind–body therapies.[49] The field of CPP would benefit from more prospective, well-powered studies that explore promising CAM therapies.

Whereas Western medicine assesses new treatments through controlled clinical trials, there are no absolute evidences that TCM is effective in the treatment of CPP. However, TCM have already been practiced extensively for over 2,000 years and offers a long history of clinical experience, and it has been shown to achieve a pain reduction in patients and may play an important role in the treatment of CPP.

REFERENCES

1. Fall, M., Baranowski, A. P., Elneil, S. *et al.* (2010). "EAU guidelines on chronic pelvic pain," *European Urology*, 57: 35–48.
2. Ghaly A. F. & Chien P. W. (2000). "Chronic pelvic pain: Clinical dilemma or clinician's nightmare," *Sexually Transmitted Infections*, 76: 419–425.
3. Mathias, S. D., Kuppermann, M., Liberman, R. F. *et al.* (1996). "Chronic pelvic pain: Prevalence, health-related quality of life, and economic correlates," *Obstetrics and Gynecology*, 87: 321–327.

4. Zondervan, K. T., Yudkin, P. L., Vessey, M. P. *et al.* (2001). "The community prevalence of chronic pelvic pain in women and associated illness behavior," *British Journal of General Practice*, 51: 541–547.
5. Grace, V. M. & Zondervan, K. T. (2004). "Chronic pelvic pain in New Zealand: Prevalence, pain severity, diagnoses and use of the health services," *Australian and New Zealand Journal of Public Health*, 28: 369–375.
6. Zondervan, K. T., Yudkin, P. L., Vessey, M. P. *et al.* (1999). "Prevalence and incidence of chronic pelvic pain in primary care: Evidence from a national general practice database," *British Journal of Obstetrics and Gynaecology*, 106: 1149–1155.
7. Simoens, S., Hummelshoj, L. & D'Hooghe, T. (2007). "Endometriosis: Cost estimates and methodological perspective," *Human Reproduction Update*, 13: 395–404.
8. Grace, V. M. & Zondervan. K. T. (2006). "Chronic pelvic pain in women in New Zealand: Comparative well-being, comorbidity, and impact on work and other activities," *Health Care for Women International*, 27: 585–599.
9. Pitts, M. K., Ferris, J. A., Smith, A. M. *et al.* (2008). "Prevalence and correlates of three types of pelvic pain in a nationally representative sample of Australian women," *Medical Journal of Australia*, 189: 138–143.
10. Gunter, J. (2003). "Chronic pelvic pain: An integrated approach to diagnosis and treatment," *Obstetrics and Gynecological Survey*, 58: 615–623.
11. Ahangari, A. (2014). "Prevalence of chronic pelvic pain among women: An updated review," *Pain Physician Journal*, 17(2): E141–E147.
12. Yosef, A., Allaire, C., Williams, C. *et al.* (2015). "Multifactorial contributors to the severity of chronic pelvic pain in women," *XXI International Federation of Gynecology and Obstetrics World Congress of Gynecology and Obstetrics*, Vancouver, British Columbia, Canada, October 4–9.
13. Royal College of Obstetrician and Gynaecologist (2012). The Initial Management of Chronic Pelvic Pain Green. Top Guideline No. 41, May.
14. American College of Obstetrician and Gynecologists (2004). Clinical Management Guidelines for Obstetrician-Gynecologists No. 51, March.
15. Howard, F. M. (2000). "The role of laparoscopy as a diagnostic tool in chronic pelvic pain," *Best Practice & Research Clinical Obstetrics & Gynaecology*, 14: 467–494.
16. Alappattu, M. J. & Bishop, M. D. (2011). "Psychological factors in chronic pelvic pain in women: Relevance and application of the fear-avoidance model of pain," *Physical Therapy*, 91(10): 1542–1550.
17. Romão, A., Gorayeb, R., Romão, G. *et al.* (2009). "High levels of anxiety and depression have a negative effect on quality of life of women with

chronic pelvic pain," *International Journal of Clinical Practice*, 63(5): 707–711.

18. Stones, R. W. & Mountfield, J. (2000). "Interventions for treating chronic pelvic pain in women," *Cochrane Database of Systematic Reviews*, (4): CD000387.
19. Andrews, J., Yunker, A., Reynolds, *et al.* (2012). *Noncyclic Chronic Pelvic Pain Therapies for Women: Comparative Effectiveness.* AHRQ Publication No. 11(12)-EHC088-EF (Agency for Healthcare Research and Quality; Rockville, MD, USA).
20. Butrick, C. W. (2007). "Chronic pelvic pain: How many surgeries are enough?" *Clinical Obstetrics and Gynecology*, 50: 412–424.
21. Lau, T. C. & Bengtson, J. M. (2010). "Management strategies for painful bladder syndrome," *Review of Obstetrics and Gynecology*, 3: 42–48.
22. Brown, C. S., Franks, A. S., Wan, J. *et al.* (2008). "Citalopram in the treatment of women with chronic pelvic pain," *Journal of Reproductive Medicine*, 53, 191–195.
23. Pérez-López, F. R. & Hita-Contreras, F. "Management of pudendal neuralgia," *Climacteric*, 17: 654–656.
24. Streuli, I., Dubuisson, J., Santulli, P. *et al.* (2014). "An update on the pharmacological management of adenomyosis," *Expert Opinion on Pharmacotherapy*, 15(16): 2347–2360.
25. Ciavattini A., Delli Carpini, G., Serri, M. *et al.* (2016). "Hypovitaminosis D and "small burden" uterine fibroids: Opportunity for a vitamin D supplementation," *Medicine (Baltimore)*, 95(52): e5698.
26. Nahin, R. L., Barnes, P. M., Stussman, B. J. *et al.* (2007). "Statistics costs of complementary and alternative medicine (CAM) and frequency of visits to CAM practitioners." US National Health Statistics Report.
27. Hawk, C., Ndetan, H. & Evans, M. W. Jr. (2012). "Potential role of complementary and alternative health care providers in chronic disease prevention and health promotion: An analysis of National Health Interview Survey data," *Preventive Medicine*, 54(1): 18–22.
28. Birdee, G. S., Kemper, K. J., Rothman, R. & Gardiner, P. (2014). "National Center for Complementary and Integrative Health. Use of complementary and alternative medicine during pregnancy and the postpartum period: An analysis of the National Health Interview Survey," *J Womens Health (Larchmt)*, 23(10): 824–829.
29. Witt, C. M., Reinhold, T., Brinkhaus, B. *et al.* (2008). "Acupuncture in patients with dysmenorrhea: A randomized study on clinical effectiveness and cost-effectiveness in usual care," *American Journal of Obstetrics and Gynecology*, 198: 166.e1–166.e8.

30. Smith, C. A., Armour, M., Zhu, X. *et al.* (2016). "Acupuncture for dysmenorrhoea," *Cochrane Database of Systematic Reviews*, (4). Art. No.: CD007854. doi: 10.1002/14651858.CD007854.pub3.
31. RCOG Guidelines. 2012, (updated 2015). Acupuncture and Chinese Herbal Medicine for Women with Chronic Pelvic Pain (Scientific Impact Paper No. 30).
32. Ozel, A., Ozel, A., Arslan, H. *et al.* (2011). "Acupuncture in the treatment of chronic pelvic pain secondary to pelvic inflammatory disease," *Acupuncture Medicine*, 29: 317318.
33. Zhi, L. X. (2007). "Randomized controlled study on superficial needling for treatment of primary dysmenorrhea," *Zhongguo Zhen Jiu*, 27: 18–21.
34. Helms, J. M. (1987). "Acupuncture for the management of primary dysmenorrhea," *Obstetrics and Gynecology*, 69(1): 51–56.
35. Huyou-Ping, Zhang, X., Zhang, L. X. *et al.* (2013). "Time-effect study on instant analgesic effect of the dragon-tiger fighting needling method on primary dysmenorrhea," *Zhongguo Zhen jiu = Chinese Acupuncture & Moxibustion*, 33(11): 1005–1009.
36. Cho, S. H. & Hwang, E. W. (2010). "Acupuncture for primary dysmenorrhoea: A systematic review," *BJOG*, 117(5): 509–521.
37. Jiang, L. Y. (2007). "Needling acupuncture for 34 cases of primary dysmenorrhea," *Journal of Emerging Traditional Chinese Medicine*, 16: 620–621.
38. Zhang, M. & Sun, S. T. (2003). "Clinical observation of acupuncture therapy for 32 cases of primary dysmenorrhea," *Journal of Chinese Science & Technology and Traditional Chinese Medicine*, 10: 322.
39. Zhou, L. S. (2003). "Clinical observation of needling acupuncture on BL32 for primary dysmenorrhea," *Journal of Chinese Medicine Hubei*, 25: 47.
40. Han, J. S., Li, B. T. & Zhao, H. R. (1998). "Acupuncture therapy for primary dysmenorrhea," *Med Aeronaut Astronaut*, 9: 26–27.
41. Liu, Y. L. (2005). "Clinical observation of acupoint injection with vitamin k3 on SP6 for primary dysmenorrhea," *Journal of Chinese Medicine Liaoning*, 32: 11856.
42. Shi, X. L., Yang, A. M. & Li, F. Z. (1994). "Effect analysis of needling acupuncture on SP6 for 120 cases of primary dysmenorrhea," *Zhongguo Zhen Jiu*, 14: 17–18.
43. Zhu, X., Hamilton, K. D. & McNicol, E. D. (2011). "Acupuncture for pain in endometriosis," *Cochrane Database of Systematic Reviews*, (9): CD007864.
44. Petrovska, B. B. (2012). "Historical review of medicinal plants' usage," *Pharmacognosy Reviews*, 6(11): 1–5.

45. Flower, A., Liu, J. P., Lewith, G. *et al.* (2012). "Chinese herbal medicine for endometriosis," *Cochrane Database of Systematic Reviews*, (5): CD006568.
46. Carinci, A., Pathak, R., Young, M. *et al.* (2013). "Complementary and alternative treatments for chronic pelvic pain," *Current Pain and Headache Reports*, 17: 316.
47. Montenegro, M. L., Mateus-Vasconcelos, E. C., Candido dos Reis, F. J. *et al.* (2010). "Thiele massage as a therapeutic option for women with chronic pelvic pain caused by tenderness of pelvic floor muscles," *Journal of Evaluation of Clinical Practice*, 16(5): 981–982.
48. Fox, S. D., Flynn, E., Allen, R. H. (2011). "Mindfulness meditation for women with chronic pelvic pain: A pilot study," *Journal of Reproductive Medicine*, 56(3–4): 158–162.
49. Adam, J. C., Ravi, P., Mark, Y. *et al.* (2013). "Complementary and alternative treatments for chronic pelvic pain," *Current Pain Headache Reports*, 17: 316.

Chapter 30

The Role of the CAG Polymorphism of the Androgen Receptor in Conditioning Male Metabolic Profile

Gianmaria Salvio, Giacomo Tirabassi, Monica Mattioli Belmonte, Roberto Di Primio and Giancarlo Balercia

1. INTRODUCTION

The effect of testosterone and its main metabolite dihydrotestosterone (DHT) on cardiovascular risk in men has been largely studied during last years,[1–5] and special attention has been paid to the CAG tract polymorphism of androgen receptor (AR). AR, in fact, is an intracellular receptor that is the specific target of testosterone and DHT and its binding is necessary for action of androgen hormones. Furthermore, AR gene is located at chromosome Xq11–12, which has 8 exons[6] and the exon 1, that encode for a protein linked to AR transcriptional activity,[7] contains a polymorphic segment. This is a sequence of CAG trinucleotide repeats that usually varies from 10 to 35 and, as supported by a large quantity of evidence,[8,9] is able to condition the peripheral effects of testosterone. In fact, many studies suggest that length of CAG repeat is negatively associated with the AR transcriptional activity and, consequently, with testosterone effect.[10–13]

Some authors,[14–16] but not others[17–19] have also reported that longer AR CAG sequences carry higher circulating levels of testosterone, suggesting that the lower AR activity could be adequately compensated by increased serum testosterone, without clinical symptoms of hypogonadism.[14]

2. SEXUAL FUNCTION

Previous studies supported the hypothesis that the length of CAG polymorphism can influence sexual function, reporting an increased risk of developing erectile dysfunction[20] and andropausal symptoms[21] in patients with normal testosterone levels and longer CAG repeats. Furthermore, a shorter CAG repeat number is associated with a better recovery of male sexual function during testosterone replacement therapy (TRT) for subjects affected by post-surgical hypogonadotropic hypogonadism[11] and late-onset hypogonadism.[22]

2.1. *Male fertility*

The correlation between the number of CAG repeats and male fertility has been largely debated. In 2010, Mifsud *et al.*[23] evaluated the correlation between sperm parameters and size of CAG sequence of AR in 357 patients of which 215 presented male infertility. They observed that some men with azoospermia had significantly longer CAG alleles than fertile controls and also reported that the CAG length was directly correlated to the severity of the spermatogenic defect, showing that ≥26 CAG repeats were associated with a sevenfold higher risk of azoospermia. Those findings were in line with previous studies[24–26] but not with others. In fact, a meta-analysis of Nenonen *et al.*[27] showed no difference in the average CAG repeat number between fertile and infertile men in the nearly 4,000 subjects evaluated, in accordance with previous *in vitro* data from the same authors.[28] Thus, more studies are required to establish the effective role of CAG repeats in male reproductive function.

2.2. *Prostate cancer*

As far as the relationship between prostate cancer and number of CAG repeats is concerned, the presence of circulating androgen hormones is necessary to stimulate the growth of an existing tumor, even if there is no evidence that they may activate the process of carcinogenesis.[29] In fact, AR can inhibit p53 accumulation in the nucleus of human prostate adenocarcinoma cells, inducing growth and survival.[13] Thus, the tissues' sensitivity to testosterone, which seems to be influenced by size of CAG sequence, should play a key role in the pathogenesis of this kind of neoplasia. For this purpose, Gu *et al.*,[30] in 2012, conducted a meta-analysis on 27 different studies, finding a possible protective effect for CAG repeat polymorphism with >20 repeats in patients aged 45 years and older.

2.3. *Bone metabolism*

The effect of CAG polymorphism on bone metabolism is unclear. Some authors reported no association between the number of CAG repeats and bone mineral density (BMD),[31] whereas others advocated an inverse correlation between the CAG sequence length and value of BMD, due to the lesser effect of testosterone on bone.[32] Furthermore, in 2014, our group found that patients treated with TRT for hypogonadotropic hypogonadism have an improvement in BMD independently associated with a shorter AR CAG tract.[33]

2.4. *Testicular cancer*

Concerning testicular cancer (TC), men with androgen insensitivity syndrome caused by AR gene mutations have a higher risk of developing TC. Jing *et al.*,[34] in a recent meta-analysis involving over 3,000 TC cases, reported an increased risk of TC in patients with longer GGN repeats in AR, whereas a significant association was found between CAG repeats and TC in the population-based, mid-latitude, high-latitude, seminoma, and nonseminoma subgroups. Furthermore, they observed that CAG repeat polymorphisms with >25 and <21 + >25 repeats were associated with an increased risk in the mid-latitude subgroup but were associated with a decreased risk of TC in the high-latitude subgroup, suggesting that latitude may play a key role in the effect of CAG polymorphism on the risk of TC. Furthermore, previous studies reported a higher risk of TC for patients with CAG sequence in AR longer than 25 repeats,[35,36] whereas others correlated the CAG repeat length with the clinical stage of TC, indicating that longer sequences are associated with advanced disease at diagnosis.[35]

2.5. *Psychiatric status*

The influence of CAG polymorphism on male psychic state is interesting. Mannin[37] suggests that, within the range of 11–30 repeats, subjects with shorter sequences present a higher speed of neuronal transmission and values of general intelligence. Furthermore, other authors[38] have recently observed that patients with intermediate levels of serum testosterone and number of CAG repeats, rather than extreme values of these parameters, show a better attitude to partnering and fathering. Moreover, levels of testosterone and the length of CAG repeats have also been correlated to symptoms of depression,[39] self-reported measures of dominance and prestige,[40] violent behavior,[41] and impulsivity.[42] In addition, shorter CAG tracts have been associated with Attention Deficit Hyperactivity Disorder and conduct disorder.[43]

2.6. *Neurodegenerative disorders*

Trinucleotide repeat expansions are implicated in many neuromuscular diseases, including the fragile X syndrome, Huntington disease, spinocerebellar ataxia type 1, dentatorubral-pallidoluysian atrophy, Machado–Joseph disease, and Friedrich ataxia.[44] In the same manner, CAG polymorphism in AR is related to spinal-bulbar muscular atrophy (SBMA), an adult-onset neurodegenerative disorder characterized by progressive muscle weakness and atrophy due to the degeneration of the motor neuron located in the spinal and bulbar regions.[45] The length of the CAG sequence is directly proportional to the severity of symptoms and to the earlier onset of disease.[46] The expansion in the AR gene seems to cause an abnormal nuclear accumulation of the AR protein, with subsequent transcriptional dysregulation, axonal transport disruption, and finally, mitochondrial dysfunction,[45] resulting in neurodegeneration.

3. METABOLIC PROFILE

The term metabolic syndrome (MetS) refers to a combination of pathological conditions, e.g., obesity, hypertension, dyslipidemia, and hyperglycemia; expression of insulin resistance; and associated to an increased cardiovascular risk.[47] The relationship between metabolic risk and CAG polymorphism is unclear, as well as the relationship between metabolic risk and testosterone. In this regard, some findings show a significant association between low total testosterone levels and the prevalence of MetS.[48,49] Recently, Canguven *et al.*[50] conducted a study on 88 male subjects affected by late-onset hypogonadism (LOH) who underwent TRT with 1,000 mg testosterone undecanoate for one year. They show a steady decrease in waist circumference greater than 4.61 cm, in total cholesterol (from 5 ± 1.22 to 4.37 ± 0.92 mmol/L), in triglycerides (from 2.03 ± 0.97 to 1.79 ± 0.91 mmol/L), and in the level of HbA1c (from 8.06 ± 2.93 to 6.92 ± 1.74%). A recent review from Anaisse *et al.*[51] highlighted the correlation between male hypogonadism and obesity, insulin resistance, dyslipidemia, hypertension, and cardiovascular disease, demonstrating that TRT has a positive effect on each factor of MetS. Furthermore, results from a study by Permpongkosol *et al.*,[52] conducted on 120 subjects with LOH treated for eight-year with long-acting testosterone undecanoate have shown a significant decrease in waist circumference, percentage of body fat, total cholesterol, LDL cholesterol, and HbA1c.

On the other hand, some authors have also reported a protective effect of hypogonadism from major adverse cardiovascular events,[53] suggesting that low testosterone levels could represent a protective mechanism in unhealthy conditions. Furthermore, in the past years, three major studies[54–56] reported an increased cardiovascular risk in subjects who underwent TRT.

Therefore, data are conflicting and, in this context, the role of CAG polymorphism in influencing metabolic profile in men has not been clearly established.

The first study showing an association between CAG repeat length and risk of MetS was the one by Skjaerpe *et al.*[57] in 2009. The study was conducted on 68 men with low levels of testosterone and 104 men with normal levels of testosterone, all of them aged between 60 and 80 years, evaluating anthropometric measures (body weight, height, waist circumference, and blood pressure) and serum glucose metabolism with serum glucose levels and oral glucose tolerance test. They found a lower number of CAG repeats in men with less favorable metabolic profile, showing an association that did not change after adjustment for testosterone levels.

Haring *et al.*,[58] instead, reported no direct association between CAG repeat length and cardiometabolic risk factors, but they also reported that CAG repeat length could be an important contributing factor in the association of low testosterone concentrations with incident MetS, since subjects with longer CAG repeats and low testosterone concentrations had the highest risk of incident MetS. In contrast, Alevizaki *et al.*[59] found an inverse association between the severity of coronary artery disease (CAD) and the number of CAG repeats, suggesting that men with more severe CAD could have an increased sensitivity to androgens.[59] Furthermore, some authors reported no association between CAG repeats and levels of gonadal steroids or lipid levels.[19]

An interesting work focused on the metabolic effects of TRT in patients with post-surgical hypogonadotropic hypogonadism, a particular type of hypogonadism. In this work, the authors reported a significant improvement in all metabolic variables after TRT and, in particular, that the shorter length of the CAG repeat polymorphism promotes the improvement of the cardiovascular risk factors after TRT.[60]

Concerning body composition, it has been reported that a lower number of CAG repeats in the AR gene could favor the fat accumulation in adolescent boys,[61] whereas in physically active adult men, the length of the CAG polymorphism seems to have little or no effect on adiposity and its regional distribution.[62] In contrast, the shorter length of the AR CAG repeat tract seems to be independently associated with abdominal fat decrease in men receiving TRT for post-surgical hypogonadotropic hypogonadism.[12] Additionally, in a study conducted on 99 healthy older men and 113 healthy postmenopausal women, GGN and CAG repeats have been combined to evaluate the relationship between those alleles and indices of obesity, and the authors found that AR gene polymorphisms are significantly related to body shape in older subjects, especially in women.[63]

Another study, instead, has shown a direct relationship between fat-free mass and CAG repeat length. Furthermore, authors also reported increasing serum testosterone levels for higher AR CAG repeat number and, consequently, between testosterone and fat-free mass,[15] as reported by others.[64]

In a study conducted on 129 elderly men aged 75–89 years, Lapauw *et al.*[65] have reported no direct association between CAG repeat length and body composition. Anyway, a deeper analysis revealed that CAG repeat number, albeit modestly, can modulate the effect of testosterone on body composition.[65]

Campbell *et al.*,[66] in 2007, conducted a study on 156 lean subjects with an average body fat of 10% and an average BMI of 17.8 ± 1.9 kg/m^2. He found that the AR CAG repeat length was significantly and related to fat-free mass and height. This last finding suggests the hypothesis that longer CAG repeats could result in less effective testosterone exposure of long bones during puberty, and, consequently, to a prolonged growth.[66]

Results from the TIMES2 (testosterone replacement in hypogonadal men with either metabolic syndrome or type 2 diabetes), a multicenter, randomized, double-blind, and placebo-controlled study, have shown that treatment with transdermal testosterone is able to reduce insulin resistance assessed by HOMA-IR after six months.[67] In a subsequent analysis from the same study, Stanworth *et al.*[16] have analyzed the effect of AR CAG in modulating the effect of TRT on insulin resistance, lipids, body composition, and other clinical parameters. The authors reported no association between the length of CAG repeats and change in waist, BMI, body fat, total cholesterol, LDL cholesterol, lipoprotein-a, and systolic pressure, but they observed a significant reduction in the levels of fasting insulin and triglycerides and in values of diastolic pressure, with a greater decrease in patients with shorter AR CAG and, consequently, a greater androgenic effect.

A study conducted on a cohort of 113 nondiabetic subjects[68] has shown no direct relationship between the AR CAG repeat length and insulin resistance as determined by HOMA-IR, in line with previous data,[14] but authors also reported that, for short CAG lengths, increasing free testosterone concentrations appeared to worsen insulin sensitivity. Furthermore, this effect was attenuated with rising CAG length, until it turned to the opposite effect for CAG length >23. At normal free testosterone concentrations, instead, the impact of the CAG length on insulin sensitivity was minimal, suggesting that modulation by the CAG repeat length could be more significant for patients with mild-to-moderate low testosterone levels, as in LOH.[68]

A study conducted in 233 men with type 2 diabetes has evaluated the relationship between CAG repeat polymorphism length, sex hormones, clinical indexes of obesity, and leptin, showing an independent association of AR CAG repeat length with waist circumference, BMI, and leptin, whereas testosterone was negatively associated with BMI, waist circumference, and leptin. Furthermore, a positive association of testosterone and LH levels with AR CAG polymorphism has been reported, suggesting a role for AR in the negative feedback of testosterone in the hypothalamic–pituitary–gonadals axis.[16]

A recent publication found no association between CAG polymorphism length and clinical parameters defined as androgen-sensitive endpoints such as body composition parameters (BMI, waist circumference, and mid-upper arm circumference), fasting plasma glucose, insulin resistance (HOMA-IR), blood pressure, and sexual, physical, or psychological function.[18] According to another study, subjects with shorter AR alleles seems to be associated with lower levels of HDL-cholesterol, but they have no increased risk for coronary heart disease or myocardial infarction in two independent case-control studies.[69] Another recent work also reported lower levels of HDL-cholesterol in subjects with <22 CAG repeats, and authors have also reported an increased risk of hypertension, maybe due to an activation of the sympathetic vasomotor tone mediated by testosterone,[70] that could impair endothelial response to ischemia, as observed by others.[32]

Zitzmann *et al.*[71] reported a modulatory effect of CAG polymorphism in the AR gene within the body composition/insulin/leptin secretion-complex: they observed that higher a CAG repeat number are associated with an impaired androgenic effect of testosterone, with adverse effects on fat mass and insulin sensitivity.[71] In a previous study, however, they reported that shorter CAG repeats are associated with decreased levels of HDL and reduced endothelial response to ischemia (assessed by flow-mediated dilatation).[32] Thus, they concluded that the CAG polymorphism probably modulates cardiovascular risk factors both adversely and beneficially, depending on co-factors.[71]

In conclusion, the influence of AR CAG polymorphism on the metabolic profile seems complicated, and actual data from the literature are, in part, conflicting. Anyway, the argument is fascinating, and further studies would be useful to elucidate this complex relationship.

REFERENCES

1. Tirabassi, G., Gioia, A., Giovannini, L., Boscaro, M., Corona, G., Carpi, A., Maggi, M. & Balercia, G. (2013). "Testosterone and cardiovascular risk," *Internal and Emergency Medicine*, 1: S65–S69.
2. Rosano, G. M., Vitale, C. & Fini, M. (2015). "Testosterone in men with hypogonadism and high cardiovascular risk," *Endocrine*, 50: 320–325.
3. Bekaert, M., Van Nieuwenhove, Y., Calders, P., Cuvelier, C. A., Batens, A. H., Kaufman, J. M., Ouwens, D. M. & Ruige, J. B. (2015). "Determinants of testosterone levels in human male obesity," *Endocrine*, 50: 202–211.
4. Buysschaert, M., Medina, J. L., Bergman, M., Shah, A. & Lonier, J. (2015). "Prediabetes and associated disorders," *Endocrine*, 48: 371–393.
5. Mitsuhashi, K., Senmaru, T., Fukuda, T. *et al.* (2016). "Testosterone stimulates glucose uptake and GLUT4 translocation through LKB1/ AMPK signaling in 3T3-L1 adipocytes," *Endocrine*, 51: 174–184.
6. Casella, R., Maduro, M. R., Lipshultz, L. I. *et al.* (2001). "Significance of the polyglutamine tract polymorphism in the androgen receptor," *Urology*, 58: 651–656.
7. Simental, J. A., Sar, M., Lane, M. V. *et al.* (1991). "Transcriptional activation and nuclear targeting signals of the human androgen receptor," *Journal of Biological Chemistry*, 266: 510–518.
8. Ding, D., Xu, L., Menon, M., Reddy, G. P. & Barrack, E. R. (2005). "Effect of GGC (glycine) repeat length polymorphism in the human androgen receptor on androgen action," *Prostate*, 62: 133–139.
9. Tirabassi, G., Biagioli, A. & Balercia, G. (2014). "Bone benefits of testosterone replacement therapy in male hypogonadism," *Panminerva Medica*, 56: 151–163.

10. Tirabassi, G., Cignarelli, A., Perrini, S. *et al.* (2015). "Influence of CAG repeat polymorphism on the targets of testosterone action," *International Journal of Endocrinology*, 29: 8107.
11. Tirabassi, G. *et al.* (2014). "Androgen receptor gene CAG repeat polymorphism independently influences recovery of male sexual function after testosterone replacement therapy in post-surgical hypogonadotropic hypogonadism," *Journal of Sexual Medicine*, 11: 1302–1308.
12. Tirabassi, G. *et al.* (2014). "Central body fat changes in men affected by post-surgical hypogonadotropic hypogonadism undergoing testosterone replacement therapy are modulated by androgen receptor CAG polymorphism," *Nutrition Metabolism*, 24: 908–913.
13. Nantermet, P. V., Xu, J., Yu, Y., Hodor, P., Holder, D., Adamski, S. *et al.* (2004). "Identification of genetic pathways activated by the androgen receptor during the induction of proliferation in the ventral prostate gland," *Journal of Biological Chemistry*, 279: 1310–1322.
14. Platt, H., Payne, D., John, S. L., Jiang, M. *et al.* (2009). "Increased estrogen rather than decreased androgen action is associated with longer androgen receptor CAG repeats," *Journal of Clinical Endocrinology and Metabolism*, 94: 277–284.
15. Walsh, S., Zmuda, J. M., Cauley, J. A., Shea, P. R., Metter, E. J., Hurley, B. F., Ferrell, R. E. & Roth, S. M. (1985). "Androgen receptor CAG repeat polymorphism is associated with fat-free mass in men," *Journal of Applied Physiology*, 98: 132–137.
16. Stanworth, R. D., Kapoor, D., Channer, K. S. & Jones, T. H. (2008). "Androgen receptor CAG repeat polymorphism is associated with serum testosterone levels, obesity and serum leptin in men with type 2 diabetes," *European Journal of Endocrinology*, 159: 739–746.
17. Ryan, C. P., McDade, T. W., Gettler, L. T., Eisenberg, D. T., Rzhetskaya, M., Hayes, M. G. & Kuzawa, C. W. (2017). "Androgen receptor CAG repeat polymorphism and hypothalamic-pituitary-gonadal function in Filipino young adult males," *American Journal of Human Biology*, 29.
18. Eendebak, R. J., Huhtaniemi, I. T., Pye, S. R. *et al.* (2016). "The androgen receptor gene CAG repeat in relation to four-year changes in androgen-sensitive endpoints in community-dwelling older European men," *European Journal of Endocrinology*, 175: 583–593.
19. Goutou, M., Sakka, C., Stakias, N., Stefanidis, I. & Koukoulis, G. N. "AR CAG repeat length is not associated with serum gonadal steroids and lipid levels in healthy men," *International Journal of Andrology*, 32: 616–622.

20. Liu, C. C., Lee, Y. C., Tsai, V. F. *et al.* (2015). "The interaction of serum testosterone levels and androgen receptor CAG repeat polymorphism on the risk of erectile dysfunction in aging Taiwanese men," *Andrology*, 3: 902–908.
21. Liu, C. C., Lee, Y. C., Wang, C. J. *et al.* (2012). "The impact of androgen receptor CAG repeat polymorphism on andropausal symptoms in different serum testosterone levels," *The Journal of Sexual Medicine*, 9: 2429–2437.
22. Tirabassi, G., Corona, G., Biagioli, A. *et al.* (2015). "Influence of androgen receptor CAG polymorphism on sexual function recovery after testosterone therapy in late-onset hypogonadism," *Journal of Sexual Medicine*, 12: 381–388.
23. Mifsud, A., Sim, C. K. S., Boettger-Tong, H. *et al.* (2001). "Trinucleotide (CAG) repeat polymorphisms in the androgen receptor gene: Molecular markers of risk for male infertility," *Fertility and Sterility*, 75: 275–281.
24. Tut, T. G., Ghadessy, F. J., Trifiro, M. A., Pinsky, L. & Yong, E. L. J. (1997). "Long polyglutamine tracts in the androgen receptor are associated with reduced trans-activation, impaired sperm production, and male infertility," *Journal of Clinical Endocrinology & Metabolism*, 82: 3777–3782.
25. Dowsing, A. T., Yong, E. L., Clark, M., McLachlan, R. I., de Kretser, D. M. & Trounson, A. O. (1999). "Linkage between male infertility and trinucleotide repeat expansion in the androgen-receptor gene," *Lancet*, 354: 640–643.
26. Patrizio, P., Leonard, D. G. B., Chen, K.-L., Hernandez-Ayup, S., Trounson, A. O. (2001). "Larger rinucleotide repeat size in the androgen receptor gene of infertile men with extremely severe oligozoospermia," *Journal of Andrology*, 22: 444–448.
27. Nenonen, H., Giwercman, A., Hallengren, E. & Giwercman, Y. L. (2011). "Nonlinear association between androgen receptor CAG repeat length and risk of male subfertility — a meta-analysis," *International Journal of Andrology*, 34: 327–332.
28. Nenonen, H., Björk, C., Skjaerpe, P. A. *et al.* (2010). "CAG repeat number is not inversely associated with androgen receptor activity *in vitro*," *Molecular Human Reproduction*, 6: 153–157.
29. Wilding, G. *et al.* (1992). "The importance of steroid hormones in prostate cancer," *Cancer Surveys*, 13: 113–130.
30. Gu, M., Dong, X., Zhang, X., Niu, W. (2012). "The CAG repeat polymorphism of androgen receptor gene and prostate cancer: A meta-analysis," *Molecular Biology Reports*, 39: 2615–2624.

31. Kenny, A. M., McGee, D., Joseph, C., Covault, J., Abreu, C., Raisz, L. G. (2005). "Lack of association between androgen receptor polymorphisms and bone mineral density or physical function in older men," *Endocrine Research*, 31: 285–293.
32. Zitzmann, M., Brune, M., Kornmann, B., Gromoll, J., Junker, R. & Nieschlag, E. (2001). "The CAG repeat polymorphism in the androgen receptor gene affects bone density and bone metabolism in healthy males," *Clinical Endocrinology*, 55: 649–657.
33. Tirabassi, G., delli Muti, N., Gioia, A. *et al.* (2014). "Effects of testosterone replacement therapy on bone metabolism in male post-surgical hypogonadotropic hypogonadism: Focus on the role of androgen receptor CAG polymorphism," *Journal of Endocrinal Investigation*, 37: 393–400.
34. Jiang, W., Zhang, J., Zhou, Q., Liu, S., Ni, M., Zhu, P., Wu, Q., Li, W., Zhang, M. & Xia, X. (2016). "Predictive value of GGN and CAG repeat polymorphisms of androgen receptors in testicular cancer: A meta-analysis," *Oncotarget*, 7: 13754–13764.
35. Giwercman, A., Lundin, K. B., Eberhard, J. *et al.* (2004). "Linkage between androgen receptor gene CAG trinucleotide repeat length and testicular germcell cancer histological type and clinical stage," *European Journal of Cancer*, 40: 2152–2158.
36. Grassetti, D., Giannandrea, F., Paoli, D. *et al.* (2015). "Androgen receptor polymorphisms and testicular cancer risk," *Andrology*, 3: 27–33.
37. Manning, J. (2007). "The androgen receptor gene: a major modifier of speed of neuronal transmission and intelligence?" *Medical Hypotheses*, 68: 802–804.
38. Gettler, L. T., Ryan, C. P., Eisenberg, D. T. *et al.* (2017). "The role of testosterone in coordinating male life history strategies: The moderating effects of the androgen receptor CAG repeat polymorphism," *Hormones & Behavior*, 87: 164–175.
39. Sankar, J. S. & Hampson, E. (2012). "Testosterone levels and androgen receptor gene polymorphism predict specific symptoms of depression in young men," *Gender Medicine*, 9: 232–243.
40. Simmons, Z. L. & Roney, J. R. (2011). "Variation in CAG repeat length of the androgen receptor gene predicts variables associated with intrasexual competitiveness in human males," *Hormones and Behavior*, 60: 306–312.
41. Rajender, S., Pandu, G., Sharma, J. D. *et al.* (2008). "Reduced CAG repeats length in androgen receptor gene is associated with violent criminal behavior," *International Journal of Legal Medicine*, 122: 367–372.
42. Aluja, A., Garcia, F. L., Blanch, A. & Fibla, J. (2011). "Association of androgen receptor gene, CAG and GGN repeat length polymorphism and

impulsive-disinhibited personality traits in inmates: The role of short-long haplotype," *Psychiatric Genetics*, 21: 229–239.

43. Comings, D. E., Chen, C., Wu, S. & Muhleman, D. (1999). "Association of the androgen receptor gene (AR) with ADHD and conduct disorder," *NeuroReport*, 10: 1589–1592.
44. Mitas, M. (1997). "Trinucleotide repeats associated with human disease," *Nucleic Acids Research*, 25: 2245–2254.
45. Katsuno, M., Banno, H., Suzuki, K., Adachi, H., Tanaka, F. & Sobue, G. (2010). "Clinical features and molecular mechanisms of spinal and bulbar-muscular atrophy (SBMA)," *Advances in Experimental Medicine and Biology*, 685: 64–74.
46. Francomano, D., Greco, E. A., Lenzi, A. & Aversa, A. (2013). "CAG repeat testing of androgen receptor polymorphism: Is this necessary for the best clinical management of hypogonadism?" *Journal of Sexual Medicine*, 10: 2373–2381.
47. Lindblad, U., Langer, R. D., Wingard, D. L., Thomas, R. G., Barrett-Connor, E. L.(2001). "Metabolic syndrome and ischemic heart disease in elderly men and women," *American Journal of Epidemiology*, 153: 481–489.
48. Corona, G., Monami, M., Rastrelli, G. *et al.* (2011). "Testosterone and metabolic syndrome: A meta-analysis study," *Journal of Sexual Medicine*, 8: 272–283.
49. Brand, J. S., van der Tweel, I., Grobbee, D. E. *et al.* (2010). "Testosterone, sex hormone-binding globulin and the metabolic syndrome: A systematic review and meta-analysis of observational studies," *International Journal of Epidemiology*, 24. doi: 10.1093/ije/dyq158.
50. Canguven, O. *et al.* (2017). "Testosterone therapy has positive effects on anthropometric measures, metabolic syndrome components (obesity, lipid profile, Diabetes Mellitus control), blood indices, liver enzymes, and prostate health in elderly hypogonadal men," *Andrologia*, e12768 (In press).
51. Anaissie, J., Roberts, N. H., Wang, P. & Yafi, F. A. (2017). "Testosterone replacement therapy and components of the metabolic syndrome," *Sexual Medicine Review*, 5: 200–210.
52. Permpongkosol, S. *et al.* (2016). "Effects of eight-year treatment of long-acting testosterone undecanoate on metabolic parameters, urinary symptoms, bone mineral density, and sexual function in men with late-onset hypogonadism," *Journal of Sexual Medicine*, 13: 1199–1211.
53. Corona, G., Rastrelli, G., Maseroli, E. *et al.* (2014). "Low testosterone syndrome protects subjects with high cardiovascular risk burden from major adverse cardiovascular events," *Andrology*, 2: 741–747.

54. Vigen, R. *et al.* (2013). "Association of testosterone therapy with mortality, myocardial infarction, and stroke in men with low testosterone levels," *JAMA*, 310: 1829–1836.
55. Finkle, W. D., Greenland, S., Ridgeway, G. K., Adams, J. L., Frasco, M. A., Cook, M. B., Fraumeni, J. F. Jr., Hoover, R. N. (2014). "Increased risk of non-fatal myocardial infarction following testosterone therapy prescription in men," *PLoS ONE*, 9: e85805.
56. Basaria, S. *et al.* (2010). "Adverse events associated with testosterone administration," *New England Journal of Medicine*, 363: 109–122.
57. Skjaerpe, P. A. *et al.* (2010). "Androgen receptor gene polymorphism and the metabolic syndrome in 60–80 years old Norwegian men," *International Journal of Andrology*, 33: 500–506.
58. Haring, R., Ernst, F., Schurmann, C. *et al.* (2012). "The androgen receptor CAG repeat polymorphism as a risk factor of low serum testosterone and its cardiometabolic effects in men," *International Journal of Andrology*, 35: 511–520.
59. Alevizaki, M., Cimponeriu, A. T., Garofallaki, M. *et al.* (2003). "The androgen receptor gene CAG polymorphism is associated with the severity of coronary artery disease in men," *Clinical Endocrinology*, 59: 749–755.
60. Tirabassi, G. *et al.* (2013). "Androgen receptor gene CAG repeat polymorphism regulates the metabolic effects of testosterone replacement therapy in men post-surgical hypogonadotropic hypogonadism," *International Journal of Endocrinology.* doi: 10.1155/2013/816740.
61. Mouritsen, A., Hagen, C. P., Sørensen, K. *et al.* (2013). "Androgen receptor CAG repeat length is associated with body fat and serum SHBG in boys: A prospective cohort study," *Journal of Clinical Endocrinology and Metabolism*, 98: E605–E609.
62. Lez, J. P. G.-G., Guadalupe-Grau, A., Rodriguez-Gonzalez, F. G. *et al.* "Androgen receptor gene polymorphisms and the fat-bone axis in young men and women," *Journal of Andrology*, 33: 644–650.
63. Gustafson, D. R. *et al.* (2003). "Androgen receptor gene repeats and indices of obesity in older adults," *International Journal of Obesity*, 27: 75–81.
64. Bhasin, S., Storer, T. W., Berman, N., Yarasheski, K. E., Clevenger, B., Phillips, J., Lee, W. P., Bunnell, T. J. & Casaburi, R. (1997). "Testosterone replacement increases fat-free mass and muscle size in hypogonadal men," *Journal of Clinical Endocrinology and Metabolism*, 82: 407–413.
65. Lapauw, B., Goemaere, S., Crabbe, P., Kaufman, J. M. & Ruige, J. B. (2007). "Is the effect of testosterone on body composition modulated by the androgen receptor gene CAG repeat polymorphism in elderly men? *European Journal of Endocrinology*, 156: 395–401.

66. Campbell, B. C., Gray, P. B., Eisenberg, D. T., Ellison, P. & Sorenson, M. D. (2007). "Androgen receptor CAG repeats and body composition among Ariaal men," *International Journal of Andrology*, 32:140–148.
67. Jones, T. H., Arver, S., Behre, H. M. & Buvat, J. *et al.* (2011). "Testosterone replacement in hypogonadal men with type 2 diabetes and/or metabolic syndrome (the TIMES2 study)," *Diabetes Care*, 34: 828–837.
68. Mohlig, M., Arafat, A. M., Osterhoff, M. A. *et al.* (2011). "Androgen receptor CAG repeat length polymorphism modifies the impact of testosterone on insulin sensitivity in men," *European Journal of Endocrinology*, 164: 1013–1018.
69. Hersberger, M., Muntwyler, J., Funke, H. *et al.* (2005). "The CAG repeat polymorphism in the androgen receptor gene is associated with DL cholesterol but not with coronary atherosclerosis or myocardial infarction," *Clinical Chemistry*, 51: 1110–1115.
70. Yang, D., Tian, J., Zhang, X. *et al.* (2017). "The polymorphic CAG repeat in exon1 of androgen receptor is associated with level of HDL-cholesterol and hypertension in Chinese middle-aged to elderly men," *Clinical Endocrinology*, 87: 29–34. doi: 10.1111/cen.13326.
71. Zitzmann, M., Gromoll, J., von Eckardstein, A. & Nieschlag, E. (2003). "The CAG repeat polymorphism in the androgen receptor gene modulates body fat mass and serum concentrations of leptin and insulin in men," *Diabetologia*, 46: 31–39.

Chapter 31

China and Traditional Chinese Medicine (TCM) Policies: Medical Education System and Vocational Training

Daniela Caruso

1. INTRODUCTION

For several centuries, Traditional Chinese Medicine (TCM) was the only official medical system of China. Starting from the second half of the 19th century, modern medicine became prevalent and, just after the proclamation of the People's Republic of China in the 1949, it was introduced the current system, in which traditional Chinese medicine is at the same and equal level with modern medicine. Hospitals specializing in Chinese medicine and, at the same time, many modern-medicine–type hospitals feature TCM coexisting and working as an integrative system. Subjects of Western medicine (WM) have been embedded within the curricula of TCM universities; similarly, most universities devoted to modern medicine also have TCM departments. Thus the two different medical systems have a symbiotic relationship within one integral healthcare system, and

TCM provides 10–20% of healthcare services in China.[1] TCM studies and research have become an important factor in the development of Chinese healthcare and international scientific relations. At the moment, more than 700,000 students presently study TCM in China. In 2015, around 5,510 of these students were international. (the majority were from other Asian nations). According to the Chinese State Administration of TCM, most international students enroll at the bachelor's level, and an overwhelming 89% of the international students fund their own education.[2] China is the only country in the world where WM and traditional medicine (TM) are practiced alongside each other at every level of the healthcare system. Until 1997, they accounted for around 40% of all healthcare delivered in China.[3] Every city had a hospital practicing traditional Chinese medicine, and there were plans for every county to have one. In 95% of the hospitals practicing WM, there are TCM departments; when patients arrive at the department, they can choose Chinese or Western treatment. The collaboration between the two systems is well illustrated by the fact that, in WM hospitals, around 40% of the medicines prescribed are traditional. Similarly, in the TM hospitals, 40% of all prescribed drugs are Western medicines. In 2006, about 12% of all licensed clinicians were TCM practitioners (TCMPs), delivering 10–20% of all healthcare in mainland China, with over 200 million and 7 million episodes of outpatient and inpatient TCM service utilization, respectively. In most health centers and clinics, TCM and WM are practiced alongside each other. About 75% of all health centers have a TCM or integrated TCM-WM department and about one third of the total service provision in these centers was provided by TCMP. Nevertheless, only 33,574 TCMP were practicing in health centers or clinics whereas 166,614 TCMP were working in hospitals. This may imply a lack of TCM primary care workforce serving the rural populations. TCM hospitals account for 13.8% of mainland China's 38,492 hospitals, of which only 1.1% were formally integrated TCM-WM hospitals.[3]

The central government continues to pursue a policy for TCM expansion. Since the CPC's 18th National Congress in 2012, the Party and the government have granted greater importance to the development of TCM and made a series of major policy decisions and adopted a number of plans in this regard. On December 6, 2016, China's State Council[9] Information Office issued a White Paper on the development of TCM in

China,[4] which represents an important step aiming to boost China's TCM policies. The importance of establishing timely TM policy was further reemphasized in the Beijing Declaration at the WHO Congress on TM; the document highlights four areas which should be placed in the attention of governments and, among these, the education, vocational training, and improvements of the physicians skills as well:

III *Governments should establish systems for the qualification, accreditation or licensing of traditional medicine practitioners. Traditional medicine practitioners should upgrade their knowledge and skills based on national requirements; and*

IV. *The communication between conventional and traditional medicine providers should be strengthened and appropriate training programs be established for health professionals, medical students and relevant researcher.*[5]

2. EDUCATION IN TCM

China's medical degree system appears complex to other countries. There are multiple tiers of healthcare providers, varied routes to accreditation, and diverse roles of personnel with medical degrees in China. This reflects the difficulties of trying to meet people's healthcare needs, tackling the major political, economic, and social change over the past 80 years. The "opening up" of China's interactions with the outside world, particularly through international trade and communications, has generated a growing awareness of the importance of medical education and cooperation in this field between China and developed countries. TCM has two models of education. One is the traditional master–apprentice model, which used to be the main method of teaching during historical times. The other is university tuition, which has become the main mode of TCM education. Chinese university education is divided into three levels: bachelor's, master's, and PhD levels. Undergraduate education for traditional Chinese doctors takes five years and contains about 5,000 hours of study. This may be followed by graduate and postgraduate studies, of three years duration each. Undergraduate TCM education is divided into majors, according to fields of specialization. The most important majors are: TCM major (with emphasis on training clinicians using herbal therapy), acupuncture-manual therapy major, traditional Chinese pharmacology major, etc. There also exist TCM vocational schools offering three-year academic programs.

Currently the education of traditional Chinese doctors in China is strongly modernized and institutionalized. Its two mainstays are university education and continuous education. Nevertheless, the traditional structures of education, and the strong emphasis on clinical practice and person-to-person teaching, which constitute an essential part of TCM, are also integrated into this system. The Chinese medical education system has been undergoing state-mandated reform since the turn of the millennium, and with greater impetus since 2008.[7] The important place of plurality in the Chinese healthcare system is pointed out by the State Council's 2015 directives on healthcare reform, which stipulates that 15% of the public hospital will subsidize by 2020 are reserved for TMs, including TCM and other minority medicines.[6] In March 2009, the Chinese Government launched a set of important health reforms, and medical education will be key for successful development of the health system.[7] Since 1998, the rapid spread of medical education might be compromising quality and producing graduates unable to find jobs. Provincial schools have experienced unprecedented expansion over the past decade. Yearly enrolment into higher medical education increased six-fold from 75,000 in 1998 to nearly 450,000 in 2008. Some institutions admit 2,000–3,000 medical students every year, numbers that necessitate compromises, such as the replacement of anatomy with multimedia learning, and a scarcity of clinical clerkships. Student–teacher ratios in higher medical education nearly tripled from 7 in 1998 to 20 in 2008, leading to concerns about quality. In 2004–2008, the number of newly employed health workers accounted for only 20–40% of medical graduates, indicating that many graduates do not enter clinical practice. This surplus of medical graduates is accompanied by an unequal distribution of health workers in urban versus rural areas.[8,10]

2.1. *The clinical professional degree stream*

The medical academic degree system in China is organized in a three-level degree system aiming to award awarding bachelor's, master's, and doctorate degrees. Medical universities provide a five-year undergraduate medical curriculum for candidates who have completed high school education and passed the National Admission Examination. Holders of the bachelor's degree who pass the National Postgraduate Entrance Examination are qualified to enter the master's degree program (professional degree or research degree) for two to three years of full-time study. After obtaining the master's degree, a student who passes the National Doctor Entrance Examination may enter a medical university or medical institute to pursue a doctorate degree. The DM is a research degree. It is awarded after successful completion of three years of further study: six-month curriculum study and 2.5-year medical research. Also, the Doctor of Clinical Medicine (DCM) is a professional degree. It is awarded after successful completion of three-year study: six-month curriculum study and 1.5-year clinical training in a hospital and one-year medical research. The graduates are required to have solid knowledge in the diagnosis and treatment of special diseases and have specific skills in a subspecialty, taking on the responsibility as chief-of-residents, supervising and training junior clinical staff. The study period between graduating from high school and obtaining DCM varies from 8 to 14 years in China. In addition to the five-year undergraduate medical curriculum, some medical universities present seven-year programs in clinical medicine leading directly to a master's level qualification, i.e., Master of Clinical Medicine (MCM). More than 40 medical schools have both five- and seven-year undergraduate medical courses in China. The top 12 leading medical schools in China have been authorized by the Ministry of Education to develop a dedicated eight-year program, leading to the DCM. Yearly enrolment into the eight-year course in the 12 medical schools is limited to 1,300 individuals. The earliest tertiary institution of TCM was the Nanjing University of Traditional Chinese Medicine, which was evolved from the Jiangsu Province Advanced School of Chinese Medicine established in 1954. The first batch of TCM tertiary institutions approved by the State Council in 1956 included four universities: Beijing University of Chinese Medicine, Chengdu University of Traditional Chinese Medicine, Shanghai University of Traditional Chinese Medicine, and Guangzhou University of Chinese Medicine. According to 2013 data from the State Administration of Traditional Chinese Medicine, People's Republic of China, 45 TCM tertiary institutions and another 215 tertiary institutions provide TCM programs/majors in mainland China. TCM tertiary institutions in mainland China usually provide programs/majors in Chinese medicine, Chinese materia medica, acupuncture, moxibustion, and tuina. There are also other TCM-related or medicine-related multidisciplinary programs/majors available, such as Health Service Management, Medical English, and Nursing. In the TCM education system, undergraduate programs generally take five years to complete. Master's and doctoral programs are both three years. Nevertheless, education reform tends to develop new models for the "cultivation of innovative talents" (培养创新人才, Péiyǎng chuàngxīn réncái).[11] During the five-year undergraduate program, the general requirements for both majors are that the student systematically master TCM's fundamental theories, basic therapeutic, and diagnostic techniques; that the student master a part of modern medicine's basic knowledge and a part of modern medicine's therapeutic and diagnostic methods; that the student become familiar with TCM clinical thinking; that the student obtain proficiency in clinical skills; that the student be able to apply the methods of both TCM and modern medicine in the treatment and prevention of common diseases; that the student learn to obtain knowledge independently and be able to participate in certain research tasks. Such students, upon successfully passing the final exams, receive the bachelor of medicine degree. For "TCM" majors, the emphasis is placed on mastering the clinical usage of herbal therapy, especially in diseases of internal medicine, but also including emergency medicine. For "acupuncture manual therapy" majors, greater emphasis is placed on acupuncture and manual therapy, especially their applications in the fields of neurology, orthopedics, and rehabilitation.[12]

REFERENCES

1. Chinese State Administration of TCM (2008). *National Yearbook of TCM Statistics* (Public Administration College of Beijing University, Beijing). Available at: http://tongji.cnki.net/overseas/engnavi/HomePage.aspx?id=N2016030084&name=YZYYJ&floor=1. Accessed 7 October 2017.
2. Chinese State Administration of TCM. Available at: www.moe.gov.cn/jyb_xwfb/xw_fbh/moe_2069/xwfbh_2016n/xwfb_161026/161026_sfcl/201610/t20161026_286184. Accessed 30 April 2017.

3. Hesketh, T. & Zhu, W. X. (1997). "Health in China — Traditional Chinese medicine: One country, two systems," *British Medical Journal*, 315: 115–117.
4. Xu, J. & Yang, Y. (2009). "Traditional Chinese medicine in the Chinese health care system," *Health Policy*, 2: 133–139.
5. The State Council, The People's Republic Of China (2016). "White Paper on Traditional Chinese Medicine in China." Available at: http://english.gov.cn/archive/white_paper/2016/12/06/content_281475509333700.htm.
6. WHO Beijing Declaration (2008). Available at: http://tongji.cnki.net/overseas/engnavi/HomePage.aspx?id=N2016030084&name=YZYYJ&floor=1. Accessed 7 October 2017.
7. Yang, L., Liu, L., Yang, L., Zhao, G. & Cao, (2012). "*Quanqiu beijing xiade zhongguo yixue jiaoyu gaige* (Medical education Reform of China in the Global Context)," *Chinese Journal of Medical Education Research*, 5: 457–459 [in Chinese].
8. Office of the State Council (2015). "State Council's Notice Regarding the Publication of the Outline of the Organization of National Medical Public Health Service System." Available at: http://tongji.cnki.net/overseas/engnavi/HomePage.aspx?id=N2016030084&name=YZYYJ&floor=1. Accessed 7 October 2017.
9. Chinese State Council (2009–2012). "Notice of the State Council on printing and distributing the plan on recent priorities in carrying out the reform of health care system," *State Council Circular*. Available at: http://www.gov.cn/zwgk/200904/07/content_1279256.htm.
10. Anand, S., Fan, V. Y., Zhang, J. *et al.* (2008). "China's human resources for health: Quantity, quality, and distribution," *Lancet*, 372: 1774–1781.
11. Yu, C. (2009). "On the cultivation of innovative talents in colleges and universities," *International Education Studies*, 2(4): 164.
12. Ministry of Education of P. R. of China-State Administration of TCM (2008). *Gaodeng xuexiao benke jiaoyu zhongyixue zhuanye shezhi jiben yaoqiu* (Basic requirements of TCM undergraduate education). Available at: http://202.205.178.7/publicfiles/business/htmlfiles/moe/s3864/201010/xxgk_109607.html [in Chinese].